Population Mental Health

Over the last century public health efforts, such as immunization, safer food practices, public health education and promotion, improved sanitation, and water purification have been tremendously successful in eradicating and controlling a host of diseases. The result has been a dramatic improvement in population health and life expectancy. However, public health has paid far less attention to the impact of mental illness on individuals and society as a whole.

This pioneering volume examines the evidence-base for incorporating mental health into the public health agenda by linking the available research on population mental health with public mental health policy and practice. Issues covered in the book include the influence of mental health policies on the care and well-being of individuals with mental illness, the interconnectedness of physical and mental disorders, the obstacles to adopting a public health orientation to mental health/mental illness, and the potential application of public health models of intervention.

Setting out a unique and innovative model for integrated public mental health care, *Population Mental Health* identifies the tools and strategies of public health practice – surveillance and screening, early identification, preventive interventions, health promotion and community action – and their application to twenty-first century public mental health policy and practice.

Neal Cohen is Distinguished Lecturer at the CUNY School of Public Health at Hunter College and the Hunter College School of Social Work in New York City. Dr. Cohen previously served as New York City's Commissioner of Health and Commissioner of the Department of Mental Health, Mental Retardation and Alcoholism Services.

Sandro Galea is the Anna Cheskis Gelman and Murray Charles Gelman Professor and Chair of the Department of Epidemiology at the Columbia University Mailman School of Public Health. Dr. Galea's research is concerned with the social and biological determinants of the mental health of populations.

Routledge studies in public health

Available titles include:
Planning in Health Promotion Work
Roar Amdam

Forthcoming titles include:
Alcohol, Tobacco and Obesity
Morality, mortality and the new public health
Edited by Kirsten Bell, Amy Salmon and Darlene McNaughton

Population Mental Health

Evidence, policy, and public health practice

Edited by Neal Cohen and Sandro Galea

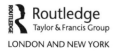

Routledge
Taylor & Francis Group

LONDON AND NEW YORK

First published 2011
by Routledge
2 Park Square, Milton Park, Abingdon, Oxon OX14 4RN

Simultaneously published in the USA and Canada
by Routledge
711 Third Avenue, New York, NY 10017

Routledge is an imprint of the Taylor & Francis Group, an informa business

British Library Cataloguing in Publication Data
A catalogue record for this book is available from the British Library

Library of Congress Cataloging in Publication Data
A catalog record for this book has been requested

ISBN: 978-0-415-77921-0 (hbk)
ISBN: 978-0-203-81861-9 (ebk)

Typeset in Sabon
by Wearset Ltd, Boldon, Tyne and Wear

Contents

Notes on contributors   viii
Acknowledgments   xi

1 Population mental health: evidence, policy, and public
   health practice   1
   NEAL COHEN AND SANDRO GALEA

PART I
Evidence   7

2 The burden of mental disorders worldwide: Results from
   the World Mental Health surveys   9
   RONALD C. KESSLER, SERGIO AGUILAR-GAXIOLA,
   JORDI ALONSO, SOMNATH CHATTERJI, SING LEE,
   DAPHNA LEVINSON, JOHAN ORMEL,
   T. BEDIRHAN ÜSTÜN, AND PHILIP S. WANG

3 Epidemiology in public mental health   38
   EZRA SUSSER AND REBECCA P. SMITH

4 Social and environmental influences on population mental
   health   51
   EMILY GOLDMANN AND SANDRO GALEA

5 Disparities in mental health status and care in the U.S. 69
   SERGIO AGUILAR-GAXIOLA, WILLIAM S. SRIBNEY,
   BONNIE RAINGRUBER, NATASHA WENZEL,
   DANA FIELDS-JOHNSON, AND GUSTAVO LOERA

6 The particular role of stigma   92
   PATRICK W. CORRIGAN AND DROR BEN-ZEEV

PART II
Policy 117

7 Social policy and the American mental health system of
   care 119
   DAVID MECHANIC AND GERALD N. GROB

8 Legislating social policy: mental illness, the community,
   and the law 139
   JOHN PETRILA AND JEFFREY SWANSON

9 Community rights, recovery, and advocacy 161
   DAVID ROE AND KIM T. MUESER

10 "No health without mental health": the global effort to
   improve population mental health 174
   MARK TOMLINSON, LESLIE SWARTZ, AND
   KAREN DANIELS

PART III
Public health practice 193

11 Mental health service utilization in the United States: Past,
   present, and future 195
   BENJAMIN G. DRUSS, PHILIP S. WANG, AND
   RONALD C. KESSLER

12 Public health approaches to improving population mental
   health: a local government perspective on integrating
   mental health promotion into general public health practice 206
   ADAM KARPATI

13 Realizing the possibilities of school mental health across
   the public health continuum 224
   CARRIE MILLS, MAURA MULLOY, AND MARK WEIST

14 Healthy aging and mental health: a public health challenge
   for the 21st century 248
   MARIANNE C. FAHS, WILLIAM CABIN, AND
   WILLIAM T. GALLO

15 Protecting urban families from community violence   283
    NEAL COHEN

16 Public health and population approaches for suicide
    prevention   303
    ERIC D. CAINE, KERRY L. KNOX, AND
    YEATES CONWELL

Conclusion   339

17 Twenty-first century public health practice: preventing mental
    illness and promoting mental health   341
    NEAL COHEN AND SANDRO GALEA

    Index   358

Contributors

Sergio Aguilar-Gaxiola, Center for Reducing Health Disparities and Clinical and Translational Science Center, School of Medicine, University of California, Davis, Sacramento, CA.

Jordi Alonso, Health Services Research Unit, IMEM (Hospital del Mar Research Institute), and CIBER en Epidemiología y Salud Pública (CIB-ERESP), Barcelona, Spain.

Dror Ben-Zeev, Institute of Psychology, Illinois Institute of Technology, Chicago, IL.

William Cabin, Richard Stockton College, Pomona, NJ.

Eric D. Caine, Department of Psychiatry and Center for the Study and Prevention of Suicide, University of Rochester Medical Center, Rochester, NY, and Center of Excellence, Canandaigua VA Medical Center, Canandaigua, NY.

Somnath Chatterji, Department of Measurement and Health Information Systems, World Health Organization, Geneva, Switzerland.

Neal Cohen, School of Public Health, School of Social Work, Hunter College, City University of New York, New York, NY.

Yeates Conwell, Department of Psychiatry and Center for the Study and Prevention of Suicide, University of Rochester Medical Center, Rochester, NY, and Center of Excellence, Canandaigua VA Medical Center, Canandaigua, NY.

Patrick W. Corrigan, Institute of Psychology, Illinois Institute of Technology, Chicago, IL.

Karen Daniels, Health Systems Research Unit, Medical Research Council, Cape Town, South Africa.

Benjamin G. Druss, Department of Health Policy and Management, Rollins School of Public Health, Emory University, Atlanta, GA.

Marianne C. Fahs, Health Policy and Management, City University of New York, School of Public Health at Hunter College and Graduate Center, New York, NY.

Dana Fields-Johnson, Center for Reducing Health Disparities, School of Medicine, University of California Davis, Sacramento, CA.

Sandro Galea, Department of Epidemiology, Mailman School of Public Health, Columbia University, New York, NY.

William T. Gallo, Health Policy and Management, City University of New York School of Public Health at Hunter College and Graduate Center, New York, NY.

Emily Goldmann, Department of Epidemiology, Mailman School of Public Health, Columbia University, New York, NY.

Gerald N. Grob, Institute for Health, Health Care Policy, and Aging Research, Rutgers University, New Brunswick, NJ.

Adam Karpati, Division of Mental Hygiene, Department of Health and Mental Hygiene, New York, NY.

Ronald C. Kessler, Department of Health Care Policy, Harvard Medical School, Boston, MA.

Kerry L. Knox, University of Rochester Medical Center, Rochester, NY, and Center of Excellence, Canandaigua VA Medical Center, Canandaigua, NY.

Sing Lee, The Chinese University of Hong Kong, Hong Kong, China.

Daphna Levinson, Research & Planning, Mental Health Services Ministry of Health, Jerusalem, Israel.

Gustavo Loera, Center for Research on Urban Education and Workforce Diversity, Mental Health America of Los Angeles, Los Angeles, CA.

David Mechanic, Institute for Health, Health Care Policy, and Aging Research, Rutgers University, New Brunswick, NJ.

Carrie Mills, Division of Child & Adolescent Psychiatry, University of Maryland School of Medicine, Baltimore, MD.

Kim T. Mueser, Departments of Psychiatry and of Community and Family Medicine, Dartmouth Medical School, Dartmouth Psychiatric Research Center.

Maura Mulloy, Center for School Mental Health, University of Maryland, Baltimore, MD.

Johan Ormel, Department of Psychiatry and Psychiatric Epidemiology, University Medical Center Groningen, University Center for Psychiatry, Groningen, the Netherlands.

John Petrila, Department of Mental Health Law & Policy, Louis de la Parte Florida Mental Health Institute, College of Behavioral and Community Sciences, College of Public Health, University of South Florida, Tampa, FL.

Bonnie Raingruber, Center for Nursing Research and School of Medicine, University of California, Davis, Sacramento, CA.

David Roe, Department of Community Mental Health, Faculty of Social Welfare & Health Sciences, University of Haifa, Haifa, Israel.

Rebecca P. Smith, New York, NY.

William S. Sribney, Third Way Statistics.

Ezra Susser, Department of Epidemiology, Mailman School of Public Health, Columbia University, College of Physicians and Surgeons and New York State Psychiatric Institute, New York, NY.

Jeffrey Swanson, Department of Psychiatry & Behavioral Sciences, Duke University School of Medicine, Durham, NC.

Leslie Swartz, Department of Psychology, Stellenbosch University, Stellenbosch, South Africa.

Mark Tomlinson, Department of Psychology, Stellenbosch University, Stellenbosch, South Africa.

T. Bedirhan Üstün, EIP/HFS, World Health Organization, Geneva, Switzerland.

Philip S. Wang, National Institute of Mental Health, Bethesda, MD.

Mark Weist, Department of Psychology, University of South Carolina, Columbia, SC.

Natasha Wenzel, College of Natural Resources and College of Letters and Science, University of California, Berkeley, Berkeley, CA.

Acknowledgments

We are grateful to all the authors who have contributed chapters to this book. We have learned a tremendous amount from them, both through our discussions as this book was taking shape and through reading the chapters themselves. We are indebted to Ms Sara Putnam and to Ms Erin Gilbert who were invaluable editorial partners in many aspects of this book's preparation.

This book is dedicated to Ilene, who has inspired so many to deliver quality mental health care in the public sector (NC).

This book is dedicated, as always, to Margaret, Oliver Luke, and Isabel Tess (SG).

Neal Cohen and Sandro Galea

1 Population mental health
Evidence, policy, and public health practice

Neal Cohen and Sandro Galea

Introduction

The past 150 years have seen dramatic and continuing improvements in health and life expectancy. In the last century alone, life expectancy increased by three decades (Centers for Disease Control and Prevention (CDC), 1999), largely due to the control of infectious diseases through a number of systematic public health efforts, including air, water, and food safety enhancements, as well as population level health education and promotion initiatives (Greene, 2001). Formulating a 21st century public health agenda to address the increasing burden of chronic diseases worldwide will require the same innovation and perseverance.

The past 20 years have seen some advances toward a population approach to mental health. For example, the issuance of the Global Burden of Disease Study (Murray & Lopez, 1996) introduced new methods for measuring the contribution of chronic diseases to human suffering and the global burden of mental illnesses. In the United States, the release of a series of Surgeon General Reports on Mental Health (U.S. Public Health Service, 1999a; 1999b; 2000; 2001) further underscored the public health significance of mental health. Additionally, in the first decade of the 21st century new models and approaches to psychiatric epidemiology are quantifying the prevalence and burden of mental disorders, the adequacy of service delivery models, and the risk factors that contribute to morbidity and premature mortality (Susser, Schwartz, Morabia, & Bromet, 2006). However, population-based research into mental health continues to receive far less attention than the clinically based discoveries that have deepened our understanding of mental illness and brought about a range of safe, effective, and well-documented treatments for most mental disorders.

Incorporating mental health into the "mainstream" public health agenda means applying the tools and strategies of the public health field (e.g., surveillance, screening and early identification, preventive interventions, health promotion, and community action) to 21st century public mental health policy and practice. Thus, the goal of this book is to place population-level mental health within a broader public health framework. Specifically, we aim to highlight the centrality of mental health to public health, with a particular focus on the relevant aspects of policy and public health practice that ameliorate the mental health of populations.

The emergence of psychiatric epidemiology and population mental health

In the early 19th century, the sociologist Emile Durkheim helped establish the early roots of psychiatric epidemiology with his seminal work *Le Suicide* (1897). Durkheim posited a link between social processes, such as poor economic conditions and community religious affiliations, and psychopathology outcomes such as suicide. In the early 20th century, Faris and Dunham (1939) looked at associations between social processes and rates of schizophrenia and substance abuse in Chicago. Psychiatric epidemiology became more fully emerged as a distinct discipline in the mid 20th century, spurred on in part by military screening for psychological symptoms and impairments during the Second World War (Tohen, Bromet, Murphy, & Tsuang, 2000). Community surveys – notably the Midtown Manhattan Study (Srole, Langer, Michael, Kirkpatrick, Opler, & Rennie, 1962) and the Stirling County Study (Leighton, 1959) – ushered in a new era of descriptive psychiatry and the assessment of psychopathology prevalence in the general population (Susser, Schwartz, Morabia, & Bromet, 2006).

However, ongoing lack of clarity about diagnostic criteria for psychopathology continued to limit the field until the publication of the third edition of the *Diagnostic and Statistical Manual of Mental Disorders* (DSM-III) (American Psychiatric Association (APA), 1980). The DSM-III was the first edition of the manual to be based on empirical data rather than theory and conjecture, allowing a clearer conceptualization of mental illness. At the same time, the first surveys specifically designed to assess mental disorders in the general population, consistent with DSM criteria, such as the Schedule for Affective Disorders and Schizophrenia, were being developed (Luppino et al., 2010; Susser et al., 2006). These instruments led to other instruments such as the Diagnostic Interview Schedule (DIS) and the Composite Internal Diagnostic Interview (CIDI), which were applied in large, national, population-based studies such as the Epidemiologic Catchment Area study (Regier et al., 1984) and the National Comorbidity Surveys (Kessler et al., 1994) that provided national estimates of psychopathology that inform population mental health research and practice to this day.

The Epidemiologic Catchment Area study, for example, estimated that the 12-month prevalence of any DIS disorder was 21.7%, with higher prevalences reported for substance use and anxiety disorders compared to other disorders (Bourdon, Rae, Locke, Narrow, & Regier, 1992). The National Comorbidity Survey, using a revised version of the CIDI, found

12-month prevalence of any measured disorder to be 29.5%, with higher prevalences reported for anxiety disorders compared to other disorders (Kessler et al., 1994). On a global scale, the World Mental Health Surveys estimated the 12-month prevalence of mental disorders for several high- and lower-income countries; estimates for any disorder ranged from 8.2 to 26.4% in high-income countries and 4.3 to 20.5% in lower-income countries. In all countries, the 12-month prevalence of anxiety disorders was greater compared to mood, impulse-control, and substance use disorders (Demyttenaere et al., 2004).

Increasingly, epidemiologists have combined efforts to document the prevalence and incidence of mental disorders with efforts to document the impairment and disability that accompanies these disorders. Two observations have emerged. First, recent work has been fruitful in drawing explicit links between psychopathology and physical illness. Although the direction of this association is still unclear, several studies indicate that mental illnesses are associated with physical illnesses, including asthma, cardiovascular disease, and obesity, among others (Kuper, Marmot, & Hemingway, 2002; Luppino et al., 2010; Oraka, King, & Callahan, 2009; Prince et al., 2007; Roy-Byrne et al., 2008). Thus, a failure to consider population-level mental illness may hinder public health efforts to improve physical health. Second, it has become clear that the disability and impairment that mental illness causes is equal to or surpasses that of many other diseases but receives far less attention on the public health agenda. In 2002, unipolar depressive disorders were the fourth leading cause of disability-adjusted life years (DALYs) worldwide; by 2030 they are expected to be the second leading cause of DALYs in the world and first in high-income countries (Mathers & Loncar, 2006). Furthermore, in 2005, 13.5% of the total DALYs were attributable to neuropsychiatric conditions, which is projected to increase to 14.4% by 2030 (Prince et al., 2007). The relationship between poor mental health and overall morbidity further highlights the importance of establishing population mental health as a core element of the public health paradigm.

Organization and content of the book

This book has been organized into three parts. In the first part, five chapters highlight the public health significance of mental health by focusing on the evidence and epidemiology of the burden, influences on population mental illness, as well as disparities and stigma. In the first chapter, Kessler and colleagues discuss morbidity attributable to mental illnesses worldwide and argue that the far-reaching health consequences of mental illness render these disabilities and disorders a central public health challenge. They argue that mental health research should be merged with public health research as a whole so that public mental health has greater connection to, and can benefit more fully from, scientific advances in public health. Next, Susser and Smith discuss the epidemiology of mental illness, highlighting the important contributions of the Epidemiological Catchment Area study and the National Comorbidity Study. He further discusses a shift in the field from classic psychiatric epidemiological measures of prevalence and incidence toward measurement of impairment and quality of life. In the next chapter, Goldmann and Galea summarize past research findings and theories on the mechanisms through which social and environmental factors influence mental illness. They discuss how changing demographics, including increased urbanization and migration, may shape future research. In the fourth chapter, Aguilar-Gaxiola and colleagues highlight differences in mental health and illness based on race/ethnicity. A focus of this chapter is the disparity in utilization of and access to mental health care. Lastly, Corrigan and Ben-Zeev conclude this section by addressing one of the consequences of stigma associated with mental illness – the underutilization of care. Recommendations and directions are given for decreasing the influence of stigma in mental health care utilization.

In the second part, four chapters address the policy aspects central to population mental health, including the mental health care system, laws and regulations, and the global effort to improve the mental health of populations. In the first chapter, Mechanic and Grob detail the history of mental health care and discuss the consequences of deinstitutionalization, particularly how social policies toward mental illness changed as a result of mental health care financing. Next, Petrila and Swanson expand on the results of deinstitutionalization, focusing on the relation between mental illness and crime and incarceration. They further discuss mandated treatment and emphasize the importance of evidence-based alternatives. In the third chapter, Roe and Mueser discuss the shift in public mental health systems from support and rehabilitation to recovery from mental illness. This chapter calls for more research on recovery and provides recommendations toward a recovery-oriented perspective. Lastly, Tomlinson, Swartz, and Daniels conclude the section by noting the implications of mental illness for worldwide disability. They call for a global initiative to address the need for a care infrastructure to respond to an increase in mental illness worldwide.

In the final part, six chapters focus on public health practice as it applies to mental health care utilization of the population as whole, as well as vulnerable subpopulations, such as children and the elderly. In the first chapter, Druss, Wang, and Kessler summarize the history of mental health care utilization from institutionalization to community and outpatient delivery systems. They discuss the current system, based on tiers of providers, as well as lack of utilization by those with mental illness. In the second chapter, Karpati considers the growing integration of public mental health into a broad public health context. He comments on both the potential future directions and limitations of this approach. Next, Mills, Mulloy, and Weist focus on the mental health of children, noting that the main population-based approach has concerned itself with healthy early development. They address the need for a comprehensive, school-based approach for improving the mental health of children. In the fourth chapter, Fahs, Cabin, and Gallo discuss the lack of attention paid to mental health care for the elderly. They address the challenges facing research focused on determinants of mental and physical well-being among the elderly, as well as the role that other systems, such as long-term care, can play in meeting the need for a more comprehensive mental health care system. Next, Cohen identifies the role of community and intimate partner violence in shaping the health of women and families. He summarizes the consequences of such stressors to inform new public mental health policy and programs that may address them. Lastly, Caine, Knox and Conwell conclude this section by focusing on the role of public health in preventing suicides. They discuss prevention strategies, in particular the use of a population-level approach in reducing the risk of suicides.

We conclude the book by remarking on key challenges in preventing mental illness and promoting mental health in a population-based framework. We aim for this book to catalyze discussion about mental health in a population health context and would like it to contribute to discussion and research in the area.

References

American Psychiatric Association. (1980). *Diagnostic and Statistical Manual of Mental Disorders* (3rd ed.). Washington, DC: American Psychiatric Association.

Bourdon, K. H., Rae, D. S., Locke, B. Z., Narrow, W. E., & Regier, D. A. (1992). Estimating the prevalence of mental disorders in U.S. adults from the Epidemiologic Catchment Area Survey. *Public Health Reports, 107*(6), 663–666.

Centers for Disease Control and Prevention. (1999). Control of infectious diseases. *Morbidity and Mortality Weekly Report, 48*(29), 621–629.

Demyttenaere, K., Bruffaerts, R., Posada-Villa, J., Gasquet, I., Kovess, V., Lepine, J. P., et al. (2004). Prevalence, severity, and unmet need for treatment of mental disorders in the World Health Organization World Mental Health Surveys. *JAMA, 291*(21), 2581–2590.

Durkeim, E. (1897). *Le Suicide.* New York: Free Press.

Faris, R., & Dunham, H. (1939). *Mental disorders in urban areas: An ecological study of schizophrenia and other psychoses.* New York: Hafner Publishing.

Greene, V. W. (2001). Personal hygiene and life expectancy improvements since 1850: Historic and epidemiologic associations. *American Journal of Infection Control, 29*(4), 203–206.

Kessler, R. C., McGonagle, K. A., Zhao, S., Nelson, C. B., Hughes, M., Eshleman, S., et al. (1994). Lifetime and 12-month prevalence of DSM-III-R psychiatric disorders in the United States: Results from the National Comorbidity Survey. *Archives of General Psychiatry, 51*(1), 8–19.

Kuper, H., Marmot, M., & Hemingway, H. (2002). Systematic review of prospective cohort studies of psychosocial factors in the etiology and prognosis of coronary heart disease. *Seminars in Vascular Medicine, 2*(3), 267–314.

Leighton, A. H. (1959). *My name is legion: Foundations for a theory of man in relation to culture* (Vol. 1.). New York: Basic Books.

Luppino, F. S., de Wit, L. M., Bouvy, P. F., Stijnen, T., Cuijpers, P., Pennix, B. W., & Zitman, F. G. (2010). Overweight, obesity, and depression: A systematic review and meta-analysis of longitudinal studies. *Archives of General Psychiatry, 67*(3), 220–229.

Mathers, C. D., & Loncar, D. (2006). Projections of global mortality and burden of disease from 2002 to 2030. *PLoS Medicine, 3*(11), e442.

Murray, C. J., & Lopez, A. D. (Eds.). (1996). *The global burden of disease: A comprehensive assessment of mortality and disability from diseases, injuries and risk factors in 1990 and projected to 2020.* Boston, MA: Harvard School of Public Health, World Health Organization, and World Bank.

Oraka, E., King, M. E., & Callahan, D. B. (2009). Asthma and serious psychological distress: Prevalence and risk factors among US adults, 2001–2007. *Chest, 137*(3), 609–616.

Prince, M., Patel, V., Saxena, S., Maj, M., Maselko, J., Phillips, M. R., & Rahman, A. (2007). Global mental health 1: No health without mental health. *Lancet, 370*(9590), 859–877.

Regier, D. A., Myers, J. K., Kramer, M., Robins, L. N., Blazer, D. G., Hough, R. L., et al. (1984). The NIMH Epidemiologic Catchment Area program: Historical context, major objectives, and study population characteristics. *Archives of General Psychiatry, 41*(10), 934–941.

Roy-Byrne, P. P., Davidson, K. W., Kessler, R. C., Asmundson, G. J., Goodwin, R. D., Kubzansky, L., et al. (2008). Anxiety disorders and comorbid medical illness. *General Hospital Psychiatry, 30*(3), 208–225.

Srole, L., Langer, T. S., Michael, S. T., Kirkpatrick, P., Opler, M., & Rennie, T. A. (1962). *Mental health in the metropolis.* New York: Harper & Row.

Susser, E., Schwartz, S., Morabia, A., & Bromet, E. J. (2006). *Psychiatric epidemiology.* New York: Oxford University Press.

Tohen, M., Bromet, E., Murphy, J. M., & Tsuang, M. T. (2000). Psychiatric epidemiology. *Harvard Review of Psychiatry, 8*(3), 111–125.

U.S. Public Health Service. (1999a). *Mental health: A report of the Surgeon General.* Washington, DC: U.S. Department of Health and Human Services.

U.S. Public Health Service. (1999b). *The Surgeon General's call to action to prevent suicide.* Washington, DC: U.S. Department of Health and Human Services.

U.S. Public Health Service. (2000). *Report of the Surgeon General's conference on children's mental health: A national action agenda.* Washington, DC: U.S. Department of Health and Human Services.

U.S. Public Health Service. (2001). *Mental health: Culture, race and ethnicity: Supplement to Mental health: A report of the Surgeon General.* Washington, DC: U.S. Department of Health and Human Services.

Part I
Evidence

2 The burden of mental disorders worldwide

Results from the World Mental Health surveys

Ronald C. Kessler, Sergio Aguilar-Gaxiola, Jordi Alonso, Somnath Chatterji, Sing Lee, Daphna Levinson, Johan Ormel, T. Bedirhan Üstün, and Philip S. Wang

Introduction

This chapter reviews epidemiologic evidence on the burden of mental disorders worldwide and focuses on estimates of the disability of commonly occurring mental disorders. Many studies in high-income countries have estimated the effects of specific disorders on disability (Berto, D'Ilario, Ruffo, Di Virgilio, & Rizzo, 2000; Maetzel & Li, 2002; Reed, Lee, & McCrory, 2004). In particular, a considerable amount of research has been carried out in the U.S. to quantify the magnitude of the short-term societal costs of mental disorders in terms of healthcare expenditures, impaired functioning, and reduced longevity (Greenberg & Birnbaum, 2005; Greenberg et al., 1999). The magnitude of the cost estimates in these studies is staggering. For example, Greenberg and colleagues (1999) estimated that over the decade of the 1990s, the annual societal costs of anxiety disorders in the U.S. exceeded $42 billion. Further, this estimate is likely conservative, as it excludes the indirect costs of early-onset anxiety disorders due to adverse life course outcomes (e.g., the effects of child-adolescent anxiety disorders on subsequent low educational attainment and consequent long-term effects on income) and to increased risk of other disorders (e.g., the effects of anxiety disorders on subsequent cardio-vascular disorder).

Comparative studies, however, are rare (Druss et al., 2008; Merikangas et al., 2007). However, data on comparative illness burden are critical for making resources allocation decisions, as these decisions inevitably require comparative assessments (Lopez & Mathers, 2007; Murray & Lopez, 1996; Murray, Lopez, Mathers, & Stein, 2001). Recognizing the importance of this information, one of the main aims of the World Health Organization's (WHO) World Mental Health (WMH) survey initiative is to produce comparative data on the prevalence and severity of mental disorders in participating WMH countries throughout the world. Although this is still a work in progress, enough useful information has been produced to warrant a review.

The World Mental Health (WMH) survey initiative

The WMH survey initiative is designed to help countries throughout the world carry out and analyze epidemiologic surveys on the prevalence and correlates of mental disorders. A key aim is to help countries that would not otherwise have the expertise or infrastructure to implement high-quality, community epidemiologic surveys, by providing centralized instrument development, training, and data analysis (www.hcp.med.harvard.edu/wmh). Twenty-four countries so far have completed WMH surveys (see Table 2.1). The vast majority of these surveys are nationally representative, although a few report data from only a single region (e.g., the São Paolo Metropolitan Area in Brazil and the Beijing, Shanghai, and Shenzhen Metropolitan Areas in the People's Republic of China) or regions (e.g., six metropolitan areas in Japan). Detailed descriptions of the field procedures (Pennell et al., 2008) and sample characteristics (Heeringa et al., 2008) of the WMH surveys are presented elsewhere.

All WMH surveys use the same diagnostic interview, the WHO Composite International Diagnostic Interview (CIDI) (Kessler & Üstün, 2004). The CIDI is a state-of-the-art, fully structured research diagnostic interview designed for use by trained lay interviewers who do not have any clinical experience. Consistent training materials, training programs, and quality control monitoring procedures are used in all WMH surveys to guarantee comparability across surveys. The same WHO translation, back-translation, and harmonization procedures for the survey and the training materials are also used across countries (Harkness et al., 2008; Pennell et al., 2008). Blinded clinician re-interviews with a probability subsample of WMH respondents confirm that the diagnoses generated by the CIDI are consistent with independent clinical diagnoses generated by culturally competent clinicians (Haro et al., 2006).

Due to our interest in disease burden, the CIDI was designed to go well beyond the mere assessment of mental disorders to include a wide range of measures about a number of correlates. Five of these are of special importance for the current report. First, the CIDI assesses disorder severity, which is important in light of the finding in previous epidemiologic surveys that quite a high proportion of the general population in many countries meets criteria set out in the *Diagnostic and Statistical Manual of Mental Disorders* (DSM) or the International Classification of Disorders (ICD) for a mental disorder (Somers, Goldner, Waraich, & Hsu, 2006; Waraich, Goldner, Somers, & Hsu, 2004; Wittchen & Jacobi, 2005). Faced with this high prevalence, mental health policy planning efforts need to consider disorder severity for treatment planning purposes, as the simple presence

Table 2.1 World Mental Health sample characteristics by World Bank Income Categories[a]

| | Survey[b] | Sample Characteristics[c] | Field Dates | Age Range | Sample Size | | Response Rate[d] |
					Part I	Part II	
I. Low/lower-middle income countries							
Colombia	NSMH	Stratified multistage clustered area probability sample of household residents in all urban areas of the country (approximately 73% of the total national population)	2003	18–65	4,426	2,381	87.7
India	WMHI	Stratified multistage clustered area probability sample of household residents in Pondicherry region. NR	2003–2005	18+	2,992	1,373	98.8
Iraq	IMHS	Stratified multistage clustered area probability sample of household residents. NR	2006–2007	18+	4,332	4,332	95.2
Nigeria	NSMHW	Stratified multistage clustered area probability sample of households in 21 of the 36 states in the country, representing 57 percent of the national population. The surveys were conducted in Yoruba, Igbo, Hausa, and Efik languages.	2002–2003	18+	6,752	2,143	79.3
PRC	B-WMH S-WMH	Stratified multistage clustered area probability sample of household residents in the Beijing and Shanghai metropolitan areas.	2002–2003	18+	5,201	1,628	74.7

continued

Table 2.1 continued

	Survey[b]	Sample Characteristics[c]	Field Dates	Age Range	Sample Size		Response Rate[d]
					Part I	Part II	
PRC	Shenzhen	Stratified multistage clustered area probability sample of household residents and temporary residents in the Shenzhen area.	2006–2007	18+	7,134	2,476	80.0
Ukraine	CMDPSD	Stratified multistage clustered area probability sample of household residents. NR	2002	18+	4,725	1,720	78.3
Total					35,562	16,053	82.6
II. Upper-middle income countries							
Brazil	São Paulo Megacity	Stratified multistage clustered area probability sample of household residents in the São Paulo metropolitan area.	2005–2007	18+	5,037	2,942	81.3
Bulgaria	NSHS	Stratified multistage clustered area probability sample of household residents. NR	2003–2007	18+	5,318	2,233	72.0
Lebanon	LEBANON	Stratified multistage clustered area probability sample of household residents. NR	2002–2003	18+	2,857	1,031	70.0

Country	Survey	Sample description	Field dates	Age range	Sample size	Part II sample	Response rate
Mexico	M-NCS	Stratified multistage clustered area probability sample of household residents in all urban areas of the country (approximately 75% of the total national population).	2001–2002	18–65	5,782	2,362	76.6
Romania	RMHS	Stratified multistage clustered area probability sample of household residents. NR	2005–2006	18+	2,357	2,357	70.9
South Africa	SASH	Stratified multistage clustered area probability sample of household residents. NR	2003–2004	18+	4,315	4,315	87.1
Total					25,666	15,240	76.6
III. High income countries							
Belgium	ESEMeD	Stratified multistage clustered probability sample of individuals residing in households from the national register of Belgium residents. NR	2001–2002	18+	2,419	1,043	50.6
France	ESEMeD	Stratified multistage clustered sample of working telephone numbers merged with a reverse directory (for listed numbers). Initial recruitment was by telephone, with supplemental in-person recruitment in households with listed numbers. NR	2001–2002	18+	2,894	1,436	45.9

continued

Table 2.1 continued

	Survey[b]	Sample Characteristics[c]	Field Dates	Age Range	Sample Size Part I	Sample Size Part II	Response Rate[d]
Germany	ESEMeD	Stratified multistage clustered probability sample of individuals from community resident registries. NR	2002–2003	18+	3,555	1,323	57.8
Israel	NHS	Stratified multistage clustered area probability sample of individuals from a national resident register. NR	2002–2004	21+	4,859	4,859	72.6
Italy	ESEMeD	Stratified multistage clustered probability sample of individuals from municipality resident registries. NR	2001–2002	18+	4,712	1,779	71.3
Japan	WMHJ2002–2006	Un-clustered two-stage probability sample of individuals residing in households in eleven metropolitan areas	2002–2006	20+	4,129	1,682	55.1
Netherlands	ESEMeD	Stratified multistage clustered probability sample of individuals residing in households that are listed in municipal postal registries. NR	2002–2003	18+	2,372	1,094	56.4
New Zealand[e]	NZMHS	Stratified multistage clustered area probability sample of household residents. NR	2003–2004	18+	12,790	7,312	73.3
N Ireland	NISHS	Stratified multistage clustered area probability sample of household residents. NR	2004–2007	18+	4,340	1,986	68.4

Portugal	NMHS	Stratified multistage clustered area probability sample of household residents. NR	2008–2009	18+	3,849	2,060	57.3
Spain	ESEMeD	Stratified multistage clustered area probability sample of household residents. NR	2001–2002	18+	5,473	2,121	78.6
United States	NCS-R	Stratified multistage clustered area probability sample of household residents. NR	2002–2003	18+	9,282	5,692	70.9
Total					60,674	32,387	65.4
IV. Total					121,902	63,680	72.0

Notes

a The World Bank. (2008), Data and Statistics. Accessed May 12, 2009 at: http://go.worldbank.org/D7SN0B8YU0

b NSMH (The Colombian National Study of Mental Health); WMHI (World Mental Health India); IMHS (Iraq Mental Health Survey); NSMHW (The Nigerian Survey of Mental Health and Wellbeing); B-WMH (The Beijing World Mental Health Survey); S-WMH (The Shanghai World Mental Health Survey); CMDPSD (Comorbid Mental Disorders during Periods of Social Disruption); NSHS (Bulgaria National Survey of Health and Stress); LEBANON (Lebanese Evaluation of the Burden of Ailments and Needs of the Nation); M-NCS (The Mexico National Comorbidity Survey); RMHS (Romania Mental Health Survey); SASH (South Africa Health Survey); ESEMeD (The European Study Of The Epidemiology Of Mental Disorders); NHS (Israel National Mental Health Survey); WMHJ2002–2006 (World Mental Health Japan Survey); NZMHS (New Zealand Mental Health Survey); NISHS (Northern Ireland Study of Health and Stress); NMHS (Portugal National Mental Health Survey); NCS-R (The US National Comorbidity Survey Replication).

c Most WMH surveys are based on stratified multistage clustered area probability household samples in which samples of areas equivalent to counties or municipalities in the US were selected in the first stage followed by one or more subsequent stages of geographic sampling (e.g., towns within counties, blocks within towns, households within blocks) to arrive at a sample of households, in each of which a listing of household members was created and one or two people were selected from this listing to be interviewed. No substitution was allowed when the originally sampled household resident could not be interviewed. These household samples were selected from Census area data in all countries other than France (where telephone directories were used to select households) and the Netherlands (where postal registries were used to select households). Several WMH surveys (Belgium, Germany, Italy) used municipal resident registries to select respondents without listing households. The Japanese sample is the only totally un-clustered sample, with households randomly selected in each of the four sample areas and one random respondent selected in each sample household. 18 of the 24 surveys are based on nationally representative (NR) household samples.

d The response rate is calculated as the ratio of the number of households in which an interview was completed to the number of households originally sampled, excluding from the denominator households known not to be eligible either because of being vacant at the time of initial contact or because the residents were unable to speak the designated languages of the survey.

e New Zealand interviewed respondents 16+ but for the purposes of cross-national comparisons we limit the sample to those 18+.

of a diagnosis may not indicate a level of need sufficient to require treatment. Consequently, all 12-month mental disorders in the WMH surveys are classified as serious, moderate, or mild. Serious disorders are defined as non-affective psychosis, bipolar I disorder, or substance dependence with a physiological dependence syndrome; making a suicide attempt in conjunction with any other disorder; reporting severe role impairment due to a mental disorder in at least two areas of functioning measured by the Sheehan Disability Scale (SDS) (Leon, Olfson, Portera, Farber, & Sheehan, 1997); or having overall functional impairment from any disorder consistent with a Global Assessment of Functioning (GAF) (Endicott, Spitzer, Fleiss, & Cohen, 1976) score of 50 or less. Disorders not classified as serious were classified as moderate if the respondent had substance dependence without a physiological dependence syndrome or at least moderate interference in the disorder-specific scale of role impairment. All other disorders were classified as mild.

Second, the CIDI includes a disorder-specific measure of role impairment administered in exactly the same way for each mental disorder assessed in the surveys, as well as for each of a number of physical disorders that are assessed for comparison purposes. This measure, the SDS, is a widely used self-report measure of condition-specific role impairment. The WMH version of the SDS consists of four questions, each asking the respondent to rate on a 0 to 10 scale the extent to which a particular disorder "interfered with" activities in one of four role domains during the month in the past year when the disorder was most severe. The four domains include

1   "your home management, like cleaning, shopping, and taking care of the (house/apartment)" (home);
2   "your ability to work" (work);
3   "your social life" (social); and
4   "your ability to form and maintain close relationships with other people" (close relationships).

The 0 to 10 response options are presented in a visual analogue format with labels for the response options (none (0), mild (1 to 3), moderate (4 to 6), severe (7 to 9), and very severe (10)). A global SDS disability score was created for each disorder assessed in the WMH surveys by assigning each respondent the highest SDS domain score reported across the four domains. We found good internal consistency reliability (Cronbach's alpha) across the SDS domains, in the range of 0.82 to 0.92 over countries and equivalent in both high-income countries (median 0.86; inter-quartile range 0.84 to 0.88) and lower-middle-income countries (median 0.90; inter-quartile range 0.88 to 0.90) (Ormel et al., 2008). Previous methodological studies have also documented good discrimination between the role functioning of cases and controls based on SDS scores in studies of a number of disorders (Connor & Davidson, 2001; Hambrick, Turk, Heimberg, Schneier, & Liebowitz, 2004; Leon et al., 1997; Pallanti, Bernardi, & Quercioli, 2006).

Third, the CIDI assesses days out of role in the 30 days before interview, making possible statistical analysis to determine which of the many mental and physical disorders assessed in the surveys are most strongly related to this important measure of role functioning. Fourth, WMH respondents were asked to describe their own overall physical and mental health during the past 30 days using a 0 to 100 visual analogue scale (VAS), where 0 represents "the worst possible health a person can have" and 100 represents "perfect health." Respondents were asked to make these global health valuations near the end of their interview, taking into consideration all the physical and mental conditions reviewed in the survey.

Days out of role and health valuations are important outcomes not only in substantive terms but also because, unlike the previous two measures (i.e., disorder severity and disorder-specific SDS scores), they are not disorder-specific measures. Instead, they are general measures of overall functioning that allow us to make even-handed comparisons of the extent to which specific disorders are independent predictors of these outcomes. This also makes possible the study of the effects of comorbidity, which is quite an important issue in light of the fact that many chronic-recurrent physical and mental disorders are highly comorbid (Merikangas et al., 2007). Importantly, comorbidity leads to overestimation of the burden of individual disorders in analyses that fail to adjust for it (Alonso et al., 2010), resulting in differential overestimation of the effects of disorders based on differences in their patterns of comorbidity.

A fifth measure, earnings in the 12 months before the interview, was also used as an outcome to evaluate the effects of mental disorders. Previous studies in the U.S. have documented strong associations of mental disorders with decrements in earnings (Harwood et al., 2000; Kessler et al., 2008; Rice, Kelman, Miller, & Dunmeyer, 1990; Rice & Miller, 1998), but we are aware of no previous cross-national study that examined this association.

Disorder prevalence estimates in the WMH surveys

The WMH surveys show clearly that mental disorders are common in all the countries studied. The proportion of respondents estimated to have any DSM-IV/CIDI disorder in the 12 months before interview averages (mean) 16.7% across surveys, with a median of 13.6% (see Table 2.2). The highest prevalence is 29.6% in São Paulo and the lowest is 6.0% in Nigeria. The inter-quartile range (IQR, 25th to 75th %iles) of prevalence estimates across surveys was 10 to 20.7%. Relative prevalence estimates are quite consistent across surveys, with anxiety disorders the most common disorders in 22 of 24 countries. The two exceptions are Israel and Ukraine, where mood disorders are estimated to be the most common

Table 2.2 Twelve-month prevalence of DSM-IV/CIDI disorders[a] in the World Mental Health surveys[a]

	Any disorder[b]		Anxiety disorders[b]		Mood disorders[b]		Impulse-control disorders[b,c]		Substance disorders[b]	
	%	(se)	%	(se)	%	(se)	%	(se)	%	(se)
I. Low/lower-middle income countries										
Colombia	21.0	(1.0)	14.4	(1.0)	6.9	(0.4)	4.4	(0.4)	2.8	(0.4)
India – Pondicherry	20.0	(1.1)	10.5	(0.8)	5.5	(0.5)	4.3	(0.7)	5.3	(0.6)
Iraq	13.6	(0.8)	10.4	(0.7)	4.1	(0.4)	1.7	(0.3)	0.3	(0.1)
Nigeria	6.0	(0.6)	4.2	(0.5)	1.2	(0.2)	0.1	(0.0)	0.9	(0.2)
PRC – Beijing, Shanghai	7.1	(0.9)	3.0	(0.5)	2.2	(0.4)	2.7	(0.6)	1.6	(0.4)
PRC – Shenzhen	16.0	(0.9)	11.4	(0.9)	4.8	(0.4)	2.9	(0.3)	0.0	(0.0)
Ukraine	21.4	(1.3)	6.8	(0.7)	10.0	(0.8)	5.1	(0.8)	6.4	(0.8)
Total	14.8	(0.4)	9.2	0.3	4.8	(0.2)	2.7	(0.2)	1.9	(0.1)
II. Upper-middle income countries										
Brazil – São Paulo	29.6	(1.0)	19.9	(0.8)	11.8	(0.7)	5.3	(0.7)	3.8	(0.4)
Bulgaria	11.2	(0.8)	7.6	(0.7)	3.2	(0.3)	0.8	(0.3)	1.2	(0.3)
Lebanon	17.9	(1.6)	12.1	(1.2)	7.0	(0.8)	2.6	(0.7)	1.3	(0.8)
Mexico	13.4	(0.9)	8.4	(0.6)	5.0	(0.4)	1.6	(0.3)	2.5	(0.4)
Romania	8.2	(0.7)	4.9	(0.5)	2.5	(0.3)	1.9	(0.7)	1.0	(0.2)
South Africa	16.9	(0.9)	8.4	(0.6)	4.9	(0.4)	1.9	(0.3)	5.7	(0.6)
Total	16.7	(0.4)	10.2	(0.3)	5.8	(0.2)	2.5	(0.2)	3.2	(0.2)

III. High income countries

Belgium	13.2	(1.5)	8.4	(1.4)	6.1	(0.8)	1.7	(1.0)	1.3	(0.4)
France	18.9	(1.4)	13.7	(1.1)	6.8	(0.7)	2.4	(0.6)	0.8	(0.3)
Germany	11.0	(1.3)	8.3	(1.1)	3.4	(0.3)	0.6	(0.3)	1.2	(0.4)
Israel	10.0	(0.5)	3.6	(0.3)	6.4	(0.4)	0.0	(0.0)	1.3	(0.2)
Italy	8.8	(0.7)	6.5	(0.6)	3.6	(0.3)	0.4	(0.2)	0.1	(0.1)
Japan	8.0	(0.7)	4.8	(0.6)	2.8	(0.4)	0.2	(0.1)	1.0	(0.3)
Netherlands	13.6	(1.0)	8.9	(1.0)	5.5	(0.7)	1.9	(0.7)	1.7	(0.5)
New Zealand	20.7	(0.6)	15.0	(0.5)	8.0	(0.4)	0.0	(0.0)	3.4	(0.3)
Northern Ireland	23.1	(1.4)	14.6	(1.0)	10.6	(0.9)	4.5	(1.0)	3.5	(0.5)
Portugal	22.9	(1.0)	16.5	(1.0)	8.3	(0.6)	3.5	(0.4)	1.6	(0.3)
Spain	9.7	(0.8)	6.6	(0.9)	4.4	(0.4)	0.5	(0.2)	0.3	(0.2)
United States	27.0	(0.9)	19.0	(0.7)	9.8	(0.4)	10.5	(0.7)	3.8	(0.4)
Total	17.7	(0.3)	11.9	(0.2)	7.2	(0.2)	2.7	(0.2)	2.2	(0.1)
IV. Total	16.7	(0.2)	10.8	(0.2)	6.2	(0.1)	2.6	(0.1)	2.4	(0.1)

Notes

a The disorders included anxiety disorders (generalized anxiety disorder, panic disorder, agoraphobia, specific phobia, social phobia, post-traumatic stress disorder, and separation anxiety disorder), mood disorders (major depressive disorder, dysthymic disorder, bipolar disorder), impulse-control disorders (attention-deficit/hyperactivity disorder, oppositional-defiant disorder, conduct disorder, intermittent explosive disorder), and substance disorders (alcohol and drug abuse with or without dependence).

b Between-country differences in prevalence are significant both for any disorder ($\chi^2_{24} = 1401.2$, $p < 0.001$) and for each class of disorder ($\chi^2_{24} = 715.4$–1099.9, $p < 0.001$).

c Prevalence of impulse-control disorders was estimated in the sub-sample of respondents who were 44 years of age or younger at the time of the interview.

disorders. Mood disorders are the next most common class of disorders in all but two other countries. The exceptions are South Africa, where substance use disorders are more common than mood disorders, and Beijing-Shanghai and the U.S., where behavior disorders are more common than mood disorders. The 12-month prevalence of having any disorder varied significantly across countries ($\chi^2_{24} = 1,401.2$, p < 0.001).

A number of recent literature reviews have presented detailed comparative data on the estimated prevalence of individual mental disorders and classes of disorder based on published community epidemiologic surveys (Somers et al., 2006; Waraich et al., 2004; Wittchen & Jacobi, 2005). Several consistent patterns that emerge in these reviews are replicated in the WMH data. First, anxiety disorders are consistently found to be the most prevalent class of mental disorders in the general population, and mood disorders are generally the next most prevalent class. Third, specific phobia is the most prevalent individual mental disorder in the general population (Silverman & Moreno, 2005). Major depression and social phobia are generally found to be the next most prevalent disorders, again consistent with WMH results. It is important to note that these relatively high prevalence estimates are, if anything, conservative, as critics argue that the diagnostic criteria in the DSM and ICD systems are overly conservative (e.g., Mylle & Maes, 2004; Ruscio et al., 2007). A related issue is that considerable evidence exists for clinically significant subthreshold manifestations of many mental disorders that are in some cases more prevalent than the disorders themselves (e.g., Brown & Barlow, 2005; Matsunaga & Seedat, 2007; Skeppar & Adolfsson, 2006).

Severity of mental disorders

While many previous epidemiologic surveys estimated disorder prevalence, the WMH surveys are the first to generate systematic estimates of disorder severity. Roughly one-quarter (24.5%) of all disorders are classified as a serious mental illness (SMI) in the WMH surveys, using the definition of SMI described in Table 2.3. The median proportion of cases with SMI across surveys is 22.3%. The range is 6.2 to 36.9%, and the IQR is 18.6 to 25.8%. A higher proportion of all disorders is classified moderate (mean 37.8%, median 38.7%), with a range of 12.5 to 50.6% and an IQR of 32.7 to 42.9%. A roughly similar proportion of all disorders was classified mild (mean and median both 37.7%), with a range of 28.3 to 74.8% and IQR of 34.9 to 42.1%.

The severity distribution among cases varies significantly across countries ($\chi^2_{48} = 352.9$, p < 0.001), although these differences are modest in substantive terms, with a Pearson contingency coefficient of 0.06 for the association between country income level and disorder severity. There are much more substantial positive associations (Pearson correlations) of overall disorder prevalence with both the proportion of cases classified as serious (0.30) and the proportion of cases classified as either serious or moderate (0.40). The positive association found between estimated prevalence and severity across countries is potentially important because it speaks to an issue raised in the methodologic literature regarding the possibility of biased prevalence estimates.

Two separate research groups found an opposite sort of pattern than the one found in the WMH surveys. The first was a study comparing results from the Korean Epidemiologic Catchment Area (KECA) Study (Chang et al., 2008) with results from parallel surveys in other countries. The authors argued that the lower estimated prevalence of major depression in the KECA than in the other surveys was due, at least in part, to a higher threshold for reporting depression among people in the Korean population. In support of this assertion, the investigators showed that Koreans diagnosed as depressed with an earlier version of the CIDI had considerably higher levels of role impairment than respondents diagnosed as depressed using the same instrument in the U.S.

The second relevant previous study was carried out as part of the WHO Collaborative Study on Psychological Problems in General Health Care (PPG) (Üstün & Sartorius, 1995). Nearly 26,000 primary care patients in 14 countries were assessed using an earlier version of the CIDI that included an evaluation of current symptoms of depression. As in the WMH surveys, substantial cross-national variation was found in the prevalence of major depression. However, the investigators found that the average amount of impairment associated with depression across countries was inversely proportional to the estimated prevalence of depression in those countries (Simon, Goldberg, Von Korff, & Üstün, 2002). This result is consistent with the possibility that the substantial cross-national variation in estimated prevalence of depression in the PPG study might be due, at least in part, to cross-national differences in diagnostic thresholds. However, we do not find results consistent with these in the WMH surveys, where the countries with the lowest prevalence estimates of DSM-IV/CIDI disorders also had the lowest reported levels of impairment associated with those disorders.

Comparative role disabilities of mental and physical disorders

As noted above, the WMH surveys assessed disorder-specific disability with the SDS. Respondents with any of the mental and physical disorders assessed in the surveys were asked to report the extent to which each such disorder interfered with their ability to carry out their daily activities in both productive roles (i.e., job, school, housework) and social roles (i.e., social and personal life). Rates of reported disability for the 10 most common physical disorders and for the 10 most common mental disorders are compared in each survey (Ormel et al., 2008).

Table 2.3 Twelve-month prevalence of DSM-IV/CIDI disorders by severity in the WMH surveys[a]

	Unconditional prevalence[b]						Conditional prevalence[c]					
	Disorders						Disorders					
	Serious		Moderate		Mild		Serious		Moderate		Mild	
	%	(se)	%	(se)	%	(se)	%	(se)	%	(se)	%	(se)
I. Low/lower-middle income countries												
Colombia	4.9	(0.5)	8.6	(0.7)	7.5	(0.5)	23.3	(2.1)	41.2	(2.6)	35.5	(2.1)
India – Pondicherry	4.3	(0.3)	7.8	(0.7)	7.9	(0.8)	21.7	(1.6)	39.0	(3.1)	39.3	(2.8)
Iraq	3.0	(0.4)	4.9	(0.4)	5.7	(0.6)	21.9	(2.3)	36.0	(2.6)	42.1	(2.9)
Nigeria	0.8	(0.3)	0.8	(0.2)	4.5	(0.5)	12.8	(3.8)	12.5	(2.6)	74.8	(4.2)
PRC – Beijing, Shanghai	1.0	(0.3)	2.3	(0.5)	3.8	(0.6)	13.8	(3.7)	32.2	(4.9)	54.0	(4.6)
PRC – Shenzhen	1.0	(0.3)	5.2	(0.5)	9.8	(0.8)	6.2	(1.6)	32.7	(2.9)	61.2	(3.6)
Ukraine	4.9	(0.4)	8.4	(0.8)	8.1	(1.0)	22.9	(1.8)	39.4	(2.9)	37.7	(3.5)
Total	2.8	(0.2)	5.3	(0.2)	6.7	(0.3)	18.8	(0.9)	35.9	(1.2)	45.3	(1.3)
II. Upper-middle income countries												
Brazil – São Paulo	10.0	(0.6)	9.8	(0.5)	9.8	(0.6)	33.9	(1.4)	33.0	(1.8)	33.2	(1.4)
Bulgaria	2.3	(0.3)	3.6	(0.5)	5.4	(0.5)	20.3	(2.8)	32.1	(3.6)	47.7	(2.7)
Lebanon	4.0	(0.7)	7.7	(1.0)	6.2	(1.2)	22.3	(3.1)	42.9	(4.9)	34.9	(5.6)
Mexico	3.5	(0.4)	4.7	(0.4)	5.2	(0.5)	26.3	(2.4)	34.8	(2.2)	38.9	(2.5)
Romania	2.3	(0.4)	2.4	(0.3)	3.5	(0.5)	27.9	(3.4)	29.3	(3.7)	42.8	(3.5)
South Africa	4.3	(0.4)	5.3	(0.5)	7.2	(0.6)	25.7	(1.8)	31.4	(2.1)	43.0	(2.1)
Total	4.7	(0.2)	5.5	(0.2)	6.5	(0.3)	28.0	(0.9)	33.1	(1.1)	39.0	(1.0)

III. High income countries

Belgium	4.3	(0.8)	5.1	(0.8)	3.8	(0.6)	32.6	(4.2)	38.7	(3.4)	28.8	(4.8)
France	3.5	(0.5)	8.1	(0.8)	7.2	(0.9)	18.6	(2.5)	43.1	(3.0)	38.3	(3.6)
Germany	2.4	(0.4)	4.8	(0.8)	3.9	(0.7)	21.6	(2.5)	43.2	(4.5)	35.2	(4.1)
Israel	3.7	(0.3)	3.5	(0.3)	2.8	(0.2)	36.9	(2.4)	34.8	(2.3)	28.3	(2.1)
Italy	1.4	(0.2)	4.2	(0.5)	3.2	(0.5)	15.9	(2.7)	47.8	(3.9)	36.3	(3.9)
Japan	1.3	(0.4)	3.8	(0.5)	2.9	(0.4)	16.1	(4.5)	47.2	(4.8)	36.7	(3.7)
Netherlands	4.2	(0.6)	4.2	(0.5)	5.2	(0.8)	31.1	(3.5)	31.1	(3.6)	37.8	(4.7)
New Zealand	5.3	(0.3)	8.6	(0.4)	6.7	(0.3)	25.8	(1.0)	41.7	(1.4)	32.5	(1.2)
Northern Ireland	6.7	(0.7)	7.7	(0.7)	8.7	(1.1)	28.8	(3.0)	33.4	(2.6)	37.8	(3.3)
Portugal	4.0	(0.4)	11.6	(0.6)	7.3	(0.5)	17.5	(1.5)	50.6	(2.0)	31.9	(1.9)
Spain	1.9	(0.2)	4.2	(0.5)	3.6	(0.6)	19.9	(2.4)	43.5	(4.1)	36.6	(4.8)
United States	6.9	(0.4)	10.7	(0.5)	9.4	(0.6)	25.5	(1.4)	39.7	(1.2)	34.8	(1.4)
Total	4.5	(0.1)	7.2	(0.2)	6.0	(0.2)	25.4	(0.6)	40.7	(0.7)	33.9	(0.7)
IV. Total	4.1	(0.1)	6.3	(0.1)	6.3	(0.1)	24.5	(0.5)	37.8	(0.5)	37.7	(0.6)

Notes

a See Table 3 footnote 1 for a list of the disorders. A respondent was defined as having a serious disorder if he either met criteria for bipolar I disorder or substance dependence with a physiological dependence syndrome; made a suicide attempt in conjunction with any DSM-IV/CIDI disorder; reported at least two areas of role functioning with severe impairment due to a mental disorder on the Sheehan Disability Scales (SDS; Leon et al, 1997); or reported an overall level of functional impairment at a level consistent with a Global Assessment of Functioning (Endicott et al, 1976) score of 50 or less in conjunction with any DSM-IV/CIDI disorder. Respondents not classified as having a serious disorder were classified moderate if they had a SDS score rated at least moderate or met criteria for substance dependence without a physiological dependence syndrome. All other respondents with DSM-IV/CIDI disorders were classified mild.

b Unconditional prevalence is prevalence in the total sample. Conditional prevalence is prevalence among cases. For example, the 4.9 percent of respondents in the Colombia survey with a 12-month serious disorder represent 23.3 percent of the 21.0 percent of respondents in the Colombia who had any 12-month DSM-IV/CIDI disorder. (The 21.0 percent total prevalence is reported in Table 2.)

c Between-country differences in prevalence are significant both for unconditional prevalence for each class of disorders ($\chi^2_{24} = 146.8 - 187.2$, $p < 0.001$) and for conditional prevalence for each class of disorders ($\chi^2_{24} = 377.9 - 741.6$, $p < 0.001$).

Table 2.4 Disorder-specific global Sheehan Disability Scale ratings for commonly occurring mental and chronic physical disorders in high-income and lower-middle-income World Mental Health Countries[a]

	Proportion rated severely disabling			
	High-income		Lower-middle income	
	%	(se)	%	(se)
I. Physical disorders				
Arthritis	23.3	(1.5)	22.8	(3.0)
Asthma	8.2*	(1.4)	26.9	(5.4)
Back/neck	34.6*	(1.5)	22.7	(1.8)
Cancer	16.6	(3.2)	23.9	(10.3)
Chronic pain	40.9*	(3.6)	24.8	(3.8)
Diabetes	13.6	(3.4)	23.7	(6.1)
Headaches	42.1*	(1.9)	28.1	(2.1)
Heart disease	26.5	(3.9)	27.8	(5.2)
High blood pressure	5.3*	(0.9)	23.8	(2.6)
Ulcer	15.3	(3.9)	18.3	(3.6)
II. Mental disorders				
ADHD	37.6	(3.6)	24.3	(7.4)
Bipolar	68.3*	(2.6)	52.1	(4.9)
Depression	65.8*	(1.6)	52.0	(1.8)
GAD	56.3*	(1.9)	42.0	(4.2)
IED	36.3	(2.8)	27.8	(3.6)
ODD	34.2	(6.0)	41.3	(10.3)
Panic disorde	48.4*	(2.6)	38.8	(4.7)
PTSD	54.8*	(2.8)	41.2	(7.3)
Social phobia	35.1	(1.4)	41.4	(3.6)
Specific phobia	18.6	(1.1)	16.2	(1.6)

Notes
* Significant difference between high income and lower-middle income countries based on 0.05-level two-sided tests
a See the text for a description of the Sheehan Disability Scale and the definition of severe disability.

Of the 100 logically possible pair-wise, disorder-specific mental-physical comparisons, the proportion of disability ratings in the severe range is higher for the mental than physical disorder in 76 comparisons in high-income countries and 84 comparisons in lower-middle-income countries (Table 2.4). Nearly all of these higher mental than physical disability ratings are statistically significant at the 0.05 level and hold in within-person comparisons (i.e., comparing the reported disabilities associated with a particular mental-physical disorder pair in the subsample of respondents who had both disorders). A similar pattern is found when treated physical disorders are compared with all (i.e., treated or not) mental disorders to address the concern that the more superficial assessment of physical than mental disorders might have led to the inclusion of subthreshold cases of physical disorders with low disability.

Days out of role associated with mental disorders

It is noteworthy that the disorder severity classification used in the WMH surveys is validated by a consistently monotonic association between reported disorder severity and mean number of days out of role associated with the disorders. This association is statistically significant in all but four surveys (Table 2.5). Respondents with serious disorders in most surveys reported at least 40 days in the past year when they were totally unable to carry out usual activities because of these disorders (IQR: 56.7 to 135.9 days). The mean days out of role for mild disorders, in comparison, is in the range 11.7 to 68.9 days, while the mean for moderate disorders is intermediate between these extremes (21.1 to 109.4 days; IQR: 39.3 to 65.3 days). When we compared between-country differences in these means with between-country differences in prevalence, using the same logic as in the previous section, we once again found a positive association between prevalence and the indicator of severity. For example, in the three WMH countries with the highest estimated overall 12-month prevalence of DSM-IV/CIDI disorders (US, Ukraine, New Zealand), the mean number of days out of role associated with disorders classified "severe" is in the range 98.1 to 142.5, compared to means in the range 48.7 to 56.7 in the three countries with the lowest 12-month prevalence estimates (Japan, Nigeria, People's Republic of China).

Another possibility is that we underestimated prevalence in some countries because the DSM-IV categories are less relevant to symptom expression in those countries. We did not investigate this in the WMH surveys, but a sophisticated analysis of this possibility was carried out as part of the PPG (Üstün & Sartorius, 1995). In that study, an analysis of cross-national variation in the structure of depressive symptoms was carried out using item response theory (IRT) methods (Simon et al., 2002). The results showed clearly that both the latent structure of depressive symptoms and the associations between specific depressive symptoms and this latent structure were very similar across the countries studied. These results do not support the suggestion that the large cross-national variation in estimated prevalence of depression is due to cross-national differences in the nature of depression. Comparable psychometric analyses have not yet been completed for other disorders, however, so it remains possible that cross-national differences exist in latent structure that might play a part in explaining the substantial differences in 12-month prevalence documented in the WMH surveys.

At the same time, it is noteworthy that the countries with the lowest disorder prevalence estimates in the WMH series also have the highest

Table 2.5 Association between severity of 12-month DSM-IV/CIDI disorders and days out of role in the World Mental Health surveys

	Serious		Moderate		Mild		Wald F[a]
	Mean	(se)	Mean	(se)	Mean	(se)	
I. WHO Region: Pan American Health Organization (PAHO)							
Colombia	53.0	(8.9)	33.7	(6.7)	15.6	(3.0)	10.8*
Mexico	42.8	(6.9)	26.3	(5.3)	11.7	(2.7)	11.7*
United States	135.9	(6.9)	65.3	(4.6)	35.7	(2.7)	126.1*
II. WHO Region: African Regional Office (AFRO)							
Nigeria	56.7	(22.3)	51.5	(18.8)	25.9	(7.4)	1.6
South Africa	73.1	(9.7)	49.3	(6.5)	32.5	(4.8)	9.1*
III. WHO Region: Eastern Mediterranean Regional Office (EMRO)							
Lebanon	81.4	(10.6)	42.0	(9.5)	13.6	(5.4)	14.4*
IV. WHO Region: European Regional Office (EURO)							
Belgium	96.1	(26.0)	59.9	(11.6)	42.5	(9.6)	3.7*
France	105.7	(14.3)	71.8	(16.5)	67.6	(17.3)	2.7
Germany	77.8	(18.1)	33.2	(8.2)	45.7	(12.1)	2.2
Israel	184.6	(12.5)	109.4	(10.1)	44.6	(9.1)	41.8*
Italy	178.5	(25.6)	55.6	(10.9)	41.7	(11.2)	11.7*
Netherlands	140.7	(19.9)	87.1	(17.1)	68.9	(22.7)	4.0*
Spain	131.5	(15.8)	56.6	(10.0)	57.4	(22.0)	8.1*
Ukraine	142.5	(14.5)	103.2	(9.2)	51.6	(9.9)	13.9*
V. WHO Region: Western Pacific Regional Office (WPRO)							
People's Republic of China	48.7	(18.4)	21.1	(5.2)	21.3	(7.2)	1.5
Japan	51.0	(17.3)	39.3	(10.6)	22.5	(6.4)	3.7*
New Zealand	98.1	(5.9)	54.6	(3.4)	36.4	(3.6)	40.7*

Notes
* Significant association between severity and days out of role at the 0.05 level.
a Results are based on simple mean comparisons. No control variables were used in the analysis.

proportions of treated cases classified as "subthreshold"; i.e., not meeting criteria for any of the DSM-IV/CIDI disorders assessed in the WMH interview. This finding at least indirectly raises the possibility that the assessments in the CIDI are less adequate in capturing the psychopathological syndromes that are common in all the WMH countries. In particular, the syndromes associated with treatment in low-prevalence countries are not well characterized by the CIDI. Additional WMH clinical reappraisal studies using flexible and culturally sensitive assessments of psychopathology are currently underway in both high-income and lower-middle-income countries.

These results involve individual-level effects; however, also instructive are examinations of societal-level effects, by which we mean effects that take into consideration not only relative impairment but also relative prevalence of different disorders. We are only beginning to do this in the cross-national WMH data, but results of this sort have been generated for the U.S. WMH survey (Merikangas et al., 2007). That analysis estimated that fully one-third of all the days out of role associated with chronic-recurrent health problems in the US population are due to mental disorders. This amounts to literally billions of days of lost functioning per year in the U.S. population. We do not yet know if comparable results will be obtained in parallel analyses of WMH surveys in other countries, but preliminary results suggest that this is likely to be the case.

Comparative health valuations of mental and physical disorders

The WMH analysis of health valuations was similar to the analysis of SDS in that both compared mental disorders to physical disorders. However, a somewhat different set of disorders was included in the two analyses – the most commonly occurring disorders in the SDS analysis and the disorders most strongly related to VAS scores in the health valuation analysis. The health valuation analysis was also more textured than the SDS analysis in that it allowed us to investigate the effects of comorbidity by examining regression equations that predicted VAS scores from information about the presence of individual disorders either considered alone or controlling for comorbid disorders. This was not possible in the SDS analysis because SDS scores were disorder-specific, whereas VAS scores were not.

Bivariate linear regression models (i.e., using only one disorder at a time to predict VAS scores) were used to study predictive associations of disorders with VAS scores. Every one of the disorders had a negative association with VAS scores (i.e., associated with reduced perceived health) (see Table 2.6). Coefficients based on the multivariate model that controlled for comorbid disorders are consistently lower than those based on bivariate models. The condition-specific ratio of the former to the latter is in the range 0.24 to 0.70 with a median IQR of 0.42 (0.31 to 0.51). Very similar results were found in lower-middle-income (0.53; 0.35 to 0.62) and high-income (0.41; 0.27 to 0.51) countries (Alonso et al., 2010). The influence of comorbidity can also be seen in the fact that the correlation across disorders between mean number of comorbid disorders and the ratio of the coefficient based on the bivariate model to the coefficient based on the multivariate model is statistically significant (–0.46). More detailed analysis showed that coefficients are generally very similar in high-income and lower-middle income-countries, with a Spearman rank-order correlation of 0.54. This is why results are presented here for high-income and lower-middle-income countries combined.

At the bivariate level, the coefficients associated with most mental disorders, in the range 7.3 to 17.8 in predicting scores on the 0 to 100 VAS health valuation scale, are larger than those associated with all but two of

Table 2.6 Individual-level condition-specific estimates of predictive associations between individual disorders and Visual Analogue Scale (VAS) health evaluations based on bivariate and the best-fitting multivariate model in the total sample[a]

	Bivariate (Bi)[b]		Multivariate (Mul)		Mul/Bi[c]	Mean comorbidity[d]
	Est	(se)	Est	(se)	Est	
I. Chronic physical conditions						
Arthritis	−9.5*	(0.5)	−4.9*	(0.4)	0.51	2.0
Cancer	−2.6*	(1.1)	−0.8	(0.9)	0.31	2.1
Cardiovascular disorders	−8.4*	(0.4)	−4.9*	(0.4)	0.59	1.8
Chronic pain conditions	−10.9*	(0.4)	−6.8*	(0.4)	0.63	1.8
Diabetes	−8.8*	(1.0)	−6.1*	(0.8)	0.70	2.0
Digestive disorders	−9.9*	(0.9)	−4.1*	(0.8)	0.41	2.3
Headaches or migraines	−9.9*	(0.4)	−4.5*	(0.4)	0.45	2.0
Insomnia	−16.0*	(0.7)	−7.9*	(0.7)	0.50	2.9
Neurological disorders	−17.8*	(1.7)	−12.0*	(1.4)	0.67	2.6
Respiratory disorders	−4.3*	(0.4)	−1.4*	(0.4)	0.31	1.6
II. Mental conditions						
Alcohol abuse	−7.3*	(1.1)	−3.2*	(1.1)	0.44	1.8
Bipolar disorder	−17.8*	(1.4)	−5.3*	(1.5)	0.30	3.9
Drug abuse	−12.4*	(1.8)	−5.2*	(1.7)	0.42	2.6
Generalized anxiety disorder	−13.4*	(1.1)	−4.5*	(1.1)	0.34	3.0
Major depressive episode	−14.8*	(0.5)	−7.6*	(0.5)	0.52	2.5
Panic disorder	−16.6*	(1.0)	−6.7*	(1.0)	0.40	3.4
Post–traumatic stress disorder	−15.3*	(1.1)	−4.7*	(0.9)	0.31	3.5
Social phobia	−11.2*	(0.8)	−2.6*	(0.9)	0.24	2.9

Notes

* Significant at the 0.05 level, two-sided test.

a These estimates have a similar interpretation to metric regression coefficients, but differ from the latter in that they are based on simulations generated from the coefficients in the nonlinear/non-additive best-fitting multivariate mode. The latter model included controls for both number and types of comorbid disorders. The model and the estimation procedure are both described in detail elsewhere (Alonso et al., 2010).

b A separate model for each condition adjusted by socio-demographic controls.

c The ratio of the estimate based on the best-fitting multivariate model to the estimate based on the bivariate model.

d Mean number of other conditions reported by respondents with the condition in the row.

the physical disorders (2.6 to 10.9). The two exceptions are insomnia (16.0) and neurological disorders (17.8), which have coefficients as large as those of the most severe mental disorders (panic disorder and bipolar disorder, with coefficients of 16.6 to 17.8). It should be noted, though, that insomnia and neurological disorders also have the highest overlap with mental disorders of all the physical disorders considered. Indeed, insomnia is a common symptom of numerous mental disorders and could arguably have been classified as a mental disorder rather than as a physical disorder. (The DSM-IV, in fact, includes a diagnosis of insomnia.) Some neurological disorders, in comparison, are so closely related and difficult to distinguish from certain mental disorders that they are often referred to as neuropsychiatric disorders. Thus, it is noteworthy that with the exceptions of insomnia and neurological disorders, the bivariate coefficients associated with all the physical disorders considered are consistently lower than those associated with the bulk of the mental disorders. These results are broadly consistent with those found in our analysis of the SDS data.

The situation is quite different, though, in the multivariate model, where the coefficients associated with mental disorders (median 4.7; IQR 3.2 to 5.3) are quite comparable in magnitude to those associated with physical disorders (median 4.9; IQR 4.1 to 6.1). This difference is due to the coefficients associated with mental disorders shrinking much more than those associated with the physical disorders in the multivariate model compared to the bivariate models. This greater shrinkage, in turn, is due to the higher comorbidity of mental disorders (median number of comorbid disorders 2.9; IQR 2.5 to 3.4) than physical disorders (median 2.0, IQR 1.8 to 2.3). When we estimated only aggregate coefficients for having any (i.e., one or more) mental disorder and any physical disorder, the coefficients (standard errors) were significantly lower ($t = 2.8$, $p = 0.004$) for any mental disorder (7.4 (0.3)) than for any physical disorder (8.6 (0.3)). The fact that the effect of mental disorders is lower than the effect of physical disorders in the aggregate multivariate analysis, whereas the effects of individual mental disorders are generally higher than those of individual physical disorders in bivariate analyses means that the indirect effects of mental disorders due to comorbidity are to some meaningful extent mediated by physical comorbidities (e.g., comorbidity of mental disorders with insomnia and neurological disorders).

The long-term adverse effects of mental disorders

All of the associations described above dealt with short-term effects of current mental disorders on various aspects of current functioning or on current perceived health. Mental disorders are also known to have long-term effects. Commonly occurring mental disorders have much earlier age-of-onset (AOO) distributions than most chronic physical disorders (Kessler et al., 2007). WMH respondents with a lifetime history of each disorder were asked to report retrospectively how old they were when the disorder first began. AOO distributions were generated from these reports and are very consistent across countries (Kessler et al., 2007). Some anxiety disorders, most notably the phobias and separation anxiety disorder (SAD), had very early AOO distributions, with median AOO in the range of seven to 14 and the vast majority of lifetime cases occurring within five to 10 years of these medians. Similarly, early onsets were typical for the externalizing disorders considered in the WMH surveys. In comparison, the other common anxiety disorders (panic disorder, generalized anxiety disorder, and posttraumatic stress disorder) and mood disorders have later AOO distributions, with median AOO in the age range 25 to 50 and a wide IQR (15 to 75). Substance use disorders have intermediate median AOO (20 to 35), with the vast majority of cases having onsets within 10 years of these medians.

WMH analyses show that early-onset mental disorders are significant predictors of the subsequent onset and persistence of a wide range of physical disorders (He et al., 2008; Ormel et al., 2007). This is part of a larger pattern of associations between early-onset mental disorders and a wide array of adverse life course outcomes that might be conceptualized as societal costs of these disorders, including reduced educational attainment, early marriage, marital instability, and low occupational and financial status (Kessler et al., 1997; Kessler, Foster, Saunders, & Stang, 1995; Kessler, Walters, & Forthofer, 1998; Lee et al., 2009). It is unclear if these associations are causal, that is, if interventions to treat early-onset mental disorders would prevent the subsequent onset of the adverse outcomes with which they are associated. From a public health perspective, carrying out long-term interventions to evaluate this issue would be valuable. Even in the absence of this evidence, though, the available data from the WMH surveys show that mental disorders, and especially early-onset mental disorders, are associated with substantially reduced life changes in terms of physical health and achievements in a variety of role domains.

The workplace costs of mental disorders to employers

A large part of the societal burden of mental disorders is the costs of mental disorders due to reduced rates of labor force participation (Zhang, Zhao, & Harris, 2009), elevated rates of unemployment among people in the labor force (Chatterji, Alegria, Lu, & Takeuchi, 2007), and underemployment among those who are employed (Kessler et al., 2008). All of these associations are documented in the WMH surveys. It is important to note that mental disorders also have costs to employers, including high rates of sporadic absenteeism (Kessler & Frank, 1997) and disability-related work leave (Kessler et al., 1999), as well as low levels of on-the-job work performance (Berndt et al., 1998). The most commonly used approach to study these labor market costs is the human capital approach (Tarricone, 2006), which is based on the observation that wages and salaries are paid in direct return for productive services. This makes earnings a good indicator of the human capital accumulated by the individual and earnings-equivalent time forgone because of an illness a good representation of the indirect costs of that illness to the employer.

Although a considerable body of empirical research has used the human capital approach to document the adverse societal effects of mental disorders, this research has been carried out largely in a small number of high-income countries (Chatterji et al., 2007; Kessler et al., 1999). However, the data on prevalence of mental disorders presented earlier in this chapter make it clear that mental disorders are common throughout the world. Based on this observation, we used the WMH data to estimate the human capital costs of specific disorders on role functioning in workplace settings (de Graaf et al., 2008; Kessler et al., 2006). The results are striking. In the U.S. WMH survey, for example, 6.4% of workers had an episode of major depressive disorder (MDD) in the year of the survey, resulting in an average of over five weeks of lost work productivity (Kessler et al., 2006). Given the salaries of these workers, the annual human capital loss to employers in the U.S. labor force associated with MDD was estimated to be in excess of $36 billion. A similar result was found in a WMH analysis that estimated the workplace costs of adult attention deficit hyperactivity disorder (ADHD) in 10 WMH surveys (de Graaf et al., 2008). ADHD was associated with an average of 22 days excess lost productivity per worker with this disorder across the ten WMH countries that assessed it. Comparable analyses for other disorders are in progress in ongoing WMH investigations.

The effects of mental disorders on earnings

We also estimated the effects of mental disorders on earnings. We focused on serious mental illness (SMI) because previous research has shown that earnings and long-term work incapacity are both much more strongly related to SMI than to less serious forms of mental illness (Kessler et al., 2008; Shiels, Gabbay, & Ford, 2004). WMH respondents were asked to report their personal earnings in the 12 months before interview. In order to facilitate pooling of results across countries, earnings reports were divided by the median earnings in the country. These transformed scores were then used as outcomes in a pooled regression model estimated simultaneously across all countries. The regression analysis used a dummy variable for SMI as the predictor of primary interest. The outcome was the continuous earnings score (appropriately transformed to address the problem of a highly skewed distribution in most countries). Control variables included sociodemographics (age, sex), country, substance disorders, and interactions between sex and all other predictors. The sex interactions were included because previous research has shown that the predictors of earnings differ betweeen males and females (Kessler et al., 2008; Rice & Miller, 1998).

SMI was associated with an enormous reduction in earnings: 32% of the median within-country earnings in high-income countries and 33% of median within-country earnings in lower-middle-income countries (Levinson et al., 2010). Decomposition showed that 39% of this total association in high-income countries and 27% in lower-middle-income countries was due to the reduced probability of having any earnings among people with SMI. That is, people with SMI were significantly less likely to be employed. A larger component of the total association, 49% of the total in high-income countries and 66% in lower-middle-income countries, was due to lower mean level of earnings among people with SMI who had any earnings. That is, employed people with SMI were found to have significantly lower earnings than other employed people. Further analysis showed that part of this effect was due to people with SMI having lower education than other people, but a significant residual association still existed between SMI and low earnings even after controlling for education.

The cost-effectiveness of treatment

Costs as large as those documented above raise the question of whether expansion of detection and treatment efforts and increases in treatment quality improvement initiatives might reduce the adverse effects of mental disorders to an extent that makes treatment cost-effective either from a societal an employer perspective. An effectiveness trial carried out in conjunction with the WMH survey in the U.S. evaluated this question experimentally (Wang, Simon et al., 2007). A large sample of workers was screened for major depressive disorder (MDD) and randomized to either a model outreach and best-practices treatment intervention or to usual care. The intervention group at six and 12 months had significantly higher job retention than controls, as well as significantly more hours worked than controls (equivalent to an annual two weeks more work). The financial benefits of these intervention effects (in terms of hiring and training costs, disability payment, and salaries paid for sickness absence days) were substantially higher than the costs of treatment, demonstrating that an expansion of workplace screening, detection, and treatment of worker mental disorders could represent a human capital investment opportunity for employers. Replications of this study are currently underway in other WMH countries. Extensions of the intervention to consider treatment of bipolar depression and adult ADHD are also underway. Ongoing analyses of the WMH data are also searching for other intervention targets that can be used to evaluate the effects of treatment in reducing the burdens associated with mental disorders.

Conclusions

The data reviewed in this chapter illustrate that mental disorders are commonly occurring in the general population, often have an early age-of-onset, and often are associated with significant adverse societal costs. We also presented some evidence that at least part of this burden can be reversed with best-practices treatment. The latter finding argues much more persuasively than the naturalistic survey findings that mental disorders are actual causes rather than merely correlates of impaired role functioning. Based on these results, we can safely conclude that mental disorders are common and consequential from a societal perspective throughout the world.

However, as reported elsewhere, the WMH data show that only a small minority of people with even seriously impairing mental disorders receive treatment in most countries and that even fewer receive high-quality treatment (Wang, Aguilar-Gaxiola et al., 2007). This situation has to change. A good argument can be made based on the WMH results that an expansion of treatment would be a human capital investment opportunity from the employer's perspective, and the same argument might be made from a societal perspective. Ongoing WMH analyses are continuing to refine the naturalistic analyses of the adverse effects of mental disorders in an effort to target experimental interventions that can demonstrate the value of expanded treatment in addressing the enormous global burden of mental disorders.

Acknowledgments

Preparation of this chapter was supported, in part, by the following grants from the U.S. Public Health Service: U01MH060220, R01DA012058, R01MH070884, R01DA016558. Portions of this paper appeared previously in Kessler, R. C., Aguilar-Gaxiola, S., Alonso, J., et al. (2009). The global burden of mental disorders: An update from the WHO World Mental Health (WMH) Surveys. *Epidemiologia E Psichiatria Sociale*, 18(1), 23–33, © 2009 Cambridge University Press, and Alonso, J., Petukhova, M., Vilagut, G., et al. (2010). Days out of role due to common physical and mental conditions: Results from the WHO World Mental Health Surveys. *Molecular Psychiatry*, doi:10.1038/mp.2010.101, © 2010 Nature Publishing Group. Both used with permission. A complete list of WMH publications can be found at www.hcp.med.harvard.edu/wmh/. The views and opinions expressed in this report are those of the authors and should not be construed to represent the views of any of the sponsoring organizations, agencies, or Governments.

Declaration of interest

Kessler has been a consultant for GlaxoSmithKline Inc., Pfizer Inc., Wyeth-Ayerst, Sanofi-Aventis, Kaiser Permanente, and Shire Pharmaceuticals; has served on advisory boards for Eli Lilly & Company and Wyeth-Ayerst; and has had research support for his epidemiological studies from Eli Lilly and Company, Pfizer Inc., Ortho-McNeil Pharmaceuticals Inc., Sanofi-Aventis, Merck, Shire, and Bristol-Myers Squibb.

References

Alonso, J., Petukhova, M., Vilagut, G., Chatterji, S., Heeringa, S., Üstün, T. B., et al. (2010). Days out of role due to common physical and mental conditions: Results from the WHO World Mental Health Surveys. *Molecular Psychiatry*, doi:10.1038/mp.2010.

Alonso, J., Vilagut, G., Chatterji, S., Heeringa, S., Schoenbaum, M., Üstün, T. B., et al. (2010). Including information about comorbidity in estimates of disease burden: Results from the WHO World Mental Health Surveys. *Psychological Medicine*. doi:10.1017/S0033291710001212.

Berndt, E. R., Finkelstein, S. N., Greenberg, P. E., Howland, R. H., Keith, A., Rush, A. J., et al. (1998). Workplace performance effects from chronic depression and its treatment. *Journal of Health Economics, 17*(5), 511–535.

Berto, P., D'Ilario, D., Ruffo, P., Di Virgilio, R., & Rizzo, F. (2000). Depression: Cost-of-illness studies in the international literature, a review. *Journal of Mental Health Policy and Economics, 3*(1), 3–10.

Brown, T. A., & Barlow, D. H. (2005). Dimensional versus categorical classification of mental disorders in the fifth edition of the Diagnostic and Statistical Manual of Mental Disorders and beyond: Comment on the special section. *Journal of Abnormal Psychology, 114*(4), 551–556.

Chang, S. M., Hahm, B. J., Lee, J. Y., Shin, M. S., Jeon, H. J., Hong, J. P., et al. (2008). Cross-national difference in the prevalence of depression caused by the diagnostic threshold. *Journal of Affective Disorders, 106*(1–2), 159–167.

Chatterji, P., Alegria, M., Lu, M., & Takeuchi, D. (2007). Psychiatric disorders and labor market outcomes: Evidence from the National Latino and Asian American Study. *Health Economics, 16*(10), 1069–1090.

Connor, K. M., & Davidson, J. R. (2001). SPRINT: A brief global assessment of post-traumatic stress disorder. *International Clinical Psychopharmacology, 16*(5), 279–284.

de Graaf, R., Kessler, R. C., Fayyad, J., ten Have, M., Alonso, J., Angermeyer, M., et al. (2008). The prevalence and effects of adult attention-deficit/hyperactivity disorder (ADHD) on the performance of workers: Results from the WHO World Mental Health Survey Initiative. *Occupational and Environmental Medicine, 65*(12), 835–842.

Druss, B. G., Hwang, I., Petukhova, M., Sampson, N. A., Wang, P. S., & Kessler, R. C. (2008). Impairment in role functioning in mental and chronic medical disorders in the United States: Results from the National Comorbidity Survey Replication. *Molecular Psychiatry, 14*(7), 728–737.

Endicott, J., Spitzer, R. L., Fleiss, J. L., & Cohen, J. (1976). The global assessment scale. A procedure for measuring overall severity of psychiatric disturbance. *Archives of General Psychiatry, 33*(6), 766–771.

Greenberg, P. E., & Birnbaum, H. G. (2005). The economic burden of depression in the US: Societal and patient perspectives. *Expert Opinion on Pharmacotherapy, 6*(3), 369–376.

Greenberg, P. E., Sisitsky, T., Kessler, R. C., Finkelstein, S. N., Berndt, E. R., Davidson, J. R., et al. (1999). The economic burden of anxiety disorders in the 1990s. *Journal of Clinical Psychiatry, 60*(7), 427–435.

Hambrick, J. P., Turk, C. L., Heimberg, R. G., Schneier, F. R., & Liebowitz, M. R.

(2004). Psychometric properties of disability measures among patients with social anxiety disorder. *Journal of Anxiety Disorders, 18*(6), 825–839.

Harkness, J., Pennell, B. E., Villar, A., Gebler, N., Aguilar-Gaxiola, S., & Bilgen, I. (2008). Translation procedures and translation assessment in the World Mental Health Survey Initiative. In R. C. Kessler & T. B. Üstün (Eds.), *The WHO World Mental Health Surveys: Global perspectives on the epidemiology of mental disorders* (pp. 91–113). New York: Cambridge University Press.

Haro, J. M., Arbabzadeh-Bouchez, S., Brugha, T. S., de Girolamo, G., Guyer, M. E., Jin, R., et al. (2006). Concordance of the Composite International Diagnostic Interview Version 3.0 (CIDI 3.0) with standardized clinical assessments in the WHO World Mental Health surveys. *International Journal of Methods in Psychiatric Research, 15*(4), 167–180.

Harwood, H., Ameen, A., Denmead, G., Englert, E., Fountain, D., & Livermore, G. (2000). *The economic cost of mental illness, 1992.* Rockville, MD: National Institute of Mental Health.

He, Y., Zhang, M., Lin, E. H., Bruffaerts, R., Posada-Villa, J., Angermeyer, M. C., et al. (2008). Mental disorders among persons with arthritis: Results from the World Mental Health Surveys. *Psychological Medicine, 38*(11), 1639–1650.

Heeringa, S. G., Wells, J. E., Hubbard, F., Mneimneh, Z., Chiu, W. T., & Sampson, N. (2008). Sample Designs and Sampling Procedures. In R. C. Kessler & T. B. Üstün (Eds.), *The WHO World Mental Health Surveys: Global perspectives on the epidemiology of mental disorders* (pp. 14–32). New York: Cambridge University Press.

Kessler, R.C., Aguilar-Gaxiola, S., Alonso, J., Chatterji, S., Lee, S., Ormel, J., et al. (2009). The global burden of mental disorders: An update from the WHO World Mental Health (WMH) Surveys. *Epidemiologia E Psichiatria Sociale, 18*(1), 23–33.

Kessler, R. C., Akiskal, H. S., Ames, M., Birnbaum, H., Greenberg, P., Hirschfeld, R. et al. (2006). Prevalence and effects of mood disorders on work performance in a nationally representative sample of U.S. workers. *American Journal of Psychiatry, 163*(9), 1561–1568.

Kessler, R. C., Amminger, G. P., Aguilar-Gaxiola, S., Alonso, J., Lee, S., & Üstün, T. B. (2007). Age of onset of mental disorders: A review of recent literature. *Current Opinion in Psychiatry, 20*(4), 359–364.

Kessler, R. C., Barber, C., Birnbaum, H. G., Frank, R. G., Greenberg, P. E., Rose, R. M., et al. (1999). Depression in the workplace: Effects on short-term disability. *Health Affairs (Millwood), 18*(5), 163–171.

Kessler, R. C., Berglund, P. A., Foster, C. L., Saunders, W. B., Stang, P. E., & Walters, E. E. (1997). Social consequences of psychiatric disorders, II: Teenage parenthood. *American Journal of Psychiatry, 154*(10), 1405–1411.

Kessler, R. C., Foster, C. L., Saunders, W. B., & Stang, P. E. (1995). Social consequences of psychiatric disorders, I: Educational attainment. *American Journal of Psychiatry, 152*(7), 1026–1032.

Kessler, R. C., & Frank, R. G. (1997). The impact of psychiatric disorders on work loss days. *Psychological Medicine, 27*(4), 861–873.

Kessler, R. C., Heeringa, S., Lakoma, M. D., Petukhova, M., Rupp, A. E., Schoenbaum, M., et al. (2008). Individual and societal effects of mental disorders on earnings in the United States: Results from the national comorbidity survey replication. *American Journal of Psychiatry, 165*(6), 703–711.

Kessler, R. C., & Üstün, T. B. (2004). The World Mental Health (WMH) Survey

Initiative Version of the World Health Organization (WHO) Composite International Diagnostic Interview (CIDI). *International Journal of Methods in Psychiatric Research, 13*(2), 93–121.

Kessler, R. C., Walters, E. E., & Forthofer, M. S. (1998). The social consequences of psychiatric disorders, III: Probability of marital stability. *American Journal of Psychiatry, 155*(8), 1092–1096.

Lee, S., Tsang, A., Breslau, J., Aguilar-Gaxiola, S., Angermeyer, M., Borges, et al. (2009). Mental disorders and termination of education in high-income and low- and middle-income countries: Epidemiological study. *British Journal of Psychiatry, 194*(5), 411–417.

Leon, A. C., Olfson, M., Portera, L., Farber, L., & Sheehan, D. V. (1997). Assessing psychiatric impairment in primary care with the Sheehan Disability Scale. *International Journal of Psychiatry in Medicine, 27*(2), 93–105.

Levinson, D., Lakoma, M., Petukhova, M., Schoenbaum, M., Zaslavsky, A. M., Angermeyer, M., et al. (2010). The associations of serious mental illness with earnings in the WHO World Mental Health surveys. *British Journal of Psychiatry, 197*, 114-121.

Lopez, A. D., & Mathers, C. D. (2007). Inequalities in health status: Findings from the 2001 Global Burden of Disease study. In S. Matlin (Ed.), *The global forum update on research for health, volume 4* (pp. 163–175). London: Pro-Brook Publishing Limited.

Maetzel, A., & Li, L. (2002). The economic burden of low back pain: A review of studies published between 1996 and 2001. *Best Practice and Research Clinical Rheumatology, 16*(1), 23–30.

Matsunaga, H., & Seedat, S. (2007). Obsessive-compulsive spectrum disorders: Cross-national and ethnic issues. *CNS Spectrums, 12*(5), 392–400.

Merikangas, K. R., Ames, M., Cui, L., Stang, P. E., Üstün, T. B., Von Korff, M., & Kessler, R. C. (2007). The impact of comorbidity of mental and physical conditions on role disability in the US adult household population. *Archives of General Psychiatry, 64*(10), 1180–1188.

Murray, C. J. L., & Lopez, A. D. (1996). *The Global Burden of Disease: A comprehensive assessment of mortality and disability from diseases, injuries and risk factors in 1990 and projected to 2020.* Cambridge, MA: Harvard University Press.

Murray, C. J. L., Lopez, A. D., Mathers, C. D., & Stein, C. (2001). *The Global Burden of Disease 2000 Project: Aims, methods and data sources.* Geneva: World Health Organization.

Mylle, J., & Maes, M. (2004). Partial posttraumatic stress disorder revisited. *Journal of Affective Disorders, 78*(1), 37–48.

Ormel, J., Petukhova, M., Chatterji, S., Aguilar-Gaxiola, S., Alonso, J., Angermeyer, M. C., et al. (2008). Disability and treatment of specific mental and physical disorders across the world. *British Journal of Psychiatry, 192*(5), 368–375.

Ormel, J., Von Korff, M., Burger, H., Scott, K., Demyttenaere, K., Huang, Y. Q., et al. (2007). Mental disorders among persons with heart disease – results from World Mental Health surveys. *General Hospital Psychiatry, 29*(4), 325–334.

Pallanti, S., Bernardi, S., & Quercioli, L. (2006). The Shorter PROMIS Questionnaire and the Internet Addiction Scale in the assessment of multiple addictions in a high-school population: Prevalence and related disability. *CNS Spectrums, 11*(12), 966–974.

Pennell, B. E., Mneimneh, Z., Bowers, A., Chardoul, S., Wells, J. E., Viana, M. C., et al. (2008). Implementation of the World Mental Health Surveys. In R. C.

Kessler & T. B. Üstün (Eds.), *The WHO World Mental Health Surveys: Global perspectives on the epidemiology of mental disorders* (pp. 33–57). New York: Cambridge University Press.

Reed, S. D., Lee, T. A., & McCrory, D. C. (2004). The economic burden of allergic rhinitis: A critical evaluation of the literature. *Pharmacoeconomics, 22*(6), 345–361.

Rice, D. P., Kelman, S., Miller, L. S., & Dunmeyer, S. (1990). *The economic costs of alcohol and drug abuse and mental illness: 1985.* Washington, DC: US Department of Health and Human Services.

Rice, D. P., & Miller, L. S. (1998). Health economics and cost implications of anxiety and other mental disorders in the United States. *British Journal of Psychiatry, Supplement*(34), 4–9.

Ruscio, A. M., Chiu, W. T., Roy-Byrne, P., Stang, P. E., Stein, D. J., Wittchen, H. U., & Kessler, R. C. (2007). Broadening the definition of generalized anxiety disorder: Effects on prevalence and associations with other disorders in the National Comorbidity Survey Replication. *Journal of Anxiety Disorders, 21*(5), 662–676.

Shiels, C., Gabbay, M. B., & Ford, F. M. (2004). Patient factors associated with duration of certified sickness absence and transition to long-term incapacity. *British Journal of General Practice, 54*(499), 86–91.

Silverman, W. K., & Moreno, J. (2005). Specific phobia. *Child and Adolescent Psychiatric Clinics of North America, 14*(4), 819–843, ix–x.

Simon, G. E., Goldberg, D. P., Von Korff, M., & Ustun, T. B. (2002). Understanding cross-national differences in depression prevalence. *Psychological Medicine, 32*(4), 585–594.

Skeppar, P., & Adolfsson, R. (2006). Bipolar II and the bipolar spectrum. *Nordic Journal of Psychiatry, 60*(1), 7–26.

Somers, J. M., Goldner, E. M., Waraich, P., & Hsu, L. (2006). Prevalence and incidence studies of anxiety disorders: A systematic review of the literature. *Canadian Journal of Psychiatry, 51*(2), 100–113.

Tarricone, R. (2006). Cost-of-illness analysis. What room in health economics? *Health Policy, 77*(1), 51–63.

Üstün, T. B., & Sartorius, N. (Eds.). (1995). *Mental illness in general health care: An international study.* New York: Wiley.

Wang, P. S., Aguilar-Gaxiola, S., Alonso, J., Angermeyer, M. C., Borges, G., Bromet, E. J., et al. (2007). Use of mental health services for anxiety, mood, and substance disorders in 17 countries in the WHO world mental health surveys. *Lancet, 370*(9590), 841–850.

Wang, P. S., Simon, G. E., Avorn, J., Azocar, F., Ludman, E. J., McCulloch, J., et al. (2007). Telephone screening, outreach, and care management for depressed workers and impact on clinical and work productivity outcomes: A randomized controlled trial. *Journal of the American Medical Association, 298*(12), 1401–1411.

Waraich, P., Goldner, E. M., Somers, J. M., & Hsu, L. (2004). Prevalence and incidence studies of mood disorders: A systematic review of the literature. *Canadian Journal of Psychiatry, 49*(2), 124–138.

Wittchen, H. U., & Jacobi, F. (2005). Size and burden of mental disorders in Europe: A critical review and appraisal of 27 studies. *European Neuropsychopharmacology, 15*(4), 357–376.

Zhang, X., Zhao, X., & Harris, A. (2009). Chronic diseases and labour force participation in Australia. *Journal of Health Economics, 28*(1), 91–108.

3 Epidemiology in public mental health

Ezra Susser and Rebecca P. Smith

Introduction

Over a period of 50 years, community surveys of mental disorders (Leighton, 1959; Robins & Regier, 1991; Srole & Fischer, 1980), culminating in the World Mental Health Initiative described in the previous chapter, have built solid evidence that mental disorders are common, often disabling, under-recognized, and under-treated. Although these surveys are sometimes criticized for overstating the significance of mental disorders in population health, a good argument can be made that they actually understate it. With notable exceptions, e.g., Rutter, Tizard, Yule, Graham, and Whitmore (1976), these surveys rarely include children or elderly people, and lifetime (as opposed to current) prevalence is seriously underestimated due to problems of recall over long periods (Susser & Shrout, 2010). With few exceptions (Phillips et al., 2009), severe but less common disorders, such as schizophrenia and autism, cannot be detected reliably by most community surveys, yet these conditions are often disabling over a long period and have an impact on the lives of the patient's family and other caregivers as well as the patients themselves.

In parallel to these community surveys, a large body of work has been developed to investigate the causes and consequences of mental disorders in the population. The approaches used now encompass a wide variety of designs, ranging from the cellular to the societal level, integrating biology and genetics with the assessment of mental states, and extending over the life course to trace the evolution and origins of mental disorders. Psychiatric epidemiologists have played an important role in expanding the repertoire of epidemiologic designs, for example, by aligning with social scientists in ecological studies that look beyond inter-individual differences to differences in health that are related to family, community, or society as a whole. A full review of the designs used in psychiatric epidemiology is beyond the scope of this chapter, but readers may refer to Susser, Schwartz, Morabia, and Bromet (2006).

Despite these advances in psychiatric epidemiology, there is much progress that remains to be made. One area that has important implications for public mental health is the use of two "bread and butter" designs of epidemiology – the cohort and the case-control study – to examine the relation of mental disorders to mortality. In this chapter we describe two landmark studies that used mortality as a key endpoint: a cohort study of cigarette smoking and a case-control study of heavy alcohol use. Results from these epidemiologic studies had far-reaching implications for public health and in particular for public mental health, but the studies were not carried out by psychiatric epidemiologists. This reflects the fact that few psychiatric epidemiologists have focused on the relationship between common mental disorders and mortality. Thus, we hope to promote wider and more effective use within our field of the methods exemplified by these studies.

Cohort study of cigarette smoking in the UK

The cohort study design

In a prospective cohort study at the time exposure status is defined, all potential subjects are free from the condition or disease that the study is investigating. The subjects in the study are then followed over time. Thus, cohort studies can more clearly establish a temporal sequence between the exposure (for example, cigarette smoking) and the outcome (for example, mortality) than can a case-control study. The design is also less vulnerable to selection bias than the case-control study (see later). It does, however, have its own vulnerabilities, including the potential for specific kinds of loss to follow-up that can introduce bias (Rothman, Greenland, & Lash, 2008; Susser et al., 2006).

Though the study described below offers an excellent illustration of what can be achieved with the prospective cohort design, it is only one type of cohort study, and all types can be used to good effect. Historical or restrospective cohort studies depend on the availability and quality of exposure and outcome data that were recorded in the past. Some studies mix features of prospective and retrospective cohort studies. "Clinical" cohort studies follow cohorts of people who already have a health outcome in order to examine survivorship, "natural history", and/or predictors of prognosis. Readers will find a wide range of cohort studies described in most epidemiology textbooks (for psychiatric epidemiology, see Susser et al., 2006).

Cohort studies over the life course

For some mental disorders, the effects on mortality may only be revealed by cohort studies that span a large part of the life course. In the study we describe here, it was only after a follow-up of 50 years that the authors could detect the full impact of lifelong cigarette smoking on mortality because the latency period between the uptake of the cigarette smoking habit and death due to a smoking-related disease can be very long, usually many decades. Life course studies are also important for studies of the causes and prevention of mental disorders. Some mental disorders – for example, schizophrenia (Keshavan, Kennedy, & Murray, 2004; Opler & Susser, 2005; Susser, St. Clair, & He, 2008) – are influenced by fetal or early childhood exposures even though they do not become manifest until young adulthood or even later in the life course. In addition, mental disorders often begin in childhood or early adulthood and persist or recur over the lifecourse (Silva & Stanton, 1997). Lifelong protective factors for mental disorders may be established in the early childhood years (Hertzman & Wiens, 1996); thus, the impact of interventions at various points in the life course to prevent mental disorders or modify their adverse consequences may not be evident until decades later.

In some instances, therefore, life course studies will be needed in order to reveal the full range of origins, consequences, and potential benefits (and harms) of interventions for mental disorders. This does not mean, however, that we should privilege long-term cohort studies (or any other design) for all purposes. In the next section, we demonstrate the power of a well-designed case-control study conducted over a short time period. We do not advocate for any particular design, but rather, for the use of designs that are tailored to answer important questions.

The British doctors study

Widely regarded as one of the most important epidemiologic studies ever conducted, the British doctors study followed smokers and non-smokers over a period of 50 years to determine the contribution of cigarette smoking to premature mortality over the life course (Doll, Peto, Boreham, & Sutherland, 2004). During the course of the study, the authors elaborated the nature of the cohort design and developed its full potential by means of extending it over the life course. The study was begun in 1951 after case-control studies had already broken ground by demonstrating that cigarette smoking was a cause of lung cancer (Davey Smith, 2004; Doll & Hill, 1950; Wynder & Graham, 1950, republished 1985). According to the originators of the cohort study, "Further retrospective studies of the same kind would seem to us unlikely to advance our knowledge materially or throw any new light on the nature of the association." (Doll & Hill, 1954). Therefore, they initiated a prospective cohort study to compare health outcomes among smokers and non-smokers.

Doll and Hill sent out 59,600 questionnaires to men and women on the "Medical Register" of the UK that listed all licensed physicians. There were several reasons for choosing to study physicians. The investigators thought that doctors would pose fewer problems in follow-up than other groups because they were easier to locate, as doctors had to be registered by the UK government. Also, they felt that by virtue of their education about and interest in health-related matters, doctors might be more likely to provide accurate responses to follow-up questionnaires. Finally, the investigators knew that if they did the study among doctors, the results were more likely to be noticed by the medical profession.

The study questionnaires established the smoking habits of the doctors in 1951 and were followed up at several time points (1957, 1966, 1971, 1978, 1991, 2000), up to the year 2000. The questionnaire was kept short and simple in order to maximize the proportion of responders. Doctors were asked to classify themselves into one of three groups: current smokers; ex-smokers; or never-smokers (i.e., never regular smokers). Current smokers were asked to report their current method of tobacco smoking, the amount they were consuming, and the method by which they were consuming it. Ex-smokers were asked similar questions, but pertaining to the time at which they had most recently given up smoking.

The first, preliminary report analyzed the results of the first 29 months of follow-up (Doll & Hill, 1954) based on sufficiently complete responses to 40,564 (68%) of the questionnaires. In this report, the researchers focused on the group they judged to be at highest risk for lung cancer, men over age 35 years (N = 24,389). The study clearly confirmed the relation of cigarette smoking to lung cancer and suggested that it might also be related to other health outcomes such as cardiovascular disease. The investigators noted that there may have been some selective loss to follow-up; doctors who were already ill from cancer might have been less likely to answer the inquiries. The resulting bias would, however, be likely to lead to an underestimate of the impact of smoking on health.

Although this preliminary report was a landmark in the history of epidemiology, its results have been eclipsed by the more recent findings from the subsequent extension of the study over a 50-year period. The original authors Doll and Hill, later joined by others, continued to trace the mortality among smokers and non-smokers up to the year 2000. Findings were published at four, 10, 20, and 40 years of follow-up. The 50-year follow-up (findings described briefly below) is based on the 34,439 male British doctors who returned sufficiently complete questionnaires in 1951. Thus, it includes men who were under age 35 at the initiation of the study (excluded in the 1954 report) but does not include women. After excluding those who were lost due to emigration or other reasons, there were 31,496 men who were followed up to the year 2000. Mortality data on this group were 99.2% complete.

Significant findings for public mental health

With 50 years of mortality over the life course laid out before them, the investigators were able to reach conclusions that have far-reaching implications for public health today and no doubt well into the future. For brevity, we draw attention to three findings. These are sufficient to demonstrate the enormous significance of the study but by no means cover the full array of what was reported, nor the depth of their analysis.

The first pertains to longevity for those who smoked over their entire adult life versus those who never smoked (a question originally posed by Pearl in 1938). A "lifelong smoker" was defined as a man who was smoking in 1951 and at every other time point at which the cohort was queried. Cigarette smoking was not common, however, until around the time of World War I (Brandt, 2007; Doll & Hill, 1954). Indeed, the distribution of free cigarettes to soldiers in World War I and World War II played a major role in establishing the habit among young men in the US and the UK. Therefore, in this cohort lifelong smokers can only be reliably identified among the generation born between 1900 and 1930. For this generation, within the cohort, the median age of initiating cigarette smoking was 18, making it likely that a man who was smoking in 1951, and smoking at every subsequent time point at which he was assessed, was smoking for most or all of his adult life. When the authors compared survival of lifelong smokers so defined with never-smokers in men born during the same time period, they found that average survival was about 10 years less for the lifelong smokers than the never-smokers. This means that the population of lifelong smokers did not have the dramatic gains in survival experienced by the general population of the UK during the 20th century. The other factors promoting survival were entirely offset by their cigarette smoking.

The second finding pertains to the proportion of deaths attributable to cigarette smoking over the adult life course. For lifelong smokers born between 1900 and 1930, the results suggested that about two-thirds of their mortality was attributable to cigarette smoking. Considering the uncertainties inherent in any observational study and the uncertainty of generalizability to women and to other populations, the authors felt that the safest and most general conclusion was that "smoking kills about one half" of lifelong smokers. Although this conclusion was probably an underestimate, it was irrefutable and large enough to portray a huge public health impact.

The third finding pertains to cessation of smoking. The authors showed that those who stopped smoking at about age 50 recovered about half of the 10-year loss in survival. Those who stopped at about age 30 recovered almost all of the loss.

Case-control study of alcohol use in Russia

The case-control design

The goal of a case-control study is to use fewer respondents to obtain the same result as in a perfect cohort study, meaning the case-control study can be used to answer a question more efficiently. Though the cost of this efficiency is a greater potential for bias, a well-designed case-control study can minimize the potential bias. (For further discussion on the advantages and disadvantages to the use of each of these designs, see Rothman et al. (2008) and Susser et al. (2006).)A case control study can be understood as an efficient way to sample an underlying cohort of exposed and unexposed people some of whom develop the disease of interest (for a full explanation see Rothman et al., 2008, Susser et al., 2006). This is most clearly seen in the context of a "nested" case-control study, where the underlying cohort is enumerated, but the same logic applies to all case-control studies. Validity depends on two critical steps:

1 Selecting controls from the same source population that gave rise to the cases.
2 Selecting controls independent of exposure status.

When these principles are applied, the controls will represent the ratio of exposed to unexposed in the population from which the cases were derived. Under these conditions, other things being equal (e.g., control of confounding, validity of exposure data), the odds of exposure for cases versus non-cases ("exposure odds ratio" from a case-control study) is equal to the odds of disease for exposed versus unexposed ("disease odds ratio" from a cohort study based in the same source population).

This equality of the exposure odds ratio in a case-control study and the disease odds ratio in the underlying cohort can be demonstrated by simple algebra. Thus, the relation of exposure to disease, in the form of an odds ratio, can be obtained from a case-control study. In a nested case-control study, when the underlying cohort can be fully enumerated, one can select controls from the source population (i.e., the underlying cohort) independent of exposure status, and thereby obtain the same odds ratio in a case-control study as in a cohort study but at much less cost and in a much shorter time. The majority of case-control studies, however, are not nested in a fully enumerated cohort. One has to conceptualize and then sample the source population that gave rise to the cases, which introduces potential for bias because there is generally some uncertainty about the source population and the best approach to sample it. In many scenarios, this potential bias can be minimized by a thoughtful design, and case-control studies will produce valid results. Similar to cohort studies, there are numerous variations of the case-control design, but they are all based on the premise that the (exposure) odds ratio from the case-control study will approximate the (disease) odds ratio that would have been obtained from a cohort study of the source population.

Case-control studies of mortality due to mental disorders

In public mental health, case-control studies of mortality can be especially useful when the presence of a mental disorder or addictive behavior has a close temporal relationship to mortality. Gathering good information on the experience of deceased persons long before their death is much more difficult than learning about their behaviors and circumstances close to the time of death. In this regard, the study of heavy alcohol use provides an informative contrast with the study of cigarette smoking. Unlike cigarette smoking, for which mortality is mainly related to long-term effects on disease risk later in life, heavy alcohol use has immediate behavioral effects that, at least in some contexts, appear to mediate much of its relationship to mortality. Under these conditions, revealing the impact of heavy alcohol use on mortality using a case-control study conducted within a very short time period is possible, as illustrated below.

The example of the Russian mortality study

A case-control study conducted by Zaridze and colleagues (2009) examined the contribution of heavy alcohol use to the increase in adult mortality rates in Russia in the 1990s. By the year 2000 in Russia, the probability that a 15-year-old man would die before age 35 was 10%, and the probability that a 35-year-old man would die before age 55 was 27%; in Western Europe, these probabilities were only 2 and 6%, respectively (United Nations Population Division, 2004; World Health Organization, 2007; Zaridze et al., 2009). This dramatic increase in mortality was unprecedented for an industrialized society (excepting periods of calamitous wars).

Prior to this study, both alcohol use and mortality had increased sharply following the collapse of communism in 1991, peaking in 1994. This suggested two possible explanations. One was that the social upheaval led to increased alcohol use, which in turn increased mortality. The other was that the social upheaval was a confounding factor, that is, it led to both increased alcohol use and increased mortality and thereby created a non-causal association between them. Previous research had suggested that alcohol consumption and mortality patterns were likely to be causally related (Leon et al., 1997; 2007), but the question was not yet resolved.

The investigators selected for their study three industrial cities in western Siberia: Tomsk, Barnaul and Biysk (2002 census populations: 0.5 million, 0.7 million, and 0.2 million, respectively). These cities had principally European Russian populations, and both the overall mortality rates and the distribution of certified causes of death were similar to those in the whole of Russia and fluctuated in a similar way, with a sudden large increase in mortality from 1992 to 1994 (Men, Brennan, Boffeta, & Zaridze, 2003). The cases and controls were selected from 0.2 million residents of these three cities who died at ages 15 to 74 between 1990 and 2001. Local records included all deaths among registered residents, but not migrants. In addition to name, age, sex, and cause of death, the address of the deceased was recorded on death records, and the investigators chose to study deaths in neighborhoods in which they were most likely to obtain high participation rates. The teams of interviewers included former physicians, and they selected areas of these towns where these physicians had worked, and were therefore familiar with the neighborhood and known to many of the residents.

The total number of deceased persons included in the investigation was 60,416, and they were classified as either cases or controls, according to the cause of death. Since the recorded causes of death did not conform to International Classification of Disorders (ICD) classifications, these codings were ignored, and ICD-10 was used to assign underlying causes from the written death certificate. Cases were defined as persons who died from causes that were suspected beforehand to be related to alcohol or tobacco, and these were the vast majority. Controls were persons who died from any other cause.

Information about alcohol use by deceased persons was obtained by visiting the addresses in the death records and conducting proxy interviews with family members. Sufficient information was obtained for 48,557 deceased persons, among whom 43,082 were cases and 5,475 were controls. Since proxy information from the family about a deceased person's alcohol use is necessarily imperfect and vulnerable to recall bias by family members, the investigators built in numerous procedures to improve accuracy and reduce bias. For example, the interviewers did not know the cause of death of the deceased and were therefore blind to case versus control status. Also, the interview covered mainly other topics, so questions about alcohol use of the deceased were unobtrusive. Interviewers were carefully trained and supervised, and one in 10 interviews was randomly chosen for repetition to monitor performance.

The questionnaire asked about usual weekly alcohol consumption patterns before and during the final year of life. The responses for these two time periods tended to be similar, and the greater of the two was used. Total weekly consumption of any kind of alcohol was converted to units equivalent to "500 ml bottles of vodka." Since there were few "never-drinkers," the reference category of "unexposed" comprised those who drank less than (the equivalent of) half a bottle of vodka per week and (to exclude binge-drinkers) always drank less than half a bottle in one day. The three exposed groups drank less than one bottle per week; one to less than three bottles per week; and three or more bottles per week.

Significant findings for public mental health

We call attention to three key results of this study. First, the authors found extremely strong and dose-related associations between heavy alcohol use and deaths suspected to be alcohol- or tobacco-related (the great majority of deaths, see above). The associations were strongest for those more likely to be related to alcohol than tobacco (e.g., alcohol poisoning and accidents).

The investigators examined and tried to quantify potential bias in their results and concluded that the potential for bias was small in relation to the large size of the effects they detected. They inferred that there was a causal relation between heavy alcohol use and mortality; further, they estimated that alcohol was responsible for about one half of deaths among men and one quarter of deaths among women in the age group 35 to 54, and was also a major cause of death among men and women in the age group 55 to 74.

Second, the largest contributors to alcohol-associated excess mortality were accidents and violence. Particularly extreme were the relative risks for death from assault and suicide in the highest male and the two highest female alcohol consumption categories. Thus, it appeared that a very large proportion of the excess deaths were related to the effects of alcohol on an individual's behavior, which suggests that public health practitioners need to be concerned with not only the physical effects of heavy alcohol use on the body (e.g., cirrhosis), but also (or perhaps more) with its mental effects on hazardous behaviors. In Russia, not only interventions that reduce alcohol consumption but also interventions that reduce the hazardous behaviors associated with alcohol consumption are required for reducing the high mortality rates. This is no doubt also true, to some degree, for many other nations.

Third, after their case-control data suggested that the association between heavy alcohol use and mortality was likely to be causal, the authors turned to another approach to help rule out alternative explanations for the association. They examined the ecological relationship between alcohol use and mortality in the 1980s in Russia, the period prior to the social upheaval that accompanied the collapse of communism. They showed that, for the period 1985 to 1987, following the short-lived restrictions placed on alcohol use under the Gorbachev regime in 1985, both alcohol use and mortality declined suddenly and sharply. This suggested that other effects of the social upheaval of 1991 were less viable explanations for the increased mortality of the 1990s and supported the view that the increased mortality was mediated by increased alcohol consumption, as suggested by their case-control study.

Uses of epidemiology in public mental health

What can we learn from these studies? First and foremost, in both studies the investigators began with a carefully specified question whose answer had profound implications for public mental health and designed studies that could answer the question. Questions of public health import may be posed at any level (e.g., inter-individual differences, cross-national differences) or across any stage of the life course (e.g., conception to birth, youth to old age), and sometimes questions can be asked that encompass more than one level or life stage. Once we have considered the level and life stage we wish to address, we can choose a design which is suitable to answer it. Too often, we resort to prevailing approaches that are most familiar to us but are not suitable to answer our questions.

Second, despite the inherent limitations of single studies, those that are well conceived and conducted can make an enormous contribution, as we have illustrated in this chapter. In fact, both of these studies, conducted in particular populations, have implications for health across the entire globe. Cigarette smoking is increasing now in low- and middle-income countries, the consequence of which (if the trend continues) will be a massive impact on global mortality later in this century (Peto et al., 1996; Peto, Chen, & Boreham, 1999). Similarly, heavy alcohol use is a global problem, although not as pervasive as cigarette smoking.

Third, these studies intentionally targeted exposures that they hypothe-sized (correctly) would have large effects on mortality. Observational studies carry inherent uncertainty, and some have argued that small relative risks (e.g., below 1.5) are simply beyond the resolving power of such studies (Shapiro, 2000). A reasonable counter-argument for studying small relative risks is that reduction of common exposures can be important for popula-tion health, even if the reduction has only a small impact on the average risk for an individual. This argument is often accompanied, however, by the sup-position that we have exhausted the detection of effects of large magnitude for common exposures. These two recent studies suggest otherwise.

Fourth, while some study designs are considered stronger than others in that they are generally more likely to reduce sources of random error and bias, it is misleading to construct a strict hierarchy among them. The strongest methodology can produce misleading results if it is not applied in a way that is adequate to answer a well-framed question. The randomized controlled trial, for example, is probably our best technology for address-ing whether a particular treatment (a form of exposure) has an effect or not, and the literature is rife with examples of randomized controlled trials that, because they did not ask or could not answer the right question, pro-duced misleading results.

Nonetheless, it is still important to acknowledge that a circumscribed and sharply focused question relating to public mental health will tend to be incomplete in terms of the breadth of knowledge required to fully address it. Generally, studies designed to answer other related questions (e.g., at other levels or life stages) will be needed to complement a discovery in order to better comprehend the causal process and the implications for public health. Important determinants of health at the societal level sometimes cannot be adequately detected in studies done at the level of the individual (Galea, 2007; Subramanian, Jones, Kaddour, & Krieger 2009; Susser & Susser, 1996a; 1996b). In addition, risk factor studies are done on the premise that behaviors (or other exposures) of individuals do not influence the behavior of other individuals, an assumption which is not always tenable (e.g., Epstein, 2007; Halloran, 1998; Koopman & Lynch, 1999).

Therefore, we should continue to broaden the traditional scope of psychiatric epidemiology. Some psychiatric epidemiologists are actively developing methods to incorporate and enhance emerging discoveries in genomics, epigenetics, and molecular biology. The principles that underlie epidemiologic research are directly relevant to genetic and biological research (Schwartz & Susser, 2010), although the specific methods often require substantial adaptation to the questions posed by these domains of research (Susser et al., 2006). Others are developing methods to illuminate the potential for macrosocial interventions to improve health (Galea, 2007). Like the studies of mortality described here, these endeavors require stretching our horizons, but ultimately, they will increase the uses of epidemiology in public mental health.

References

Brandt, A. (2007). *The cigarette century: The rise fall and deadly persistence of the product that defined America.* New York: Basic Books.

Doll, R., & Hill, B. (1954). The mortality of doctors in relation to their smoking habits. *British Medical Journal, 1,* 1451–1455. doi:10.1136/bmj.1.4877.1451.

Doll, R., & Hill, B. (1950). Smoking and carcinoma of the lung: A preliminary report. *British Medical Journal, 221,* 739–748. doi:10.1136/bmj.2.4682.739.

Doll, R., Peto, R., Boreham, J., & Sutherland, I. (2004). Mortality in relation to smoking: 50 years' observations on male British doctors. *British Medical Journal, 328,* 1519–1527. doi:10.1136/bmj.38142.554479.AE, (Published 22 June 2004).

Epstein, H. (2007). *The invisible cure: Africa, the West, and the fight against AIDS.* New York: Farrar, Straus and Giroux.

Galea, S. (2007). *Macrosocial determinants of population health.* New York: Springer.

Halloran, M. E. (1998). Concepts of infectious disease epidemiology. In K. Rothman & S. Greenland (Eds.), *Modern Epidemiology, 2nd ed.* (529–554). Philadelphia, PA: Lippincott Williams & Wilkins.

Hertzman, C., & Wiens, M. (1996). Child development and long-term outcomes: A population health perspective and summary of successful interventions. *Social Science Medicine, 43,* 1083–1095.

Keshavan, M. S., Kennedy, J. L., & Murray, R. (2004). *Neurodevelopment and schizophrenia.* Cambridge, UK: Cambridge University Press.

Koopman, J. S., & Lynch, J. W. (1999). Individual casual models and population system models in epidemiology. *American Journal of Public Health, 89,* 1170–1174. doi:10.2105/AJPH.89.8.1170.

Leighton, A. H. (1959). *My name is Legion: Foundations for a theory of man in relation to culture. Vol I: The Stirling County study of psychiatric disorder and sociocultural environment.* New York: Basic Books.

Leon, D. A., Chenet, L., Shkolnikof, V. M., Zakharov, S., Shapiro J, Rakhmanova G., et al. (1997). Huge variation in Russian mortality rates 1984–1994: Artefact, alcohol or what? *Lancet, 350,* 383–388. doi:10.1016/S0140–6736(97)033606.

Leon, D. A., Saburova, L., Tomkins, S., Andreev, E., Kiryanov, N., McKee, M., & Shkolnikov, V. M. (2007). Hazardous alcohol drinking and premature mortality in Russia: A population based case-control study. *Lancet.* 369, 2001–09. doi:10.1016/S0140–6736(07)60941–6.

Men, T., Brennan, H., Boffeta, H., & Zaridze, D. (2003). Russian mortality trends since 1991–2001: Analysis by cause and region. *British Medical Journal, 327,* 964–969. doi:10.1136/bmj.327.7421.964.

Opler, M., & Susser, E. (2005). Fetal environment and schizophrenia. *Environmental Health Perspectives, 113,* 1239–1242. doi:10.1289/ehp. 7572.

Pearl, R. (1938). Tobacco smoking and longevity. *Science, 87,* 216–217.

Peto, R., Lopez, A. D., Boreham, J., Thun, M., Heath, C., & Doll, R. (1996). Mortality from smoking worldwide. *British Medical Bulletin, 52,* 12–21.

Peto, R., Chen, Z. M., & Boreham, J. (1999). Tobacco—the growing epidemic. *Natural Medicine, 5,* 15–21.

Phillips, M. R., Zhang, J., Shi, Q., Song, Z., Ding, Z., Pang, S., et al. (2009). Prevalence, treatment, and associated disability of mental disorders in four provinces in China during 2001–05: An epidemiological survey. *Lancet, 373,* 2041–2053.

Robins, L. N., & Regier, D. A. (1991). *Psychiatric disorders in America: The epidemiological catchment area study.* New York: Free Press.

Rothman, K. J., Greenland, S., & Lash, T. L. (2008). *Modern epidemiology* (3rd ed.). Philadelphia: Wolters Kluwer Health/Lippincott Williams & Wilkins.

Rutter, M., Tizard, J., Yule, W., Graham, P., & Whitmore, K. (1976). Research report: Isle of Wight studies, 1964–1974. *Psychological Medicine, 6,* 313–332. doi:10.1017/S003329170001388X.

Schwartz, S., & Susser, E. (2010). Invited editorial. GWAS Does only size matter? *American Journal of Psychiatry, 167,* 741–744.

Service, S., & Blower, S. M. (1995). HIV Transmission in sexual networks: An empirical analysis. *Proceedings of the Royal Society of London, Series B, Biological Sciences, 260,* 237–244. doi:10.1098/rspb.1995.0086.

Shapiro, S. (2000). Bias in the evaluation of low-magnitude associations: An empirical perspective. *American Journal of Epidemiology, 151,* 939–945.

Silva, P. A., & Stanton, W. R. (1997). *From child to adult: The Dunedin multidisciplinary health and development study.* New York: Oxford University Press.

Srole, L., & Fischer, A. K. (1980). The Midtown Manhattan longitudinal study vs 'the mental paradise lost' doctrine. A controversy joined. *Archives of General Psychiatry, 37,* 209–221.

Subramanian, S. V., Jones, K., Kaddour, A., & Krieger, N. (2009). Revisiting Robinson: The perils of individualistic and ecologic fallacy. *International Journal of Epidemiology, 38,* 342–360. doi:10.1093/ije/dyn359.

Susser, E., Baumgartner, J. N., & Stein, Z. (in press). Sir Arthur Mitchell: Standing on the shoulders of giants? *International Journal of Epidemiology.*

Susser, E., Schwartz, S., Morabia, A., & Bromet, E. J. (2006). *Psychiatric epidemiology: Searching for the causes of mental disorders.* New York, NY: Oxford University Press.

Susser, E., & Shrout, P. E. (2010). Commentary: Two plus two equals three? Do we need to think lifetime prevalence? *Psychological Medicine, 40,* 895–897. doi:10.1017/S0033291709991504.

Susser, E., St. Clair, D., & He, L. (2008). Latent effects of prenatal malnutrition on adult health: The example of schizophrenia. *Annals of New York Academy of Sciences, 1136,* 185–192.

Susser, M., & Susser, E. (1996a). Choosing a future for epidemiology: I. Eras and paradigms. *American Journal of Public Health, 86,* 668–673. doi:10.2105/AJPH.86.5.668.

Susser, M., & Susser, E. (1996b). Choosing a future for epidemiology: II. From black box to Chinese boxes and eco-epidemiology. *American Journal of Public Health, 86*, 674–677. doi:10.2105/AJPH.86.5.674.

United Nations Population Division (UNDP). (2004). World Population Prospects (2004 revision: ST/ESA/SER.A/244). New York: United Nations.

World Health Organization (WHO). (2007). WHO Statistical Information System (WHOSIS), from Geneva http://www.who.int/whosis/en.

Wynder, E. L., & Graham, E. A. (1950). Tobacco smoking as a possible etiologic factor in bronchiogenic carcinoma: A study of six hundred and eighty-four proved cases. *Journal of the American Medical Association, 143*, 329–336; republished as a landmark article *Journal of the American Medical Association, 253*, 2986–2994.

Zaridze, D., Brennan, P., Boreham, J., Boroda, A., Karpov, R., Lazarev, A., et al. (2009). Alcohol and cause-specific mortality in Russia: A retrospective case–control study of 48,557 adult deaths. *Lancet, 373*, 2201–2214.

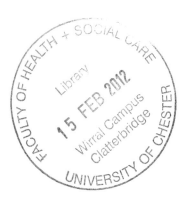

4 Social and environmental influences on population mental health

Emily Goldmann and Sandro Galea

Introduction

There has long been substantial interest in the influence of social and environmental factors on mental health. Landmark studies in the 19th and early 20th century laid the groundwork for a considerable amount of subsequent research on social and environmental determinants of mental health. In the late 1800s, Emile Durkheim (1897) explored the influence of religious beliefs on suicide rates, finding lower rates of suicide in countries that were predominantly Catholic than in predominantly Protestant countries. A 1932 study of hospital admissions for psychosis in Minnesota documented a relationship between migration and mental health, noting that hospitalization rates for psychosis were twice as high among Norwegian migrants to Minnesota as they were among Minnesota natives and individuals still living in Norway (Ødegård, 1932). A few years later, the Chicago School of Social Ecology conducted studies on characteristics of residential neighborhoods and mental disorder and found a greater burden of schizophrenia and substance abuse disorder in Chicago neighborhoods lacking social integration compared to more "socially organized" neighborhoods (Faris & Dunham, 1939; Silver, Mulvey, & Swanson, 2002). The Stirling County Study of the 1950s linked characteristics of social disintegration, such as hostility, inadequate leadership, and poverty, to increased psychiatric risk (Leighton, Harding, Macklin, Hughes, & Leighton, 1963). At the individual level, Hollingshead and Redlich (1958) found an inverse association between social class and mental illness.

In this chapter we provide a conceptual overview of social and environmental influences on population mental health. This chapter is not meant to be a systematic review of the literature on this subject; we refer the reader to other formal reviews of the topic (Galea & Steenland, in press). Rather, we have the following three objectives:

1 To define "social and environmental influences" in the context of population mental health and outline possible mechanisms through which these factors might influence psychopathology.

2   To discuss key social trends, at both the domestic and global level, and their potential effect on population mental health.
3   To consider the challenges we face in our study of the social and environmental influences on mental health.

The overall goal of this chapter is to review the current understanding of how mental health is influenced by the world around us – acknowledging that our world is constantly changing – in an effort to inform further study and create strategies to improve mental health.

Mechanisms: How the social environment may influence population health

The term "social and environmental factors" typically refers both to characteristics of individuals and their roles and relationships with others in society and to features of society for which there is no individual analog. We can consider these factors on three different levels: the individual, inter-individual, and ecologic or group-level (Galea & Steenland, in press). At the individual level, relevant factors include socioeconomic position (SEP), which is often described using measures of income, educational attainment, occupational status (Lynch & Kaplan, 2000), marital status, and race/ethnicity. Inter-individual factors include social support, discrimination, and interpersonal violence. Examples of factors at the ecologic level are: Condition of the built environment; social capital, defined as the presence of social networks between individuals within a population, as well as shared norms and mutual trust (Sampson, 2003); various measures of area SEP, such as median household income and proportion of the population below the poverty line; and racial/ethnic distribution. (For a review of the literature on the relation between these factors and mental health, see Galea & Steenland, in press.)   Borrowing theory from the field of sociology, we have previously described five different concepts that are useful in thinking about how social and environmental factors influence population mental health: social disorganization or strain, social resources, social contagion, spatial segregation, and the physical environment (Galea, Bresnahan, & Susser, 2006). In this section, we use these concepts to describe ways in which social factors at the individual, inter-individual, and ecologic level may affect mental health, largely through their influence on everyday stress, exposure to traumatic or stressful events, and ability to mitigate the psychological consequences of stress (Pearlin, Lieberman, Menaghan, & Mullan, 1981).

Social disorganization or strain

Features of the social environment may be associated with population mental health through their effect on community social organization and social strain. The theory of social disorganization was developed by

Chicago sociologists Clifford Shaw and Henry McKay in the 1920s and 1930s, in the context of studying criminal behavior. They hypothesized that the social characteristics of a community, such as low SEP, ethnic heterogeneity, and residential mobility, disrupt community social organization (Shaw & McKay, 1942; Sampson & Groves, 1989), which is the ability of the community as a whole to achieve common goals and regulate residents' behavior based on community values (Sampson, 2003). Therefore, greater social disorganization is associated with increased levels of crime.

General strain theory was developed by sociologist Robert Agnew, as a revision to original strain theory. This theory, like social disorganization theory, connects community social characteristics to delinquency. Original strain theory posited that delinquency results from the frustration of being unable to attain valued economic goals through legal channels (Merton, 1938). Agnew, however, argued that this strain or frustration is actually created when individuals (often, adolescents) are unable to escape painful or adverse environments. Agnew theorized that living in certain types of neighborhoods, interacting with certain groups of people, or even attending a particular school may be considered "adversive" to an individual. The individual then tries to escape his or her adversity using deviancy or, in anger at being unable to escape his or her environment, participates in delinquent behaviors (Agnew, 1985).

Both social disorganization theory and social strain theory connect features of the social and environmental context to levels of crime and delinquency. High-crime environments can, in turn, promote mental disorder in two ways. First, living in a high-crime neighborhood can create chronic fear and stress (Ross & Jang, 2000), which may manifest as symptoms of psychopathology (Pearlin et al., 1981). Second, an individual in this type of environment may be more likely to experience stressful or traumatic life events, such as assaultive violence, which can trigger symptoms of mental disorder such as anxiety (McLaughlin, Conron, Koenen, & Gilman, 2009) and depression (Kessler, 1997). Several studies have linked chronic fear of crime (White, Kasl, Zahner, & Will, 1987) and exposure to community violence (Curry, Latkin, & Davey-Rothwell, 2008; Shields, Nadasen, & Pierce, 2009; Zinzow et al., 2009; Kelly & Hall, 2010; Mitchell et al., 2010) to poor mental health outcomes.

Social resources

Availability of social resources can also influence mental health. This concept plays a key role in the "differential vulnerability" hypothesis, which has been used to explain the consistent finding of a greater burden of mental illness among low-SEP compared to high-SEP individuals (Dohrenwend & Dohrenwend, 1969; Kohn, Dohrenwend, & Mirotznik, 1998; Hudson, 2005). The differential vulnerability hypothesis argues that persons with lower SEP are exposed to more life stressors than individuals with high SEP and also have fewer resources with which to cope with these circumstances, making them more vulnerable to the psychological consequences of stressors (Kessler, 1997). McLeod and Kessler (1990) divide the resources involved in this vulnerability into two categories: financial and coping. Persons with low SEP, for example, may not have the financial resources to obtain mental health services. They may also suffer from chronic financial stress that makes them more likely to develop psychopathology. In addition, these individuals may lack coping resources such as resilient personality characteristics and social support, which can help prevent the development of mental disorder.

Evidence from studies of social support, in particular, strongly suggest a relation between social support and mental health. Social support can be defined as the emotional and instrumental help obtained from others, such as being made to feel worthwhile or cared for and being provided with assistance (Taylor & Seeman, 1999). Social support is generally considered from a structural perspective or from a functional perspective. The structural perspective defines social support in terms of the structure of relationships and social networks, for example, using marital status or the number of close relationships a person has to assess social support. The functional perspective focuses on whether relationships function in certain ways, for example, if they make the individual feel loved or that assistance is available if needed (Cohen and Syme 1985). Social support can influence mental health directly regardless of exposure to stressors, or it can mitigate the psychological consequences associated with stressful life events (Cohen & Syme, 1985; Dalgard, Bjork, & Tambs, 1995).

Availability of coping resources that influence mental health may also be determined by features of the social context, such as the presence of community social ties and networks (social capital) and neighborhood social cohesion. Lin and colleagues describes a two-tiered "support system" in which an outer structural layer of support, represented by social ties, networks, and community participation, promotes an inner layer, composed of the more functional aspects of social support. The inner layer influences mental health directly, while the outer layer affects mental health both directly and indirectly through its influence on the functional features of social support (Lin, Ye, & Ensel, 1999). Community-level social support, such as informal ties with neighbors and cohesiveness, may also mitigate the negative psychological consequences of environmental stressors such as fear of crime, low area SES, and physical disorder (Ross & Jang, 2000; Dupere & Perkins, 2007; Fone et al., 2007).

Social contagion

Contagion theory provides a third mechanism through which we might consider the influence of social and environmental characteristics on population mental health. While the concept of contagion has been used predominantly to describe the spread of infectious disease, there is evidence that ideas and behaviors, and perhaps mental illness, may also spread between individuals (Patten & Arboleda-Florez, 2004). Studies have used this concept to explain the "contagion" of behaviors such as violence (Patten & Arboleda-Florez, 2004), conduct disorder (Jones & Jones, 1994), and suicide (Hacker, Collins, Gross-Young, Almeida, & Burke, 2008) within a population. The "Werther effect" – named for the subsequent imitation of the suicide of Werther, a fictional character in an 18th century Geothe novel, by readers in Europe – describes how representations of suicides in the media may increase the risk of suicides in the population (Phillips, 1974). More recently, "suicide contagion" has described how exposure to suicide or to suicidal behavior of others serves as a persuasive model (Gould, 2001) that encourages individuals to attempt suicide (O'Carroll & Potter, 1994).

Various social and environmental features may promote the "contagiousness" of psychopathology. For instance, there is evidence that large, high-density populations facilitate the spread of not only infectious disease, but also mental illness (Freedman, Birsky, & Cavoukian, 1980). Studies have found that characteristics of media coverage of suicides, such as the placement and number of articles, impact subsequent suicidal behavior (Phillips, 1974). Research documenting posttraumatic stress disorder (PTSD) symptoms following the World Trade Center attacks on September 11, 2001, provides an example of how characteristics of the social context can influence the spread of psychopathology. These studies found that individuals who were not directly "exposed" to the attacks – that is, they did not witness them or lose loved ones – reported symptoms of PTSD after the attacks (Schlenger et al., 2002; Galea et al., 2003). The density of New York City, which facilitated the spread of information about the event, coupled with the ubiquitous media coverage of the event, may have encouraged the spread of psychological distress in its aftermath (Galea et al., 2006).

Spatial segregation

The social and environmental context can be structured in such a way as to create spatial segregation, which can in turn influence mental health. There may be several dimensions of segregation, but the most commonly considered is segregation by race/ethnicity or SEP. While the concept often has a negative connotation, spatial segregation can have both detrimental and salutary influences on mental health. Due to redlining and other discriminatory real estate practices, poor minority neighborhoods historically have been created in urban centers (Zenou & Boccard, 2000; Chow, Johnson, & Austin, 2005), isolated from the rest of the city. These places of concentrated poverty or disadvantage frequently have more violence, greater social disorganization and physical deterioration, and a lack of resources available in other areas, which produce stress and can contribute to mental disorder among residents (Sampson, Morenoff, & Gannon-Rowley, 2002; Chow et al., 2005). Indeed, studies have noted a greater burden of mental illness and substance abuse in these areas, compared to other areas (Glover, Leese, & McCrone, 1999; Boardman, Finch, Ellison, Williams, & Jackson, 2001). On the other hand, racial/ethnic or socio-economic homogeneity might reduce exposure to discrimination (Krieger, 2000) and social strain among area residents and promote greater social cohesion, which has also been linked to better mental health outcomes (Aneshensel & Sucoff, 1996).

Social and environmental processes can promote or discourage segrega-tion, which can in turn influence population mental health. For example, discriminatory real estate practices may isolate individuals into certain neighborhoods based on race/ethnicity or SEP, while gentrification tends to increase (at least initially) ethnic and socioeconomic heterogeneity in an area, often bringing resources and social networks that may benefit low-SEP individuals, though possibly at the expense of social cohesion (Freeman, 2006). Additionally, migration can result in spatial segregation, as individuals with shared nationality, culture, and/or language cluster into particular neighborhoods where they may have friends and family, which can promote a socially cohesive environment.

Physical environment

The physical or built environment may also influence mental health. Researchers have hypothesized that characteristics of the physical environ-ment affect psychological well-being directly and indirectly through social features of the environment (Evans, 2003; Kruger, Reischl, & Gee, 2007). Kruger and colleagues (2007) employ two models – the environmental stress model and the neighborhood disorder model – to explain how the physical environment influences mental health. The environmental stress model considers the influence of external and internal building quality and other physical characteristics of the environment, such as air quality and population density, on mental health. Poor building condition, pollution, and chronic loud noise can be experienced as daily stressors for residents, which can in turn influence their mental health (Wandersman & Nation, 1998). The neighborhood disorder model, also discussed above, connects area characteristics, such as the presence of deteriorating and abandoned buildings, to poor mental health through their influence on crime and fear of crime (Taylor, Shumaker, & Gottfredson, 1985). The presence of phys-ical deterioration can encourage crime by giving a sense that the area is vulnerable to crime or that residents would not try to stop a crime in progress (Taylor & Harrell 1996). High levels of crime induce stress and increase the risk of exposure to stressful or traumatic events, which can increase risk of mental disorder (Taylor & Harrell, 1996).

Evans (2003) provides a review of studies that have linked a variety of characteristics of the physical environment to psychological well-being. For example, living in high-rise, multi-unit residences has been associated with poor mental health among mothers of young children, likely through social isolation created by the living environment. Other researchers have found that living in poor-quality housing is associated with chronic stress and feelings of helplessness due to insecurity, crowding, noise, and lack of quality indoor air and light, which can promote or exacerbate psychopathology (Evans, 2003). These physical characteristics can also influence mental health by creating a social environment in which residents lack personal control, social support, and the ability to recover from cognitive fatigue and stress.

Features of the social environment that may influence population mental health in the 21st century

In this section, we focus on three social processes – urbanization, migration, and globalization – that may shape global population mental health in the 21st century. We first describe current and future trends in these processes. We then consider how these trends may influence psychological health by considering these processes in light of the mechanisms discussed above. We acknowledge that the relationship between these social processes and mental health is complex and can involve some and even all of the above mechanisms, with significant overlap. The goal of this section, however, is to offer a preliminary framework from which we can systematically study how changes in the social environment influence the mental health of populations.

Urbanization

The world is becoming an increasingly urban place. In 1950, urban residents made up just over 25% of the world's population. Today, more than half of the world's population – approximately three billion people – live in urban areas, and the world's urban population continues to grow. By 2050, almost 70% of the population will reside in urban areas (United Nations Population Division, 2008). Developing countries are experiencing even more rapid urbanization than developed countries (Cohen, 2006). Over the next 30 years, virtually all of global population growth is expected to be concentrated in urban areas in the developing world, and by 2017, half of the population of the developing world will live in urban areas (Cohen, 2006). This global population trend will likely influence many aspects of population health including, and perhaps centrally, mental health.

There is a rich tradition of research that has considered whether urban living is associated with mental health. In the early part of the 20th century, a seminal study by Faris and Dunham (1939) at the Chicago School of Social Ecology comparing mental health in urban and suburban areas found a greater prevalence of schizophrenia in urban areas but more manic depression in the suburbs. Around the same time, a British study demonstrated what researchers named "suburban neurosis," finding rates of mental illness higher in suburban areas than in urban ones, due to loss of familiar surroundings (when moving to the suburbs), long distances to employment in urban areas, and social isolation (Taylor, 1938; Dalgard & Tambs, 1997). A later review of the literature on urban-rural differences in mental health concluded that the large majority of studies found greater mental disorder in urban compared to rural areas (Dohrenwend & Dohrenwend, 1974), while other researchers pointed out that studies in various developed countries failed to find a significant urban-rural difference (Cheng, 1989). In the 1980s, research using data from the Epidemiologic Catchment Area study found significantly higher prevalence of major depressive disorder in urban areas than in rural areas (Blazer et al., 1985), although this finding was not replicated in the National Comorbidity Survey (a more recent population-based study) (Blazer, Kessler, McGonagle, & Swartz, 1994).

There are several explanations for differences across studies. For example, urban-rural differences may vary by country or region, and studies often employ different definitions of "urban" (Blazer et al., 1994; Harpham, 1994). Indeed, the definition of urban used by many global population researchers is country-specific (Hinrichsen, Salem, & Blackburn, 2002). Perhaps more saliently, urbanization likely has both positive and negative effects on population mental health. Urban areas have been linked with greater resources and availability of health services compared to rural areas (Moore, Gould, & Keary, 2003). Urbanization, then, may increase the number of individuals in need who obtain treatment for psychological distress. However, urbanization also brings with it a host of challenges, such as shortages in housing and greater exposure to air pollution, crime, and other environmental stressors (Hinrichsen, Salem, & Blackburn, 2002), which are associated with poor mental health outcomes (Evans, 2003; Kruger et al., 2007). Urbanization can also increase population density, producing crowded and congested living environments, which could cause social strain or facilitate the spread of certain behaviors or psychological symptoms (Freedman et al., 1980). Urban poverty has also increased with urban growth as individuals migrate from rural areas and move into poor, substandard housing in growing slums. Living in slums is associated with greater exposure to accidents, drug abuse, violence, and crime, which can promote psychological illness (Muggah & Alvazzi del Frate, 2007; Yusuf, Nabeshima, & Ha, 2007).

Thus, urbanization has the potential to influence population mental health by creating larger concentrations of poverty; exposing more people to a poor physical environment, violence, crime, and other environmental stressors; and promoting social strain or tension, and subsequent crime, through greater crowding and segregation into impoverished areas. These issues will be particularly relevant in low-income countries, where most urban population growth will take place in the coming years and adequate resources to deal with soaring urban populations are often lacking (Cohen, 2006). Although relatively few, studies of the influence over time of urbanization on mental health (Harpham, 1994) in high-income (Dekker, Peen, Koelen, Smit, & Schoevers, 2008) and low-income (Rahim & Cederblad, 1986; Guiness, 1992) countries have reported an association between greater urbanization and increasing risk of psychopathology.

Migration

In 2005, almost 200 million people (approximately 3% of the world's population) were living outside of their native country (United Nations Population Fund, 2002). This number continues to grow as people leave their homes in search of economic opportunities and refuge from conflict or disasters, and the availability of high-speed communication, inexpensive travel, and access to information about other places improves. The number of migrants is expected to reach 230 million globally by 2050 (United Nations Population Fund, 2002). Migrants tend to move from low-income to high-income countries and currently make up a larger proportion of populations in high-income than low-income countries. Migration to high-income regions is expected to continue at an average rate of 2 per 1,000 population for the next 40 years, while migration to low-income regions will continue to decrease at an average rate of 0.3 per 1,000 (United Nations Population Division, 2008).

Migration may influence population mental health in several ways. First, migration can alter an area's sociodemographic composition, with potential effects on the psychological well-being of its new and existing residents. The integration of immigrants into a less-than-welcoming population can create environments with high social disorganization and strain and low social cohesion; the link between these conditions and poor mental health has been described above.

Second, migrants may experience a great deal of stress during and after the migration process (Patino & Kirchner, 2010). Persons who have migrated to escape conflict, disasters, or have been tricked or forced into servitude by traffickers may bring with them psychological wounds relating to traumatic experiences in their countries of origin or face traumatic events in their new environments (United Nations Population Fund, 2002; Norredam, Garcia-Lopez, Keiding, & Krasnik, 2009). Additional stressors, such as discrimination and the need to adapt to a new environment, could also negatively impact their mental health (Wang, Li, Stanton, & Fang, 2010). Immigrants may be kept apart from others, segregated geographically into peripheral areas with poor housing conditions (Huttman, Blauw, & Saltman, 1991; United Nations Population Fund, 2002; Asselin et al.,

2006), putting them at greater risk of psychological distress. Difficulty with assimilation has also been found to encourage psychopathology (Bhugra, 2003; Hwang, Cao, & Xi, 2010). At the same time, migrants may choose to congregate in certain areas with people of similar culture, ethnicity, nationality, or religion (United Nations Population Fund, 2002; Asselin et al., 2006), potentially creating socially cohesive and supportive environments that promote good mental health outcomes.

Third, migrants may lose social support resources as they leave friends and family behind, potentially increasing vulnerability to poor mental health outcomes (Hwang et al., 2010). Adolescent migrants who are separated from parents are even more vulnerable (Derluyn, Mels, & Broekaert, 2009). Also important to note is that internal migration from rural areas to cities contributes to the rapid urbanization we see in developing countries (United Nations Population Fund, 2002), bringing along with it some of the mental health issues discussed in the previous section.

Studies have examined the impact of migration on overall mental health, as well as on specific disorders such as depression (Bhugra, 2003), substance use (Lu, 2010), and schizophrenia (Bhugra, 2000). While many have found greater psychological symptoms among international immigrants compared to native residents (Schrier et al., 2009) and among rural-to-urban migrants compared to their urban and rural counterparts (Li et al., 2009; Wang et al., 2010), the association between migration and mental health is not always clear (Bhugra, 2003). Future studies that address various methodological issues (discussed in the last section) are warranted.

Globalization

Globalization is a complex social and economic force that has facilitated closer connections between people and communities and the spread of information and ideas around the world. This process has contributed to many changes happening around the world – for example, increasingly rapid communication; commercial deregulation; faster and less expensive transportation; the greater mobility of people, goods, and ideas; the spread of norms, values, and customs; and growing global labor markets (United Nations Population Fund, 2002; Okasha, 2005; Bhavsar & Bhugra, 2008). There are, however, several elements of globalization that suggest it will also influence population health. For example, the spread of fast food chains, lifestyle choices, and eating behaviors around the globe has contributed to epidemics of obesity in many countries (Bornstein, Ehrhart-Bornstein, Wong, & Licinio, 2008).

Globalization has implications for mental health as well, although its impact is context-dependent rather than entirely positive or negative (Martin, 2005). Bhavsar and Bhugra (2008) provide a useful review, linking globalization to mental health in four ways. First, globalization has been linked to greater global and domestic income and wealth inequalities through its impact on labor markets and wages (Katz & Darbishire, 2000; Kelly, 2003; Bhavsar & Bhugra, 2008). Studies (though not consistently) have linked inequality to poor mental health outcomes, through its influence on community social trust and cohesion, negative feelings about worth, and feelings of loss of control (Charlesworth, Gilfillan, & Wilkinson, 2004; Marmot, 2004; Wilkinson, 2005; Bhavsar & Bhugra, 2008). Second, the authors posit that globalization can change work environments, which can create stress and affect mental health. Third, the spread of ideas and culture has influenced identities and behavioral norms. This is often accompanied by the stress of feeling pulled between traditional and modern values, particularly among young people, as well as loss of social capital in communities, resulting in psychological distress. Fourth, globalization encourages migration and the consequent stress of adapting to new environments discussed above. Additionally, there is limited evidence that increased exposure to information in the media from Western countries has "spread" mental disorders, such as anorexia, to cultures that until recently had not experienced these illnesses (Watters, 2010). On the positive side, it is important to note that globalization has the potential to promote mental health through facilitating discussion of "best practices" between practitioners all over the world, as well as improving access to data that can increase understanding, prevention, and treatment of mental illness (Bhavsar & Bhugra, 2008).

Challenges in the field

The study of social and environmental influences on population mental health, in particular the macrosocial processes we have discussed in this chapter, is complex and poses substantial methodological challenges. First and foremost is the lack of available and reliable data on social and environmental characteristics and mental disorder, particularly in low-income countries. Growing recognition of the importance of studying mental health in low-income countries (Patel, 2007), coupled with large-scale efforts on the part of organizations like the World Health Organization to collect data (through the World Mental Health survey initiative), are important steps in facilitating further study of global population mental health. A related issue is the identification and classification of mental disorders across populations. Persons in different areas across the world with different cultures, religions, and languages may not express symptoms of psychological distress in the same way. Thus, obtaining information on the culture being studied and utilizing culturally-relevant valid instruments for symptom identification is critical.

Second, research in the area continues to suffer from concerns about causality versus selection (Dohrenwend, 1966). To illustrate, if a study finds that psychopathology is significantly more prevalent in urban areas compared to non-urban areas, is it because living in urban areas exposes an individual to greater environmental stressors (Dekker et al., 2008) or is it that individuals who are mentally ill or more vulnerable to mental illness tend to live in urban areas where mental health services are more available (Dalgard & Tambs, 1997)? Studies with longitudinal designs that collect information on mental health at baseline can provide us with evidence of a causal relation between social and environmental factors and psychopathology.

Third, the choice of area-level social and environmental factors to be studied complicates research. For example, studies comparing mental health in cities versus more rural areas often use competing definitions of "city". What are the correct administrative boundaries (Cohen, 2006)? What definition of "area" or "neighborhood" is correct (Mair, Diez Roux, & Galea, 2008)? Researchers must clearly define the area of interest and provide justification for choosing that area. Studies must also have adequate heterogeneity in the area-level exposure of interest in order to demonstrate any real effects. Additionally, basic ecologic models fail to yield unbiased estimates of both contextual- and individual-level effects because they lack data at the individual level. Instead, when examining area- or neighborhood-level effects, we can use multilevel studies, which also control for individual-level effects (Greenland, 2001). Finally, places do not exist in a vacuum. It is possible that individuals are influenced not only by the area in which they live, but also by adjacent areas. Spatial modeling and the use of techniques such as agent-based modeling may be useful in this context.

Conclusion

The ultimate goal of studying the social and environmental determinants of population mental health is to advance our understanding of how mental health is shaped by the world around us. This is particularly relevant in the context of considerable ongoing changes in the social environment at home and abroad. This chapter has focused on three major social processes that we feel play a key role in how society is changing and the mechanisms through which they may influence population mental health. However, there remains a paucity of evidence on how these processes affect mental health and, in particular, how we may intervene to improve population mental health. The ongoing study of social and environmental risk factors that may influence the health of populations, concurrent with effort to tackle the key methodological challenges in the field, will play a role in future efforts to prevent illness and promote healthy communities.

References

Agnew, R. (1985). A revised strain theory of delinquency. *Social Forces, 64,* 151–167.
Aneshensel, C. S., & Sucoff, C. A. (1996). The neighborhood context of adolescent mental health. *Journal of Health and Social Behavior, 37,* 293–310.

Asselin, O., Dureau, F., Fonseca, L., Giroud, M., Hamadi, A., Kohlbacher, J., et al. (2006). Social integration of immigrants with special reference to the local and spatial dimension. In R. Penninx, M. Berger, and K. Kraal (Eds.), *The Dynamics of International Migration and Settlement in Europe*. Amsterdam, Netherlands: Amsterdam University Press.

Bhavsar, V., & Bhugra, D. (2008). Globalization: Mental health and social economic factors. *Global Social Policy, 8*, 378–396.

Bhugra, D. (2000). Migration and schizophrenia. *Acta Psychiatrica Scandinavica, Supplement*(407), 68–73.

Bhugra, D. (2003). Migration and depression. *Acta Psychiatrica Scandinavica, Supplement*(418), 67–72.

Blazer, D., George, L. K., Landerman, R., Pennybacker, M., Melville, M. L., Woodbury, M., et al. (1985). Psychiatric disorders. A rural/urban comparison. *Archives of General Psychiatry, 42*, 651–656.

Blazer, D. G., Kessler, R. C., McGonagle, K. A., & Swartz, M. Z. (1994). The prevalence and distribution of major depression in a national community sample: The National Comorbidity Survey. *American Journal of Psychiatry, 151*, 979–986.

Boardman, J. D., Finch, B. K., Ellison, C. G., Williams, D. R., & Jackson, J. S. (2001). Neighborhood disadvantage, stress, and drug use among adults. *Journal of Health and Social Behavior, 42*, 151–165.

Bornstein, S. R., Ehrhart-Bornstein, M., Wong, M. L., & Licinio, J. (2008). Is the worldwide epidemic of obesity a communicable feature of globalization? *Experimental and Clinical Endocrinology & Diabetes, 116*, S30–S32.

Charlesworth, S. J., Gilfillan, P., & Wilkinson, R. (2004). Living inferiority. *British Medical Bulletin, 69*, 49–60.

Cheng, T. A. (1989). Urbanization and minor psychiatric morbidity: A community study in Taiwan. *Social Psychiatry and Psychiatric Epidemiology, 24*, 309–316.

Chow, J. C., Johnson, M. A., & Austin, M. J. (2005). The status of low-income neighborhoods in the post-welfare reform environment. *Journal of Health & Social Policy, 21*, 1–32.

Cohen, B. (2006). Urbanization in developing countries: Current trends, future projections, and key challenges for sustainability. *Technology in Society, 28*, 63–80.

Cohen, S., & Syme, S. L. (1985). Issues in the study and application of social support. In S. Cohen & S. L. Syme (Eds.), *Social support and health*. New York: Academic Press, Inc.

Curry, A., Latkin, C., & Davey-Rothwell, M. (2008). Pathways to depression: The impact of neighborhood violent crime on inner-city residents in Baltimore, Maryland, USA. *Social Science and Medicine, 67*, 23–30.

Dalgard, O. S., Bjørk, S., & Tambs, K. (1995). Social support, negative life events and mental health. *British Journal of Psychiatry, 166*, 29–34.

Dalgard, O. S., & Tambs, K. (1997). Urban environment and mental health: A longitudinal study. *British Journal of Psychiatry, 171*, 530–536.

Dekker, J., Peen, J., Koelen, J., Smit, F., & Schoevers, R. (2008). Psychiatric disorders and urbanization in Germany. *BMC Public Health, 8*, 17.

Derluyn, I., Mels, C., & Broekaert, E. (2009). Mental health problems in separated refugee adolescents. *Journal of Adolescent Health, 44*, 291–297.

Dohrenwend, B. P. (1966). Social status and psychological disorder: An issue of substance and an issue of method. *American Sociological Review, 31*, 14–34.

Dohrenwend, B. P., & Dohrenwend, B. S. (1969). *Social status and psychological disorder*. New York: Wiley.

Dohrenwend, B. P., & Dohrenwend, B. S. (1974). Psychiatric disorders in urban settings. In S. Arieti & S. Caplan (Eds.), *American Handbook of Psychiatry*. New York: Basic Books.

Dupere, V., & Perkins, D. D. (2007). Community types and mental health: A multilevel study of local environmental stress and coping. *American Journal of Community Psychology, 39*, 107–119.

Durkheim, E. (1897). *Le suicide: Étude de sociologie*. Paris, France: F. Alcan.

Evans, G. W. (2003). The built environment and mental health. *Journal of Urban Health, 80*, 536–555.

Faris, R. E. L., & Dunham, H. W. (1939). *Mental disorders in urban areas: An ecological study of schizophrenia and other psychoses*. Chicago, IL: The University of Chicago Press.

Fone, D., Dunstan, F., Lloyd, K., Williams, G., Watkins, J., & Palmer, S. (2007). Does social cohesion modify the association between area income deprivation and mental health: A multilevel analysis. *International Journal of Epidemiology, 36*, 338–345.

Freedman, J. L., Birsky, J., & Cavoukian, A. (1980). Environmental determinants of behavioral contagion: Density and number. *Basic and Applied Social Psychology, 1*, 155–161.

Freeman, L. (2006). *There goes the hood: Views of gentrification from the ground up*. Philadelphia, PA: Temple University Press.

Galea, S., Bresnahan, M., & Susser, E. (2006). Mental health in the city. In N. Freudenberg, S. Galea, & D. Vlahov (Eds.), *Cities and the Health of the Public*. Nashville, TN: Vanderbilt University Press.

Galea, S., & Steenland, M. (in press). The social determinants of mental health. In L. B. Cottler (Ed.), *Mental health in public health*. New York: Oxford University Press.

Galea, S., Vlahov, D., Resnick, H., Ahern, J., Susser, E., Gold, J., et al. (2003). Trends of probable post-traumatic stress disorder in New York City after the September 11 terrorist attacks. *American Journal of Epidemiology, 158*, 514–524.

Glover, G. R., Leese, M., & McCrone, P. (1999). More severe mental illness is more concentrated in deprived areas. *British Journal of Psychiatry, 175*, 544–548.

Gould, M. S. (2001). Suicide and the media. *Annals of the New York Academy of Sciences, 932*, 200–221.

Greenland, S. (2001). Ecologic versus individual-level sources of bias in ecologic estimates of contextual health effects. *International Journal of Epidemiology, 30*, 1343–1350.

Guiness, E. (1992). Patterns of mental illness in the early stages of urbanization. *British Journal of Psychiatry, 160*, 8.

Hacker, K., Collins, J., Gross-Young, L., Almeida, S., & Burke, N. (2008). Coping with youth suicide and overdose: One community's efforts to investigate, intervene, and prevent suicide contagion. *Crisis, 29*, 86–95.

Harpham, T. (1994). Urbanization and mental health in developing countries: A research role for social scientists, public health professionals and social psychiatrists. *Social Science and Medicine, 39*, 233–245.

Hinrichsen, D., Salem, R., and Blackburn, R. (2002). *Meeting the Urban Challenge. Population Reports*, Series M, No. 16. Baltimore: The Johns Hopkins Bloomberg School of Public Health, Population Information Program.

Hollingshead, A. D. B., & Redlich, F. C. (1958). *Social Class and Mental Illness: A Community Study*. New York: Wiley.

Hudson, C. G. (2005). Socioeconomic status and mental illness: tests of the social causation and selection hypotheses. *American Journal of Orthopsychiatry, 75*, 3–18.

Huttman, E. D., Blauw, W., & Saltman, J. (1991). *Urban housing segregation of minorities in western Europe and the United States*. Durham, NC: Duke University Press.

Hwang, S. S., Cao, Y., & Xi, J. (2010). Project-induced migration and depression: A panel analysis. *Social Science and Medicine, 70*, 1765–1772.

Jones, M. B., & Jones, D. R. (1994). Testing for behavioral contagion in a case-control design. *Journal of Psychiatric Research, 28*, 35–55.

Katz, H. C., & Darbishire, O. (2000). *Converging divergences: Worldwide changes in employment systems*. Ithaca, NY: ILR Press.

Kelly, B. (2003). Globalisation and psychiatry. *Advances in Psychiatric Treatment, 9*, 464–474.

Kelly, S., & Hall, L. (2010). Measuring anxiety in adolescents exposed to community violence: a review, comparison, and analysis of three measures. *Issues in Mental Health Nursing, 31*, 28–38.

Kessler, R. C. (1997). The effects of stressful life events on depression. *Annual Review of Psychology, 48*, 191–214.

Kessler, R. C., Aguilar-Gaxiola, S., Alonso, J., Chatterji, S., Lee, S., Ormel, J., & Wang, P. S. (2009). The global burden of mental disorders: An update from the WHO World Mental Health (WMH) surveys. *Epidemiologia e Psichiatria Sociale, 18*, 23–33.

Kohn, R., Dohrenwend, B. P., & Mirotznik, J. (1998). Epidemiological findings on selected psychiatric disorders in the general population. In B. P. Dohrenwend (Ed.), *Adversity, stress, and psychopathology*. New York: Oxford University Press.

Krieger, N. (2000). Discrimination and health. In L. F. Berkman & I. Kawachi (Eds.), *Social Epidemiology*. New York: Oxford University Press.

Kruger, D. J., Reischl, T. M., & Gee, G. C. (2007). Neighborhood social conditions mediate the association between physical deterioration and mental health. *American Journal of Community Psychology, 40*, 261–271.

Leighton, D. C., Harding, J. S., Macklin, D. B., Hughes, C. C., & Leighton, A. H. (1963). Psychiatric findings of the Stirling Country study. *American Journal of Psychiatry, 119*, 1021–1026.

Li, X., Stanton, B., Fang, X., Xiong, Q., Yu, S., Lin, D., & Wang, B. (2009). Mental health symptoms among rural-to-urban migrants in China: A comparison with their urban and rural counterparts. *World Health & Population, 11*, 24–38.

Lin, N., Ye, X., & Ensel, W. M. (1999). Social support and depressed mood: A structural analysis. *Journal of Health and Social Behavior, 40*, 344–359.

Lu, Y. (2010). Mental health and risk behaviours of rural-urban migrants: Longitudinal evidence from Indonesia. *Population Studies (Cambridge), 64*, 147–163.

Lynch, J., & Kaplan, G. (2000). Socioeconomic position. In L. F. Berkman & I. Kawachi (Eds.), *Social Epidemiology*. New York: Oxford University Press.

Mair, C., Diez Roux, A. V., & Galea, S. (2008). Are neighbourhood characteristics associated with depressive symptoms? A review of evidence. *Journal of Epidemiology and Community Health, 62,* 940–946.

Marmot, M. G. (2004). *The status syndrome: How social standing affects our health and longevity.* New York: Times Books.

Martin, G. (2005). Globalization and health. *Global Health, 1,* 1.

McLaughlin, K. A., Conron, K. J., Koenen, K. C., & Gilman, S. C. (2009). Childhood adversity, adult stressful life events, and risk of past-year psychiatric disorder: A test of the stress sensitization hypothesis in a population-based sample of adults. *Psychological Medicine,* 1–12 [Epub].

McLeod, J. D., & Kessler, R. C. (1990). Socioeconomic status differences in vulnerability to undesirable life events. *Journal of Health and Social Behavior, 31,* 162–172.

Merton, R. (1938). Social structure and anomie. *American Sociological Review, 3,* 672–682.

Mitchell, S. J., Lewin, A., Horn, I. B., Valentine, D., Sanders-Phillips, K., & Joseph, J. G. (2010). How does violence exposure affect the psychological health and parenting of young African-American mothers? *Social Science and Medicine, 70,* 526–533.

Moore, M., Gould, P., & Keary, B. S. (2003). Global urbanization and impact on health. *International Journal of Hygiene and Environmental Health, 206,* 269–278.

Muggah, R., & Alvazzi del Frate, A. (2007). *More slums equals more violence: Reviewing armed violence and urbanization in Africa.* United Nations Development Programme. Retrieved from http://www.genevadeclaration.org/fileadmin/docs/regional-publications/Armed-Violence-and-Urbanization-in-Africa.pdf

Norredam, M., Garcia-Lopez, A., Keiding, N., & Krasnik, A. (2009). Risk of mental disorders in refugees and native Danes: A register-based retrospective cohort study. *Social Psychiatry and Psychiatric Epidemiology, 44,* 1023–1029.

O'Carroll, P. W., & Potter, L. B. (1994). Suicide contagion and the reporting of suicide: Recommendations from a national workshop. United States Department of Health and Human Services. *Morbidity and Mortality Weekly Report Recommendations and Reports, 43,* 9–17.

Ødegård, Ø. (1932). *Emigration and Insanity.* Copenhagen, Denmark: Levin & Munksgaard.

Okasha, A. (2005). Globalization and mental health: A WPA perspective. *World Psychiatry, 4,* 1–2.

Patel, V. (2007). Mental health in low- and middle-income countries. *British Medicine Bulletin, 81–82,* 1–16.

Patino, C., & Kirchner, T. (2010). Stress and psychopathology in Latin-American immigrants: The role of coping strategies. *Psychopathology, 43,* 17–24.

Patten, S. B., & Arboleda-Florez, J. A. (2004). Epidemic theory and group violence. *Social Psychiatry and Psychiatric Epidemiology, 39,* 853–856.

Pearlin, L. I., Lieberman, M. A., Menaghan, E. G., & Mullan, J. T. (1981). The stress process. *Journal of Health and Social Behavior, 22,* 337–356.

Phillips, D. P. (1974). The influence of suggestion on suicide: Substantive and theoretical implications of the Werther effect. *American Sociological Review, 39,* 340–354.

Rahim, S. I., & Cederblad, M. (1986). Effects of rapid urbanization on child behaviour and health in a part of Khartoum, Sudan–II. Psycho-social influences on behavior. *Social Science and Medicine, 22,* 723–730.

Ross, C. E., & Jang, S. J. (2000). Neighborhood disorder, fear, and mistrust: The buffering role of social ties with neighbors. *American Journal of Community Psychology, 28,* 401–420.

Sampson, R. J. (2003). Neighborhood-level context and health: Lessons from sociology. In I. Kawachi & L. F. Berkman (Eds.), *Neighborhoods and Health.* New York: Oxford University Press.

Sampson, R. J., & Groves, W. B. (1989). Community structure and crime: Testing social-disorganization theory. *American Journal of Sociology, 94,* 774–802.

Sampson, R. J., Morenoff, J. D., & Gannon-Rowley, T. (2002). Assessing "neighborhood effects": Social processes and new directions in research. *Annual Review of Sociology, 28,* 443–478.

Schlenger, W. E., Caddell, J. M., Ebert, L., Jordan, B. K., Rourke, K. M., Wilson, D., et al. (2002). Psychological reactions to terrorist attacks: Findings from the National Study of Americans' Reactions to September 11. *Journal of the American Medical Association, 288,* 581–588.

Schrier, A. C., de Wit, M. A., Rijmen, F., Tuinebreijer, W. C., Verhoeff, A. P., Kupka, R. W., et al. (2009). Similarity in depressive symptom profile in a population-based study of migrants in the Netherlands. *Social Psychiatry and Psychiatric Epidemiology,* [Epub ahead of print].

Shaw, C., & McKay, H. (1942). *Juvenile Delinquency and Urban Areas.* Chicago, IL: University of Chicago Press.

Shields, N., Nadasen, K., & Pierce, L. (2009). Posttraumatic stress symptoms as a mediating factor on the effects of exposure to community violence among children in Cape Town, South Africa. *Violence and Victims, 24,* 786–799.

Silver, E., Mulvey, E. P., & Swanson, J. W. (2002). Neighborhood structural characteristics and mental disorder: Faris and Dunham revisited. *Social Science and Medicine, 55,* 1457–1470.

Taylor, R. B., & Harrell, A. V. (1996). Physical environment and crime: A final summary report presented to the National Institute of Justice. U.S. Department of Justice.

Taylor, R. B., Shumaker, S. A., & Gottfredson, S. D. (1985). Neighborhood-level links between physical features and local sentiments: Deterioration, fear of crime, and confidence. *Journal of Architectural and Planning Research, 2,* 261–275.

Taylor, S. (1938). Surburban neurosis. *Lancet, 231,* 759–762.

Taylor, S. E., & Seeman, T. E. (1999). Psychosocial resources and the SES-health relationship. In N. E. Adler, M. G. Marmot, B. S. McEwen, & J. Stewart (Eds.), *Socioeconomic status and health in industrialized nations: Social, psychological, and biological pathways.* New York: New York Academy of Sciences.

United Nations Population Fund (UNFPA). (2004). *Meeting the challenges of migration: Progress since the ICPD.* Retrieved from http://www.unfpa.org/public/publications/pid/2069

United Nations Population Division. (2008). *World Population Prospects: The 2008 revision, population database.* Retrieved from http://esa.un.org/unpp/index.asp?panel=1

Wandersman, A., & Nation, M. (1998). Urban neighborhoods and mental health: Psychological contributions to understanding toxicity, resilience, and interventions. *American Psychology, 53,* 647–656.

Wang, B., Li, X., Stanton, B., & Fang, X. (2010). The influence of social stigma and discriminatory experience on psychological distress and quality of life among rural-to-urban migrants in China. *Social Science and Medicine, 71,* 84–92.

Watters, E. (2010). *Crazy like us: The globalization of the American psyche.* New York: Free Press.

White, M., Kasl, S. V., Zahner, G. E. P., & Will, J. C. (1987). Perceived crime in the neighborhood and mental-health of women and children. *Environment and Behavior, 19.* 588–613.

Wilkinson, R. G. (2005). *The impact of inequality: How to make sick societies healthier.* New York: New Press.

Yusuf, S., Nabeshima, K., & Ha, W. (2007). What makes cities healthy? *World Bank Policy Research Working Paper, 4107.* Retrieved from http://econ.worldbank.org

Zenou, Y., & Boccard, N. (2000). Racial discrimination and redlining in cities. *Journal of Urban Economics, 48,* 260–285.

Zinzow, H. M., Ruggiero, K. J., Resnick, H., Hanson, R., Smith, D., Saunders, B., & Kilpatrick, D. (2009). Prevalence and mental health correlates of witnessed parental and community violence in a national sample of adolescents. *Journal of Child Psychology and Psychiatry, 50,* 441–450.

5 Disparities in mental health status and care in the U.S.

Sergio Aguilar-Gaxiola, William S. Sribney, Bonnie Raingruber, Natasha Wenzel, Dana Fields-Johnson, and Gustavo Loera

Disclaimer: The views and opinions expressed in this chapter are those of the authors and should not be construed to represent the views of any of the sponsoring organizations, agencies, or the University of California.

Introduction

For decades, the disparity in access to and quality of health care in the U.S. has been an ongoing problem, especially for minority populations with a need for mental healthcare. Such disparity has severe medical, social, and economic consequences. So why has not much progress been made in eliminating or reducing disparities? What are the strategies needed to respond effectively to these disparities? What is clear is that the population in the U.S. is increasing, and if the sociocultural, socioeconomic and policy barriers in the healthcare system are not eliminated, health disparities will continue to persist and diminish quality of life for all people.

Eliminating or reducing racial and ethnic and socioeconomic disparities, especially for historically underserved minority groups (e.g., African Americans, Latinos, etc.), has long been considered a critical factor in improving access to quality healthcare. There is evidence that significant disparities in access to and use and quality of care are linked to severe medical, social and economic consequences (e.g., Schnittker & McLeod, 2005; Smedley, Stith, & Nelson, 2003). Other work contends that, although the quality care gap seems to be narrowing, the disparities in access to care for some minority populations have worsened, especially for Latinos (Agency for Healthcare Research and Quality, 2006; 2008; 2009). The medical consequences of these disparities are associated with significantly reduced life expectancy (National Center for Health Statistics, 2009), and the economic consequences of health disparities translate into astronomical costs, primarily due to lost productivity and healthcare costs. A joint Center for Political and Economic Studies commissioned report calculated the combined costs of health inequalities and premature death in the nation to be $1.24 trillion between 2003 and 2006 (LaVeist, Gaskin, & Richard, 2009).

Similar to the overall health system, the mental health system is plagued by inequities in access, utilization, treatment, and outcomes for minority populations. According to the Surgeon General's *Mental health: Culture, race, and ethnicity – A supplement to mental health* (U.S. Department of Health and Human Services, 2001), there are differences in available treatment options for minority groups, and when they seek treatment, they are more likely to receive poor quality care. In addition, racial and ethnic minorities experiencing mental health disorders often have more persistent disorders than those of whites (Breslau, Borges, Hagar, Tancredi, & Gilman, 2009).

These ongoing health system challenges, coupled with changing demographic patterns in the U.S., evidence an urgent need for action and reform and will force policy discussions about reducing racial and ethnic health inequities across the health system. The new healthcare reform law, which calls for a strong foundation to eliminate persistent racial disparities in the U.S. health system (Andrulis, Siddiqui, Purtle, & Duchon, 2010), offers a unique opportunity to advance health equity for racially and ethnically diverse populations. There are three possible scenarios for the response to the lingering mental health disparities:

1   Maintain the status quo and continue to have the health of minority populations worsen.
2   Make general improvements in the overall health system, hoping that this one-size-fits-all strategy will reduce disparities in the mental health system.
3   Improve access to quality mental health care by targeting and tailoring specific treatment options and outreach efforts toward minority populations.

The data and discussion in this chapter will explore the viability of each of these scenarios and their likelihood for success.

Some researchers have suggested that improvements to access and quality of care will likely improve the mental health status of ethnic minorities. This is based on a sort of cross-cultural "one-size-fits-all" psychiatry, wherein improvements to services that have been largely developed for white, middle-class, U.S.-born persons, are assumed equally effective for other populations (McGuire & Miranda, 2008). It should be obvious, however, that the dissimilar rates of mental illness within different minority groups (e.g., Latinos) and subgroups (e.g., Mexican Americans) speak to numerous patient variables (e.g., historical traumas; behavioral norms; conceptions of mental illness). Consider, for example, that stigma and shame are thought to be the primary causes of lower utilization rates among Asian Americans and that lack of culturally and linguistically appropriate mental health services (e.g., language skills) keep one half of all Asian/Pacific Islanders with mental disorders from seeking services (U.S. Department of Health and Human Services, 2001). Failure to acknowledge this heterogeneity is referred to as a *category fallacy*, where an assumption is made that psychiatric disorders "normed" within one cultural group, and then carried over to a new cultural context remain the same. Thus, an over-generalized approach would be dangerous, if not counterproductive. Historical issues of mistrust and mental health stigma provide powerful barriers for racial and ethnic minorities with mental health disorders that frequently result in them seeking mental health support from non-medical sources such as religious institutions and/or complementary alternative medicine (CAM).

This chapter provides an overview of disparities in access to and use of mental healthcare for racial and ethnic minorities in the U.S. Specifically, it examines the complex relationships at different poverty levels and nativity status through an analysis of the Collaborative Psychiatric Epidemiological Surveys (CPES) dataset (Alegria et al., 2007). Our current knowledge is limited regarding how race, ethnicity, and immigrant status combine to affect levels of mental health. Further, little is known about the extent to which, for example, the pattern for Latinos compares to that of Asians and how this varies for subgroups within each of these subpopulations. Issues surrounding availability, access, utilization, and quality of care for racial and ethnic minorities are multifaceted and require close examination and contextualization as we design research and policy and identify viable strategies that would address these disparities.

Demographic structure of the U.S.

The total U.S. population is expected to increase from 296 million in 2005 to 438 million in 2050, with increases in Latino and Asian populations being the primary drivers of growth. According to projections, the Latino population will triple in size from 42 million (14% of the population) in 2005 to 128 million (29%) in 2050. Between 2000 and 2006, the Latino population grew almost four-times faster (24%) than the total U.S. population (6%). Latinos will account for 60% of the nation's population growth from 2005 to 2050. The Asian population, 14 million (5% of the U.S. population) in 2005, will experience growth rates similar to that of Latinos, more than tripling in size by 2050 to 41 million (9%). In 2005, a sizable proportion of Asians in the U.S. were born outside of the country (58%), but by 2050 fewer than half (47%) will be foreign-born. Other racial and ethnic groups will not see these increases. Though the African American population will grow from 38 million in 2005 to 59 million in 2050, the proportion of the total U.S. population will remain stable at 13%. The white, non-Hispanic population, 199 million in 2005, will grow to 207 million in 2050; only a 4% increase. Projections indicate that by 2050, non-Hispanic whites will become a "minority" population: 47% of the U.S. population will be non-Hispanic white, compared with 67% in 2005 (Passel & Cohn, 2008).

Overall, estimates suggest that between 2005 and 2050, the U.S. population will increase by 142 million, of which 67 million will be immigrants and 50 million U.S.-born children or grandchildren of immigrants. Immigrants will comprise 19% of the total U.S. population in 2050, compared to 12% in 2005 (Ortman & Guarneri, 2009).

Mental health and immigrant populations

The growing size and diversity of the U.S. immigrant population will have important implications for mental health planning and service delivery. Traditional approaches toward immigrants with mental health conditions have worked on the "principle of exclusion," whereby security and disease control became legal justifications for segregation and prohibition (World Health Organization [WHO], 2010), which has led to mistrust (Elliott et al., 2009). Today, immigrants must overcome access barriers such as limited English-language proficiency, increased poverty levels, geographic and social isolation, and lack of insurance. Gender, education level, and age at time of arrival in the U.S. are also powerful factors that affect both treatment-seeking behaviors and access to treatment.

Transition from life in a foreign country to life in the U.S. is often a complex trajectory involving an acculturation process that simultaneously dissolves family values, cultural traditions, and solidarity, while substituting these support systems with behaviors that increase risk of psychiatric disorders (e.g., illicit drug abuse and interpersonal violence) (Alderete, Vega, Kolody, & Aguilar-Gaxiola, 2000). Termed the "immigrant paradox," newly arrived immigrants have better mental and physical health than U.S.-born persons of the same age. However, the protective social and cultural factors from their countries of origin decrease as immigrants reside longer in the U.S. The decline in health status of immigrants over time in the U.S. is associated with higher social acculturation, including changes in lifestyle, cultural practices, increased stress, and adoption of new social norms (Alegria et al., 2008). For Mexican immigrants, rates of mental disorders increase according to time spent in the U.S.; individuals living in the U.S. longer than 13 years have higher prevalences than those living in the U.S. less than 13 years (Vega, Kolody, Aguilar-Gaxiola, Alderete, Catalano, & Caraveo-Anduaga, 1998).

There is also an association between age of immigration and mental health treatment seeking: Latinos and Asian Americans who came to the U.S. at 12 years of age or younger reported higher rates of specialty service use (13.4%) than did African American and Caribbean black immigrants (5.8%). In contrast, African Americans, Asian Americans, Latinos, and Caribbean black immigrants who arrived in the U.S. at 13 to 17 years of age reported lower rates of specialty service use. Those arriving between ages 18 and 34 had even lower utilization rates.

The theory of selective migration proposes (Alegria et al., 2008) that persons who are "psychologically hardy" would be more likely to immigrate.

However, Vega and colleagues (1998) examined rates of disorders from the *Diagnostic and Statistical Manual of Mental Disorders, Third Edition – Revised* (DSM-III-R) in a sample of residents in Mexico City compared to recently immigrated residents in Fresno County, California, and their findings revealed strong similarities in prevalence between the two samples, suggesting that selective migration is not the cause of the immigrant paradox. Understanding the immigrant paradox is further complicated by the heterogeneous nature of the various immigrant populations in that different racial and ethnic groups (and subpopulations within subgroups) may experience mental health issues dissimilarly (Takeuchi, Alegria, Jackson, & Williams, 2007), and this dissimilarity affects the frequency and manner in which mental health services are utilized.

Mental health status

Latino mental health

Recent studies revealed that most minority groups, except for Puerto Ricans, report lower rates of lifetime mental disorders than whites. Latinos, for example, report a 30% lifetime prevalence for any psychiatric disorder compared to 43% in whites (Alegria et al., 2008). Lower lifetime rates but similar past-year rates imply that disorders are more persistent among Latinos; those who have a disorder tend to have it over many years, compared to whites, who are more likely to have a disorder for a shorter time period. This is consistent with the finding of Breslau et al. (2006), that when Latinos do develop a psychiatric illness they tend to have more persistent illnesses, with symptoms that may be more severe and disabling. Overall difference in mental health becomes more complex when the category "Latinos" is disaggregated into subgroups, and significant differences by nativity[1] (Vega et al., 1998), time of residence in the United States (Alegria et al., 2008; Vega et al., 1998), and age of migration (Alegria et al., 2008) are revealed. Puerto Ricans in particular tend to have the highest lifetime prevalence rates of mental disorders (37.4%), followed by Mexicans (29.5%), Cubans (28.2%), and other Latinos (27%) (Alegria et al., 2008). Additionally, U.S.-born Latinos have higher rates (37.1%) of mental disorders compared to immigrants (24.9%) (Alegria et al., 2008; Kessler et al., 2005; Vega et al., 1998).

African American mental health

African Americans are less likely than whites to have psychiatric disorders during their lifetimes, but they are more likely to have very severe and disabling disorders when they occur (Williams, Gonzalez, Neighbors, Nesse, Abelson, Sweetman, & Jackson, 2007). U.S.-born African Americans have the highest prevalence rates for mood and anxiety disorders (16%), almost identical to their immigrant counterparts who migrated to the U.S. before age 13 (13%). However, those immigrants who migrated after age 13 show significantly lower prevalences (8%) (Breslau et al., 2009), consistent with the "immigrant paradox" theory.

Williams and colleagues (2007) reported that Caribbean black immigrant men were at lower risk for mental health and substance abuse disorders than were U.S.-born men. Immigrant Caribbean black women were at lower risk for substance abuse than U.S.-born women. Immigrants who have lived in the U.S. for 21 years or longer showed similar prevalence rates for mental and substance abuse disorders to U.S.-born individuals. Men who immigrated between the ages of 13 and 17 showed less risk for mood and anxiety disorders, and women who immigrated at the same age had lower rates of substance abuse disorders compared to U.S.-born individuals. Third-generation Caribbean black men and women had elevated rates of mental health and substance abuse disorders compared with first-generation immigrants. From these findings, the authors concluded that acculturation may well have been associated with an increased risk of substance abuse and mental health problems.

Mental health among Asian Americans and Pacific Islanders

Prevalences among Asian Americans and Pacific Islanders are lower overall compared to their white counterparts. The most common diagnosis is major depression (14% to 38%), followed by schizophrenia (ranging from 11% to 26%), except for Filipinos who, like African Americans, had higher rates of schizophrenia than depression (24% and 16%, respectively) (Barreto & Segal, 2005). Barreto and Segal (2005) separate their data into the subgroups East Asian, Southeast Asian, Filipino, and Other Asian; of these, the Southeast Asian and Other Asian subpopulations show prevalence rates similar to other minority groups. Both the Southeast Asian and Other Asian subgroups were at higher risk for major depressive disorder, 38% and 27% respectively. Further, differences in prevalences occur across ethnic subgroups of Asian Americans (e.g., Hmong, Vietnamese, and Japanese), of which nativity status and generational status emerge as the most important indicators of within-group differences (Abe-Kim et al., 2007). Abe-Kim and colleagues also found that Asian men who arrived in the U.S. between the ages of 18 and 34 were less likely to have a substance abuse disorder than U.S.-born men. Also, second-generation and third-generation Asian women were more likely than first-generation women to have a substance abuse disorder.

Disparities in mental healthcare

There is a growing body of research providing evidence of pervading disparities for racial and ethnic minorities in access to and quality of care within the U.S. mental health system. While racial and ethnic minorities generally have equal or better mental health status than their white counterparts, available data indicate differential patterns of utilization, participation, and treatment within the mental healthcare system for African Americans, Latinos, and Asians (McGuire & Miranda, 2008). For example, Jackson and colleagues (2007) reported that U.S.-born blacks were more likely to receive mental health services than Caribbean-born blacks. Immigrants who had lived more than 21 years in the U.S. reported using more mental health services than those who had lived in the U.S. for a shorter period. Arriving in the U.S. at age 12 or younger was associated with a greater likelihood of receiving services (Jackson et al., 2007). Third-generation Caribbean blacks were more likely to use mental health services than first-generation immigrants.

Although the existence of disparities in care is well documented, the root causes remain unclear. To better understand the factors that determine the efficacy of the mental healthcare system, especially in terms of access and quality for minority populations, Echeverry (1997) highlights two categories that influence access to and acceptance of professional help: patient variables and organizational/structural variables. Patient variables include demographic characteristics (e.g., age, gender, educational status) and cultural factors (e.g., beliefs about mental illness and treatment, language, acculturation); these are usually mediated on the patient-provider level. Organizational/structural variables include insurance coverage and lack thereof and fragmentation of care, both of which constitute major systemic impediments to mental health service access.

Analysis of U.S. national data: The collaborative psychiatric epidemiological surveys

Our analysis of mental health status and service use is based on the Collaborative Psychiatric Epidemiology Surveys (CPES) dataset from three national surveys that was collected from 2001 to 2003 (Alegria et al., 2007):

1 The National Latino and Asian American Study (NLAAS).
2 The National Survey of American Life (NSAL).
3 The National Comorbidity Survey Replication (NCS-R).

Each of these surveys employed the World Health Organization Composite International Diagnostic Interview (WHO-CIDI) (Kessler & Üstün, 2004) to determine diagnoses according to DSM-IV criteria and also service-use history. Using data from these merged surveys, the final sample consisted of 15,120 adults of whom 3,246 had past-year DSM-IV disorders.

Prevalence of past-year mental disorders by ethnicity and nativity

Past-year mental disorder prevalence is greatest among U.S.-born whites (22%), with U.S.-born Latinos (19%) only slightly lower. U.S.-born

African Americans (15%) and immigrant Latinos (14%) have similar prevalence of past-year disorders, while immigrant African Americans (11%) and both U.S.-born Asians (12%) and immigrant Asians (9%) have the lowest prevalence (see Table 5.1). This trend by ethnicity and nativity is also seen when looking at depressive, anxiety, and substance-use disorders separately. The most notable difference among these groups when looking at classes of disorders is the low prevalence of alcohol or drug abuse or dependence among immigrants (Latino immigrants 1.1%, Asian immigrants 0.6%, and African American immigrants 0.1%).

Table 5.2 reveals four important points. First, disparities are greater for medical doctor (MD) visits and medications than they are for non-MD clinicians or other human services. Second, there are no statistically significant differences between U.S.-born Latinos and U.S.-born whites (except for internet support groups), nor between U.S.-born Asians and U.S.-born whites; the greatest disparities are those for immigrants of all ethnicities compared to U.S.-born whites and U.S.-born African Americans compared to U.S.-born whites. Third, by far the greatest disparity is that for Caribbean black immigrants, whose receipt of mental health services in a medical setting (MDs and medication) is less than one-third that of U.S.-born whites, and their receipt of clinician and other human services is only slightly more than one-third that of U.S.-born whites. Fourth, despite the large combined sample size of these three national surveys (over 15,000 participants), no large numbers of Latinos, Asians, and immigrant African Americans with past-year disorders were available to analyze; sample sizes for groups other than U.S.-born whites and U.S.-born African Americans range from 75 (U.S.-born Asians) to 351 (U.S.-born Latinos). At best these large studies can only show broad differences; fine differences among these groups remain shrouded in statistical uncertainty, and determining what associated factors might be casually related to differences in service use is yet more problematic. These three large surveys represent the best national data that exist, yet the statistical sampling error alone makes conclusions difficult to draw – to say nothing of possible response bias (e.g., those with untreated mental disorders being less likely to be represented in the sample). Therefore, how certain can we be about the extent of mental health disparities in the U.S.?

Table 5.3 shows that women are more likely than men to get care in medical settings, and younger (<35 years old) and older adults (≥65 years old) are less likely to get mental healthcare in these settings. With regard to the link between health insurance and medical care, participants with public insurance are more likely to receive care when compared to participants with private insurance or no insurance. Persons with comorbid mental disorders (either both substance and non-substance disorders or both depressive and anxiety disorders) and persons with functioning difficulties due to mental health problems are more likely to receive medical care. After controlling for age and sex differences in this model,

Table 5.1 Prevalence[1] of past-year mental disorders[2] for US adults[3] by ethnicity and nativity[4]

	White	African American		Latino		Asian	
	US born	US born	Immigrant	US born	Immigrant[5]	US born	Immigrant
Sample size (N)	4,174	4,380	1,132	1,370	1,888	476	1,700
Past-year mental disorder prevalence							
Depressive disorders[6]	10 (0.5)	6 (0.4)***	6 (1)**	9 (0.9)	8 (0.6)*	5 (1)***	5 (0.8)***
Anxiety disorders[7]	15 (0.7)	11 (0.6)***	7 (1)***	11 (1)**	9 (0.9)***	8 (2)***	6 (0.8)***
Alcohol or drug abuse or dependence	4.2 (0.4)	3.1 (0.4)*	0.1 (0.1)***	4.5 (0.7)	1.1 (0.2)***	2.7 (0.6)*	0.6 (0.2)***
Any of above	22 (0.8)	15 (0.7)***	11 (2)***	19 (1)	14 (1)***	12 (2)***	9 (0.9)***

Source: CPES surveys 2001–2003.

Notes

$*p<0.05$, $**p<0.01$, $***p<0.001$, for test of difference with US-born whites.
1 All data, except sample size, are weighted age–sex adjusted percentages with standard errors shown in parentheses.
2 Disorders (DSM-IV criteria) include depressive disorders, anxiety disorders, and alcohol or drug abuse or dependence.
3 Aged 18 years or older.
4 Foreign-born whites and other ethnicities not shown in table omitted because of small sample size.
5 Foreign-born Latinos include persons born in Puerto Rico.
6 Includes major depressive episodes and dysthymia; excludes mania and bipolar.
7 Includes agoraphobia, panic disorder, generalized anxiety disorder, posttraumatic stress disorder, and social phobia.

Table 5.2 Prevalence[1] of past-year mental health service use[2] among those with past-year disorders[3] for US adults[4] by ethnicity and nativity[5]

	White	African American		Latino		Asian	
	US born	US born	Immigrant	US born	Immigrant[6]	US born	Immigrant
Number of persons with past-year mental disorders (N)	1,389	844	130	351	318	75	139
Medical doctors or medications							
Psychiatrists and mental health hospitalizations	15 (1)	14 (1)	4 (3)***	10 (2)	15 (2)	23 (9)	7 (2)**
Other medical doctors	23 (1)	15 (2)**	6 (2)***	22 (3)	15 (3)**	23 (8)	7 (2)***
Medications[7]	37 (2)	21 (2)***	11 (4)***	29 (4)	26 (3)**	24 (8)	14 (4)***
Any of above 3 categories	45 (1)	32 (2)***	14 (4)***	38 (4)	32 (3)***	42 (9)	20 (4)***
Non-MD clinicians or other human services							
Psychologists, social workers, counselors, mental health hotline, nurses, occupational therapists, or other health professionals	19 (1)	15 (2)	4 (2)***	20 (3)	14 (2)	31 (9)	14 (5)
Religious or spiritual advisors	7 (1)	9 (1)	4 (1)*	7 (2)	6 (2)	15 (8)	3 (1)**
Self-help groups[8]	5 (1)	3 (1)	3 (3)	3 (2)	5 (2)	2 (2)	6 (3)
Internet support groups	2.5 (0.4)	0.6 (0.4)**	0.2 (0.2)***	1.0 (0.5)*	0.1 (0.1)***	3.8 (3.1)	4.4 (3.2)
Any of above 4 categories	25 (1)	23 (2)***	9 (3)***	25 (3)	19 (3)***	34 (8)	19 (5)
Any mental health service use	53 (2)	41 (2)***	19 (5)***	45 (4)	39 (3)***	51 (8)	34 (5)***

Source: CPES surveys 2001–2003. *$p < 0.05$, **$p < 0.01$, ***$p < 0.001$, for test of difference with US-born whites.

Notes
1 All data, except sample size and number of persons with disorders, are weighted age–sex adjusted percentages with standard errors shown in parentheses.
2 Questions on all types of service use were asked in the context of helping with "problems with your emotions or nerves or your use of alcohol or drugs."
3 Disorders (DSM-IV criteria) include depressive disorders, anxiety disorders, and alcohol or drug abuse or dependence. See footnotes 6 and 7 of Table 5.1.
4 Aged 18 years or older.
5 Foreign-born whites and other ethnicities omitted because of small sample size.
6 Foreign-born Latinos include persons born in Puerto Rico.
7 Medications include sleeping pills or other sedatives, anti-depressant medications, tranquilizers, amphetamines or other stimulants, and anti-psychotic medications.
8 Self-help group question omitted explicit mention of alcohol or drug use; question was "Did you go to a self-help group for help with your emotions or nerves?" However, 47 percent of persons responding yes to this question responded in a follow-up question that they had attended groups for people with substance problems such as Alcoholics Anonymous or Rational Recovery.

Table 5.3 Logistic regression models of past-year mental health service use for US adults with any past-year DSM-IV disorder[1]

	Medical doctors or medications	Non-MD clinicians or other human services
Female	1.7 [1.3, 2.2]***	1.2 [1.0, 1.5]*
Age (y)		
18–24	0.4 [0.2, 0.7]**	1.1 [0.7, 1.9]
25–34	0.4 [0.3, 0.6]***	1.0 [0.7, 1.4]
35–44	0.9 [0.6, 1.3]	1.2 [0.9, 1.8]
45–54	1	1
55–64	1.1 [0.6, 1.9]	0.8 [0.5, 1.5]
≥65	0.4 [0.2, 0.8]**	0.3 [0.2, 0.7]**
Marital status		
Married	1	1
Divorced, separated, widowed	1.1 [0.8, 1.5]	1.7 [1.3, 2.4]***
Never married	0.9 [0.7, 1.2]	1.3 [0.9, 1.7]
Education		
Some high school or less	1.0 [0.7, 1.5]	0.8 [0.5, 1.2]
High school graduate	1	1
Some college	1.3 [1.0, 1.6]	1.2 [0.9, 1.6]
College degree or more	1.2 [0.9, 1.6]	1.4 [1.1, 1.9]*
Insurance		
Private	1	1
Public	2.1 [1.6, 2.7]***	1.3 [0.8, 2.2]
None	0.5 [0.3, 0.7]***	0.8 [0.6, 1.1]
Comorbid with disorder of another class[2]	2.0 [1.6, 2.6]***	1.8 [1.4, 2.2]***
Unable to function 1 or more days out of past 30 days due to mental health problems	2.2 [1.7, 2.9]***	2.5 [1.8, 3.4]***
Ethnicity		
White, US born	1	1
African American, US born	0.5 [0.4, 0.7]***	0.7 [0.5, 1.0]
African American, foreign born	0.2 [0.1, 0.4]***	0.2 [0.1, 0.4]***
Latino, US born	0.8 [0.5, 1.1]	0.9 [0.6, 1.3]
Latino, foreign born	0.7 [0.5, 1.0]*	0.9 [0.5, 1.4]
Asian, US born	0.6 [0.3, 1.1]	1.0 [0.6, 1.8]
Asian, foreign born	0.4 [0.2, 0.6]***	0.7 [0.3, 1.3]

Source: CPES surveys 2001–2003. $*p < 0.05$, $**p < 0.01$, $***p < 0.001$.

Notes
1 See footnotes 2–7 from Table 5.1.
2 Person has past-year substance and nonsubstance disorders or past-year mood and anxiety disorders.

the differences among the ethnicity and nativity groups seen among the prevalence estimates of care still remain. Immigrant Latinos, immigrant Asians, U.S.-born African Americans, and immigrant African Americans all have significantly lower odds for receipt for medical mental health care relative to U.S.-born whites.

With regard to receipt of non-MD clinicians or other human services, women were again more likely to receive care, older persons ($\geq$65 years old) were less likely, and those with comorbidity or functioning problems were more likely. Being divorced, separated, or widowed was strongly associated with receipt of this modality of care. The obvious possibility here is that the event of becoming divorced, separated, or widowed may have been the primary trigger for seeking these services. Overall, there were no significant ethnic by nativity group differences, with the notable exception of immigrant African Americans, suggesting that they are at the bottom by a large margin for receipt of both medical services and non-medical human services.

An analysis of the percentage of persons with past-year mental disorders who had any past-year mental health service by poverty level showed no differences. For each of the ethnicity by nativity groups, differences by poverty level are small, and there is no significant association between poverty level and service use.

Persons with public insurance are by far the most likely to get mental health services. For example, 73% of U.S.-born whites with public insurance reported receiving services as compared to 52% with private insurance and 44% with no insurance. These results are not unique to just U.S.-born whites; other groups share a similar pattern. For African American immigrants, we found little to no significant relationship between insurance status and service use (see Table 3). Those with public insurance reported higher rates of service compared to those with private or no insurance. Similarly, with Latino immigrants we found little to no significant difference between those with public insurance (62%) and those with private insurance (47%), but those with no insurance had much lower rates of use (17%). For Asian immigrants, there was also little to no significant association between insurance status and service use. Thus, although income does not affect treatment receipt, type of insurance does, especially for the U.S.-born. The evolution of the health insurance system in the U.S., especially on the eve of healthcare reform, will have major implications for mental healthcare.

Discussion

Disparities in prevalence of mental disorders among ethnicity and nativity groups

Any discussion of disparities in mental health involves two separate yet related questions. First, are there differences in the prevalence, severity and life consequences of mental disorders among different racial, ethnic, nativity, or other social or demographic groups? Second, for those with mental disorders, are there differences in receipt of treatment among different groups, and if so, what is the cause? Much work has been done to attempt to answer these questions, but due to limitations in study design (e.g., inclusion of a truly representative sample of persons with mental disorders) and sample size (e.g., disparities may be greatest among some ethnic by nativity by age by income subgroups, requiring a very large sample to observe), it is difficult or impossible to answer these questions with great precision. A degree of uncertainty, however, should not preclude or delay policy recommendations. There are findings that have sufficient certainty to inform policy.

Consistent with previous work on the "immigrant paradox" (McGuire & Miranda, 2008; Primm, Vasquez, Mays, Sammons-Posey, McKnighty-Eily, Presley-Cantrell, et al., 2010), our analysis of the CPES data shows that mental disorder prevalence determined from self-reported symptomatology is greater among U.S.-born individuals than immigrants. Prevalence of substance abuse or dependence in particular is substantially lower among immigrants than among U.S.-born whites. We also report that for Latino and Asian immigrants (but not for African American immigrants) poverty level is not associated with disorder prevalence – in contrast to its strong association among all U.S.-born groups.

Alegria and colleagues (2003) have commented that "defining disparities in mental health status for minorities requires a broad definition of psychopathology, one that moves beyond psychiatric disorders to include mental health symptoms and behavioral problems" (p. 52). Studies like these national surveys that do not include broader mental health questions may under-report disparities in the prevalence of mental illness. It is also important to consider that whites commonly report symptoms of mental disorders when they are first noticed, while minorities report the same symptoms only when severely ill (Alegria et al., 2003). As McGuire and Miranda (2008) emphasized, it is likely that disparities exist that are not reflected in diagnoses.

Disparities in mental health treatment among ethnicity and nativity groups

Our results are consistent with observations reported by Primm and colleagues (2010) that immigrant groups are less likely to use medications for mental health issues than their U.S.-born counterparts. Given that our analysis was based on existing national data, we were limited in our investigation of additional critical factors with regard to providers' knowledge or bias about immigrant groups, cost of medications, and cultural beliefs toward the chronic medication use.

Our analysis also indicated that immigrant groups are less likely to see medical doctors for their mental health issues than are their U.S.-born counterparts. It is unclear whether this is due to lack of access to primary care physicians, stigma about mental health issues, or lack of time or understanding from primary care physicians. Our regression analysis in Table 5.3 shows that it is not simply a matter of insurance or education status for immigrants (and U.S.-born African Americans) that causes receipt of treatment to be lower among these groups. Given that it may be a complex interplay among individual behaviors, access to care, how care is delivered, and provider characteristics which causes lower treatment rates among immigrants and U.S.-born African Americans, it is not clear whether future surveys based on self-reported experiences would be able to fully delineate the causes.

Our findings that medical care for mental health issues is less likely for individuals with private insurance compared to those with public insurance is of interest given that the data were obtained before passage and implementation of mental health disparity laws. Our regression analysis in Table 5.3 shows a difference by type of insurance while controlling for severity of mental illness; hence, it does not seem likely that the difference by type of insurance is merely due to individuals with public insurance having more severe and persistent mental health issues. We believe that the explanation is more likely due to differences in access and delivery of care. One factor that may influence lower rates of care among those with private insurance might be the two layers of screening needed for individuals with mental health issues who have private insurance through a health maintenance organization (HMO) and who first must seek treatment through their primary care physician. Individuals with private HMO insurance are required to visit a primary care doctor, receive a referral, complete a telephone screening, and then be assigned to see a mental health provider. This process typically delays being seen by several weeks to a month. Whether differences between HMO and preferred provider option (PPO) private insurance affect treatment rates is an important question for the design of new insurance coverage plans in the U.S., especially as regards the implementation of healthcare reform.

Disparities and income

CPES results indicate that being below 200% of the Federal Poverty Line (FPL) had a significant effect on prevalence of past-year mental disorders except for Latino and Asian immigrants. These results are consistent with those of Muntaner, Eaton, Diala, Kessler, and Sorlie (1998), who found psychiatric disorders were higher for those in lower-income strata. CPES analyses also reveal that the percentage of individuals with mental disorders in the past year who received any treatment during that time span was not influenced by poverty level. This finding is significant because it makes it unlikely that income is the primary cause of disparities among ethnic and nativity groups. Improving treatment rates among these groups will necessitate changes to healthcare in the U.S. that are based on the cultural, linguistic and social characteristics of these groups and how healthcare delivery systems and providers interface with them. Institutional policies need to be adopted that expand hours of service, encourage flexible scheduling options, and allow time for family meetings within appointment time frames.

The finding that persons with mental health disorders in the past year, with an income below 200% of the poverty level have the same rates of any treatment in the past year as persons with income above 200% of the poverty level as well as the finding that persons with public health insurance have higher rates of any treatment leads to an obvious question: Is the quality of care received the same?

Disparities in quality of care

Quality of care is multi-dimensional, and its many aspects make it hard to evaluate. Surveys of individuals of course only assess quality of care using self-report. Different modalities of care may have been received, each requiring a different assessment of quality. In an analysis of self-reported degree of help (with choices: not at all, a little, some, and a lot) from psychiatrists, other medical doctors, and non-MD clinicians (not shown here), we saw no evidence that the degree of help differed by provider type or income. Nor were there any dramatic differences by ethnicity and nativity. Statistical power was, however, an issue for these analyses; not all persons saw each type of provider, so sample sizes for these analyses were appreciably lower than they were for the other analyses we presented here.

The category of non-MD clinician was defined in a broad manner in these surveys, mixing providers who can provide therapy (psychologists, social workers, counselors, masters-level nurses) with other types of treatment providers who do not typically do therapy (mental health hotline workers, registered nurses, and occupational therapists). This made it difficult to discern any differences in use of medication management versus therapy among immigrant and U.S.-born populations. An important distinction to clarify in future studies is the perspectives of immigrant versus U.S.-born groups in terms of preference for and use of case management, medication management, inpatient care, and outpatient therapy for mental health issues.

Implications for mental healthcare policy and practice

The results from the study emphasize the complex relationship between racial and ethnic disparities in mental healthcare access and use. The preceding discussion of the data provides important insights and implications for future policy and actions to improve the mental healthcare system. Clearly, multifaceted help-seeking strategies that promote social inclusion are essential to eliminating or reducing disparities. Data gaps and ambiguity exist, highlighting the need for future research and the need to look at opportunities to improve data collection. Yet even with the data challenges, there are clear implications coming from the dataset that are discussed in detail below.

The status of mental healthcare for all Americans remains uncertain, even in the face of sweeping healthcare policy reforms such as the Patient Protection and Affordable Care Act. The biggest dedicated federal mental health program, at $440 million, is the Substance Abuse and Mental Health Service Administration's (SAMHSA) Community Mental Health Services Block Grant, which is dedicated to improving mental health service systems across the country. Through the Community Mental Health Services Block Grant, a joint Federal-State partnership, SAMHSA's Center for Mental Health Services (CMHS) supports existing public services and encourages the development of creative and cost-effective systems of community-based care for people with serious mental disorders. With the current changes in the healthcare delivery system, improving access to community-based systems is especially important. Organizational responsibility for mental healthcare in the public sector resides primarily with states, and then counties. Inasmuch as mental illness is not treated the same as other illnesses in this regard, it has a "second-class status" in public healthcare. Further, vast differences in mental healthcare and access exist depending on specific states' and counties' budgets. Future studies should analyze the impact of state-wide and county-wide treatment availability and type. In addition, a comprehensive, national approach to provision of and funding for mental healthcare should be introduced and discussed in legislative sessions, for example, recognizing Medicaid's cost-shifting opportunities to maximize federal matching funds and its consequences to serving historically underserved populations with severe mental illness.

Government mental health policy in the medical sector can be loosely separated into targeted medical policy, such as Medicaid and Medicare, or broad social policies, such as Section 8 Housing vouchers, which can have an unintended effect on mental health status. Common targeted policies that address service disparities in mental health concentrate on health insurance, reforms to Medicaid and Medicare, and employer-based mandates such as mental health parity. Establishing policies that ensure a geographically available, culturally and linguistically competent and diverse workforce trained to provide mental healthcare are necessary to address lack of access. In order to increase trust among minority populations and help them overcome cultural and linguistic barriers so that they are successful in establishing meaningful partnerships with their mental health provider, it is critical that incentives be available for ethnically diverse students in mental health training programs. Ensuring a diverse workforce is a key strategy to reducing and eliminating racial and ethnic disparities in healthcare.

Considering different cultural expressions of mental health is also important in clinical settings. For example, routine screenings for mental health issues that allow for a variety of culturally appropriate responses could be administered to diverse populations while they wait to see health-care providers. This would help clinicians identify mental health issues their clients had not yet mentioned. It would also help educate diverse patients about U.S. perspectives regarding mental health and mental illness, so they would be in a better position to effectively communicate with their healthcare provider. Further, there is a need for increased funding for interventions designed to evaluate outreach and treatment options that specifically target minority populations if culturally relevant programs are to be developed.

Policies that have separated mental healthcare provided in an inpatient setting from general medical care have resulted in transfers to medical hospitals of individuals who need dressing changes, catheters, intravenous medications or hydration, or other medical interventions along with mental healthcare. Staff working in medical hospitals are often less familiar and less comfortable with providing mental healthcare. The person's medical condition is treated first, while their mental health needs are put on the back burner. Only after the medical treatment has concluded is the person to be transferred to a mental health or substance abuse treatment facility or outpatient mental health provider. This fragmentation of care has added to the reluctance that many ethnically diverse and immigrant individuals feel about seeking care. Reimbursement and licensing policies that support the fragmentation of mental health and medical care should be revised to correspond to patient-centered priorities that support holistic, integrated care, particularly that delivered in primary care settings. Starfield's (1992) four core dimensions provide a clear and helpful direction to tailor care, especially for underserved populations:

1 Providing first-contact access.
2 Ensuring continuity of care that ensures whole-person knowledge.
3 Providing effective care coordination.
4 Providing comprehensive care for a broad array of medical problems and health conditions.

Whole-person knowledge is particularly highly valued by patients, and it has been strongly associated with patients' adherence to physicians' advice and satisfaction with care (Safran et al., 2001; 1998).

Educational policies that align mental health content with medical and nursing school curricula are needed to ensure a well-trained workforce is in place to provide individuals with competent care in any type of facility. Moreover, policies that allow for different staffing ratios and professional pay scales between medical and mental health hospitals need to be revised. Otherwise, care that is provided in inpatient mental health settings will continue to be poor in quality. Offering masters-level social workers, mental health nurses, clinical psychologists, and psychiatrists loan forgiveness programs to work in diverse, low-income communities is critical if we are to increase access to care. Providing incentives for those who wish to specialize in child/adolescent and geriatric mental healthcare is also important to ensure an adequate number of providers are available. This is particularly necessary since age of immigration and generational status are key factors in mental healthcare.

Mental health promotion activities are critical. Broad educational programs in schools and public service advertisements on television are needed to introduce positive coping mechanisms and health promotion concepts. Programs such as anger management, coping with stress, getting adequate sleep, and the value of exercise in modulating mood are important. Building on and encouraging prevention and wellness is an important focus for health policy intervention, as is the management of mental health problems. Promoting health and wellness and encouraging healthy environments and communities may turn out to be as effective (or even more effective) in maintaining or restoring health as treating mental illness.

Funding for mental health research that targets resilient populations is also needed if we are to understand and enhance factors that promote health. Typically, funding opportunities have targeted individuals with a mental health diagnosis, which provides an incomplete understanding of the protective and positive factors that contribute to mental health. If immigrants truly do have a lower prevalence of mental disorder, then future studies, as Williams and Jackson (2005) pointed out, should examine what protective factors in the cultural background of immigrant and ethnic groups explain this phenomenon. Not only might full acculturation into mainstream U.S. society not be the best goal for ethnic immigrant groups, but U.S.-born populations may do well to adopt some of the protective factors of immigrant cultures. Indeed, U.S.-born whites may have something to learn from immigrant cultures in terms of mental health.

The concept of a "medical home" should be incorporated into mental healthcare to enhance the level of familiarity, and therefore comfort, that a patient feels with a provider; such a model also facilitates access to needed medications, diagnostic testing, therapy, and inpatient care from one location. Policies that support a mental health "home" would minimize fragmentation of care, decrease unnecessary referrals, and likely enhance access to care and improve outcomes among diverse populations.

With the increasing movement toward electronic medical records, safeguarding mental health and substance abuse treatment records is a priority if we are to address issues of trust within ethnically diverse and immigrant communities. No one should fear the loss of a job based on seeking treatment for mental health or substance abuse. National policies that ensure confidentiality of electronic medical records are a necessity.

Other policy opportunities to expand access and utilization of mental health services and improve their quality are tied to the evolution of Medicaid and Medicare programs. Medicaid and Medicare can serve as vehicles for low-income families and special populations to not only utilize mental health services, but also to reduce their fear of treatment. The current programs have systematic challenges that negatively impact the role of states in the provision of mental health services. While Medicaid and Medicare have managed to assist a large portion of Americans with mental health disorders, the system itself has dramatically shifted the economic responsibility of mental healthcare from the states to the federal government, creating a dearth of funding and services for individuals who fall outside of Medicaid and Medicare, and arguably meaning lower-quality care for some persons in the programs.

Before the advent of Medicaid and Medicare, most mental health services were provided in mental institutions run by states, and during the establishment of the public health insurance programs, the mental hospitals were considered custodial institutions of the state and received no federal aid (Cunningham, 2003). The direct consequence of this arrangement was that Medicaid and Medicare payments could not be made for inpatient treatment in state psychiatric hospitals though such treatment was reimbursable in a general hospital. In other words, spending was shifted away from historically underserved populations with severe mental disorders. This phenomenon – sometimes called "Medicaiding it" – speaks to aggressive pursuit of federal matching funds by states (Frank, Goldman, & Hogan, 2003), resulting in shifting state-run mental health services under the Medicaid and Medicare umbrella. The state has largely become a contracting and regulatory agency, a role that has superseded its position as a public and social entity with access to specialized expertise and the resources for treating people with mental illness. The resulting changes in public mental healthcare have contributed to ongoing disparities in the overall mental health system.

Opportunities in healthcare reform

With a burgeoning economic crisis and growing rates of unemployment in the U.S., the ranks of the 46 million uninsured in the U.S. are growing. Adding to those stressors are revenue shortages and inadequate funding that adversely impact Medicaid and community mental health programs. However, the Patient Protection and Affordable Care Act of 2010 offers specific provisions aimed at removing barriers for uninsured Americans (Andrulis et al., 2010). Included in healthcare reform are key provisions that will enhance mental health benefits that address access and quality of mental health services. Such provisions provide for expanded coverage through Medicaid; expanded medication coverage; a demonstration program in up to eight states that will allow Medicaid coverage of acute inpatient care provided in private psychiatric hospitals for non-elderly adults; a new state plan option that allows enrollees with at least two chronic conditions, including serious mental illness, to designate a provider (may be a community health center) as a "health home" to better coordinate and integrate access to primary care; increased coverage of wellness and preventive services, such as adult depression screening; enrollment assistance; and outreach programs to enroll vulnerable populations in Medicaid and the Children's Health Insurance Program, including individuals with mental illness.

There are also provisions in the healthcare reform law that will work at the federal level to address workforce development and training for healthcare professionals. Federal grants will be established to educate primary care providers on chronic disease management, mental health and substance abuse services, and evidence-based care guidelines. Loan repayment incentives have been included for specialties such as child and adolescent mental health and substance abuse, and grants will be offered to schools of social work, graduate psychology programs, nursing programs, and professional and paraprofessional training in child and adolescent mental health. In addition, there are provisions that promote the integration of primary and mental healthcare services in community-based mental health settings and provide funding through SAMHSA, for example, to develop innovative interventions for depression. These provisions should be used to improve the diversity and cultural competence of the heathcare workforce.

The new healthcare reform law is ambitious and seeks to provide a vehicle for eliminating ongoing racial and ethnic disparities in overall physical and mental health. Provisions that address healthcare access and quality may do much to improve flaws in the current system, but attention should be given to specific culturally and linguistically appropriate interventions that address the needs of the subgroups of racial and ethnic minorities related to their mental health if health equity is to be achieved.

Note

1 Nativity refers to whether a person is native or foreign-born (Grieco, 2009).

References

Abe-Kim, J., Takeuchi, D. T., Hong, S., Zane, N., Sue, S., Spencer, M. S., et al. (2007). Use of mental health-related services among immigrant and US-Born Asian Americans: Results from the National Latino and Asian American Study. *American Journal of Public Health, 97*, 91–98.
Agency for Healthcare Research and Quality. (2006). *National healthcare disparities report 2006* (AHRQ Publication, no. 07–0012). Rockville, MD: U.S. Department of Health and Human Services, Agency for Healthcare Research and Quality.

Agency for Healthcare Research and Quality. (2008). *National healthcare dispari-ties report 2007* (AHRQ Publication, no. 08–0041). Rockville, MD: U.S. Dept. of Health and Human Services, Agency for Healthcare Research and Quality.

Agency for Healthcare Research and Quality. (2009). *National healthcare disparities report 2008* (AHRQ Publication, no. 09–0002). Rockville, MD: U.S. Department of Health and Human Services, Agency for Healthcare Research and Quality.

Alderete, E., Vega, W. A., Kolody, B., & Aguilar-Gaxiola, S. (2000). Effects of time in the United States and Indian ethnicity on DSM-III-R psychiatric disorders among Mexican origin adults. *Journal of Nervous and Mental Disease,188*, 90–100.

Alegria, M., Canino, G., Shrout, P., Woo, M., Duan, N., Vila, D., et al. (2008). Prevalence of mental illness in immigrant and non-immigrant U.S. Latino groups. *American Journal of Psychiatry.* 165, 359–369.

Alegria, M., Perez, D. J., & Williams, S. (2003). The role of public policies in redu-cing mental health status disparities for people of color. *Health Affairs*, 22, 51–64.

Alegria, M., Jackson, J., Kessler, R. C., & Takeuchi, D. (2007). Collaborative Psy-chiatric Epidemiology Surveys (CPES), 2001–2003. (ICPSR20240-v5). Ann Arbor, MI: Institute for Social Research, Survey Research Center. Ann Arbor, MI: Inter-university Consortium for Political and Social Research, 2008–06–19. Retrieved from www.icpsr.umich.edu/CPES/data.html

Andrulis, D. P., Siddiqui, N. J., Purtle, J. P., & Duchon, L. (2010). *Patient Protec-tion and Affordable Care Act of 2010: Advancing Health Equity for Racially and Ethnically Diverse Populations.* Washington, DC: Joint Center for Political and Economic Studies.

Barreto, R. M., & Segal, S. P. (2005). Use of mental health services by Asian Amer-icans. *Psychiatric Services, 56*, 746–748.

Breslau J., Borges G., Hagar Y., Tancredi, D., & Gilman, S. (2009). Immigration to the USA and risk for mood and anxiety disorders: Variation by origin and age at immigration. *Psychological Medicine, 39*, 1117–1127.

Breslau, J., Aguilar-Gaxiola, S., Kendler, K. S., Su, M., Williams, D., & Kessler, R. C. (2006). Specifying race-ethnic differences in risk for psychiatric disorder in a USA national sample. *Psychological Medicine, 36*, 57–68.

Cunningham, R. (2003). The Mental Health Commission tackles fragmented serv-ices: An interview with Michael Hogan. *Health Affairs, Jul-Dec*(Suppl Web Exclusives), W3–440–448.

Echeverry, J. J. (1997). *Treatment barriers: Assessing and accepting mental health.* In G. Garcia and M. C. Zera (Eds.). *Psychological interventions and Research with Latino Populations* (pp. 94–124). Boston: Allyn and Bacon.

Elliott, K., Sribney, W. M., Deeb-Sossa, N., Giordano, C., Sala, M., King, R. T., & Aguilar-Gaxiola, S. (2009). *Building partnerships: Conversations with com-munities about mental health needs and community strengths.* UC Davis Center for Reducing Health Disparities. Sacramento, CA: UC Davis.

Frank, R. G., Goldman, H. G., & Hogan, M. (2003). Medicaid and mental health: Be careful what you ask for. *Health Affairs, 22*, 101–113.

Grieco, E. M. (2009). Race and Hispanic origin of the foreign-born population in the United States: 2007. *American Community Survey Reports*, ACS-11.U.S. Census Bureau, Washington, DC.

Jackson, J. S., Neighbors, H. W., Torres, M., Martin, L. A., Williams, D. R., & Baser, R. (2007). Use of mental health services and subjective satisfaction with treatment among Black Caribbean Immigrants: Results from the National Survey of American Life. *American Journal of Public Health, 97*, 60–67.

Kessler, R. C., Berglund, P., Demler, O., Jin, R., Merikangas, K. R., & Walters, E. E. (2005). Lifetime prevalence and age-of-onset distributions of DSM-IV disorders in the National Comorbidity Survey Replication. *Archives of General Psychiatry, 62*, 593–602.

Kessler, R. C., & Üstün, T. B. (2004). The World Mental Health (WMH) Survey Initiative Version of the World Health Organization (WHO) Composite International Diagnostic Interview (CIDI). *International Journal of Methods Psychiatry Research, 13*, 93–121.

LaVeist, T. A., Gaskin, D. J., & Richard, P. (2009). Joint Center for Political and Economic Studies (U.S.). *The economic burden of health inequalities in the United States*. Washington, D.C: Joint Center for Political and Economic Studies.

McGuire, T. G., & Miranda, J. (2008). New evidence regarding racial and ethnic disparities in mental health: Policy implications. *Health Affairs, 27*, 393–403.

Muntaner, C., Eaton, W. W., Diala, C., Kessler, R. C., & Sorlie, P. D. (1998). Social class, assets, organizational control and the prevalence of common groups of psychiatric disorders. *Social Science and Medicine, 47*, 2043–2053.

National Center for Health Statistics. (2009). *Health, United States, 2008*. Hyattsville, MD: U.S. Government Printing Office.

Ortman, J., & Guarneri, C. (2009). *United States Population Projections: 2000 to 2050*. Washington, DC: Bureau of the Census, U.S. Department of Commerce.

Passel, J., & Cohn, D. (2008). *U.S. Population Projections: 2005–2050* (Pew Hispanic Center Report). Washington, DC: Pew Research Center.

Primm, A. B., Vasquez, M. J. T., Mays, R.A., Sammons-Posey, D., McKnighty-Eily, L. R., Presley-Cantrell, L. R., et al. (2010). The role of public health in addressing racial and ethnic disparities in mental health and mental illness. *Preventing chronic disease: Public health research, practice and policy, 7*, 1–7.

Safran, D.G., Montgomery, J.E., Chang, H., Murphy, J., & Rogers, W.H. (2001). Switching doctors: predictors of voluntary disenrollment from a primary physician's practice. [see comment]. *Journal of Family Practice, 50*, 130–136.

Safran, D.G., Taira, D.A., Rogers, W.H., Kosinski, M., Ware, J.E., & Tarlov, A.R. (1998). Linking primary care performance to outcomes of care. *J Fam Pract. 47*, 213–220.

Schnittker, J., & McLeod, J. D. (2005). The social psychology of health disparities. *Annual Review of Sociology, 31*, 75–103.

Smedley, B. D., Stith, A. Y., & Nelson, A. R. (Eds.). (2003). *Unequal treatment: Confronting racial and ethical disparities in health care*. Washington, DC: National Academy Press.

Starfield, B. (1992). *Primary care: Concept, evaluation, and policy*. New York: Oxford University Press.

Takeuchi, D. T., Alegria, M., Jackson, J. S., & Williams, D. R. (2007). Immigration and mental health: Diverse findings in Asian, Black, and Latino Populations. *American Journal of Public Health, 97*, 11–12.

U.S. Department of Health and Human Services. (2001). *Mental health: Culture, race, and ethnicity—A supplement to mental health: A report of the surgeon general*. Rockville, MD: U.S. Department of Health and Human Services, Substance Abuse and Mental Health Services Administration, Center for Mental Health Services.

Vega, W. A., Kolody, B., Aguilar-Gaxiola, S., Alderete, E., Catalano, R., & Caraveo-Anduaga, J. (1998). Lifetime prevalence of DSM-III-R psychiatric disorders among urban and rural Mexican Americans in California. *Archives of General Psychiatry, 55*, 771–778.

Williams, D. R., Gonzalez, H. M., Neighbors, H., Nesse, R., Abelson, J. M., Sweetman, J., & Jackson, J. S. (2007). Prevalence and distribution of major depressive disorder in African Americans, Caribbean blacks, and non-Hispanic whites: Results from the National Survey of American Life. *Archives of General Psychiatry, 64*, 305–315.

Williams, D. R., & Jackson, P. B. (2005). Social sources of racial disparities in health. *Health Affairs, 24*(2), 325–334.

World Health Organization (WHO). (2010). *Health of Migrants – The Way Forward: Report of a Global Consultation.* France: WHO Press.

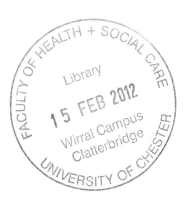

6 The particular role of stigma

Patrick W. Corrigan and Dror Ben-Zeev

Introduction

Challenges posed by mental illness are not limited to distress and disability, but also include the community's reaction to these disabilities and the prejudice and discrimination directed against people who are mentally ill. For example, employers might not employ people with serious mental illness, nor might landlords not rent property to them, and healthcare providers may offer a lower standard of care to people with serious mental illness, all because of stigmatizing attitudes. This chapter examines the intersection of stigma and populations by first reviewing the underutilization of mental health services by populations in need, reviewing meaningful distinctions in definitions of stigma, and proffering a social cognitive model to explain these differences. We then consider strategies meant to decrease stigmatizing attitudes and discriminatory behaviors and suggest areas for future research in the field.

Underutilization of mental health services

The quality and effectiveness of mental health treatments and services have improved dramatically over the past 50 years. Yet despite the abundance of viable evidence-based interventions, researchers are familiar with a number of disconcerting realities: many people who might benefit from mental health services often have difficulties obtaining them, do not fully adhere to treatment regimens, or choose never to seek services in the first place.

Large-scale epidemiologic research has provided evidence that supports these trends. Research from the 1980s Epidemiologic Catchment Area (ECA) study showed that less than 30% of people with mental illness ever seek treatment (Regier, Narrow, Rae, Manderscheid, Locke, & Goodwin, 1993). These low treatment rates are not limited to people with relatively minor or brief adjustment disorders; rather, ECA data showed that 40% of people with serious disorders, such as schizophrenia, fail to obtain treatment (Regier et al., 1993), and people with serious mental illness are no more likely to participate in treatment than those with relatively minor disorders (Narrow, Regier, Norquist, Rae, Kennedy, & Arons, 2000). The National Comorbidity Survey (NCS), conducted from 1990 to 1992, showed that less than 40% of respondents with psychiatric disorders in the past year received stable treatment (Kessler et al., 2001). Data from the subsequent 2001–2003 National Comorbidity Survey Replication (NCS-R) showed that only approximately half of people with serious mental illnesses received any treatment and that less than half of those treated received stable interventions consistent with evidence-based guidelines (Wang, Demler, & Kessler, 2002; Wang, Lane, Olfson, Pincus, Wells, & Kessler, 2005). The Substance Abuse and Mental Health Services Administration (SAMHSA) conducted a national survey that found equally sobering results: less than 10% of people with psychiatric disabilities receive such clinically indicated services as vocational rehabilitation, case management, or day treatment (Willis, Willis, Male, Henderson, & Manderscheid, 1998).

More promising findings emerge when framing the question differently. Just over 80% of NCS respondents reported they would seek professional help for a serious mental illness; the NCS-R showed similar positive findings, with about 83% of participants reporting that they would seek professional help when in need (Mojtabai, 2007). Hence, the data is somewhat mixed about treatment seeking, but a conservative estimate is that one out of five people are not seeking treatment when indicated.

Even for those who are in treatment, there remain concerns around service underutilization and poor treatment adherence. Findings from a national survey conducted by the Schizophrenia Patient Outcome Research Team showed that, although more than 90% of individuals in the survey were receiving maintenance neuroleptic treatment, participation in evidence-based psychosocial treatments was far lower (Lehman, Steinwachs, Dixon, Goldman, Osher, Postrado, 1998). Less than half of survey participants reported participation in appropriate psychotherapies, less than a quarter were involved in family therapy, and approximately 10% received intensive case management. These problems are further exacerbated by the number of people who obtain mental health services but fail to fully adhere to component prescriptions. Many patients drop out of psychosocial interventions before finishing the complete course of treatment (Tarrier, Yusupoff, Kinney, McCarthy, Gledhill, Haddock, & Morris, 1998). A review of 34 studies of compliance with psychiatric medication found, on average, that more than 40% of persons receiving antipsychotic medication failed to fully comply with prescribed regimens (Cramer & Rosenbeck, 1998), and newer evidence suggests this low rate of compliance still prevails (Julius, Novitsky, & Dubin, 2009). In an earlier study, failure to adhere to antipsychotic regimens increased re-hospitalization by three-fold, accounting for an $800 million increase in hospital costs worldwide (Weiden & Olfson, 1995).

Stigma

Stigma associated with mental illness has been identified as one of a number of primary reasons that people in need underutilize services (Link & Phelan, 2006). The World Health Organization (WHO) dedicated its 2001 annual report to global mental health issues and outlined a vicious cycle of stigma, discrimination, and neglect affecting the lives of millions of people suffering from psychiatric disorders (Bebbington, 2001). In the report, stigma and the associated discrimination against persons with mental illness were identified as the most important community barriers to overcome in order to promote mental health worldwide (WHO, 2001). In 2005, the WHO European Ministerial Conference on Mental Health in Helsinki generated an action plan that explicitly proposed to instigate activities to counter stigma. However, in order to combat stigma and reduce its negative impact, we must first understand the different manifestations of stigma associated with mental illness.

Stigma's many faces

Goffman (1963) originally adopted the term "stigma" from the Greeks, who used it to represent bodily signs indicating something bad about the moral character of the bearer. This mark can be obvious (such as skin color) or subtle (such as in people who are homosexual or people with mental illness). This type of moral imputation has egregious negative effects at a number of levels, which we have characterized as: public stigma, self-stigma, label avoidance, and structural stigma (Corrigan, Markowitz, & Watson, 2004; Corrigan & Watson, 2002). "Public stigma" is the phenomenon of large social groups endorsing stereotypes about, and subsequently acting against a stigmatized group: in this case, people with mental illness. "Self-stigma" is the loss of self-esteem and self-efficacy that occurs when people internalize public stigma. "Label avoidance" occurs when people choose not to pursue mental health services because they do not want to be labeled a "mental patient" or suffer the prejudice and discrimination that the label entails. "Structural stigma" refers to the policies of private and governmental institutions that intentionally restrict the opportunities of people with mental illness or policies that are not intended to discriminate but whose consequences nevertheless hinder the options of this population.

Below, we discuss public stigma, self-stigma, and label avoidance in the context of four micro-level, individual social cognitive processes: cues, stereotypes, prejudice, and discrimination. We discuss structural stigma separately later in the chapter from a macrosocial perspective, viewing stigma as a social phenomena.

Stigma as an individual process

In the first stage of stigmatization, mental illness is inferred from explicit cues: psychiatric symptoms, social-skills deficits, physical appearance, and common diagnostic labels (Corrigan, 2000; Penn & Martin, 1998). Many of the symptoms of severe mental illnesses like psychosis (e.g., inappropriate affect and bizarre behavior) are manifest indicators of psychiatric conditions that produce negative reactions (Link, Cullen, Frank, & Wozniak, 1987; Penn, Guynan, Daily, Spaulding, Garbin, & Sullivan, 1994; Socall & Holtgraves, 1992). Moreover, poor social skills that result from some psychiatric illnesses (Bellack, Mueser, Morrison, Tierney, & Podell, 1990; Mueser, Bellack, Douglas, & Morrison, 1991) and poor personal appearance also may lead to stigmatizing attitudes; for example, "That unkempt person on the park bench must be a mental patient" (Eagly, Ashmore, Makhijani, & Longo, 1991; Penn, Mueser, & Doonan, 1997). Eccentric behavior can also easily be misunderstood as mental illness.

Just as these signs may yield false positives, so may their absence lead to false negatives. Many people are able to conceal their experiences with mental illness without their peers being aware. This then begs the question: What else serves as a mark that leads to stigmatizing responses? Several studies suggest labeling as an important candidate (Link, 1987; Markowitz, 2001; Moses, 2009; Scheff, 1974). Labels may be given formally by others (e.g., a psychiatrist can inform someone that a patient is mentally ill) (Ben-Zeev, Young, & Corrigan, 2010), or labels can be obtained by association (e.g., a person observed coming out of a psychologist's office may be assumed to be mentally ill).

In the second stage, stigmatizing cues elicit stereotypes – knowledge structures that the general public or individuals with mental illness learn about a marked social group (Corrigan, 2007; Krueger, 1996; Lauber & Rossler, 2007). Stereotypes are especially efficient means of categorizing information about various groups. Stereotypes are considered "social" because they represent collectively agreed notions about groups of people. They are "efficient" because people can quickly generate impressions and expectations of individuals who belong to a stereotyped group. Commonly held stereotypes about people with mental illness include violence ("People with mental illness are dangerous"), incompetence ("They are incapable of independent living or real work"), and fault ("Because of weak character, they are responsible for the onset and continuation of their disorders") (Corrigan, River, Lundin, Uphoff-Wasowski, Campion, & Mathisen, 2000; Link, Phelan, Bresnahan, Stueve, & Pescosolido, 1999).

Knowledge of a set of stereotypes, however, does not necessarily constitute agreement with them (Devine, 1995; Jussim, Nelson, Manis, & Soffin, 1995). The third stage of stigma occurs when people who are prejudiced endorse the negative stereotypes ("People with mental illness are violent and incompetent") and generate negative emotional reactions as a result ("I am afraid of them") (Corrigan, Larson, & Rusch, 2009; Devine, 1995). In contrast to stereotypes, which are beliefs, prejudicial attitudes involve an evaluative (generally negative) component (Allport, 1954; Eagley & Chaiken, 1993). Prejudice, which is fundamentally a cognitive and affective response, leads to the behavioral reaction of discrimination (Crocker, Major, & Steele, 1998). One way discriminatory behavior manifests itself is as public stigma, when members of the public take negative action against the identified out-group; for example, employers may avoid hiring people with mental illness, and landlords may refuse to rent to them (Corrigan, Kerr, & Knudsen, 2005a).

Another way discriminatory behavior can have negative impact is when it is directed inward, resulting in self-stigma. Upon receiving a diagnosis (cue), the beliefs associated with mental illness (stereotypes) are activated. Living in a culture steeped in stigmatizing images, persons with mental illness may accept these notions as facts (Corrigan, 1998; Holmes & River, 1998). Individuals who agree with prejudice concur with the stereotype: "That's right, I am weak and unable to care for myself!" Self-prejudice leads to negative reactions; prominent among these is low self-esteem, typically operationalized as diminished views about personal worth (Corrigan, Faber, Rashid, & Leary, 1999; Rosenberg, 1965), and low self-efficacy, defined as the expectation that one cannot competently perform a behavior in a specific situation (Bandura, 1989; Corrigan, Watson, & Barr, 2006).

Self-stigma that negatively impacts self-esteem and self-efficacy may result in a "Why try?" effect in individuals with mental illness (Corrigan, Larson, & Rusch, 2009). People who agree with stigma and apply it to themselves may feel unworthy or unable to tackle the exigencies of specific life goals and decide to not even attempt to pursue them. A person who has internalized stereotypes such as "The mentally ill have no worth because they have nothing to offer and are only drains on society," will struggle to maintain a positive self-concept. Low self-esteem ("Why should I even try to live independently? Someone like me is just not worth the investment") and poor self-efficacy ("Why should I even try to get help? Someone like me could not successfully complete treatment") are examples of applying a derogatory stereotype to one's self even before engaging in goal-oriented activities (Corrigan et al., 2009).

Given the potential harm that can occur as a result of a diagnosis, many people may decide they do not want to be deemed a "mental patient" or suffer the prejudice and discrimination that the label entails. This form of label avoidance is perhaps the most insidious way in which stigma impedes care-seeking. Research has suggested that people with concealable labels (e.g., people of minority faith-based communities who identify as homosexual or people with mental illness) often decide to avoid harm due to stigma by keeping their true identity secret and "staying in the closet" (Corrigan & Matthews, 2003). These individuals may opt to avoid the stigma by denying their group status altogether and by not affiliating themselves with the institutions that mark them in any way (i.e., gay community activities, mental healthcare).

Figure 6.1 illustrates how various forms of stigma may affect individuals who underutilize mental health treatment services.

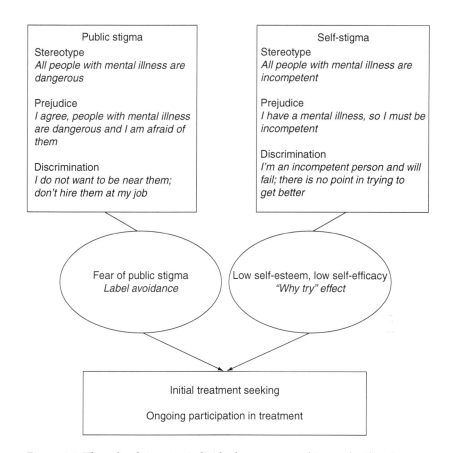

Figure 6.1 The role of sigma in individual treatment seeking and utilization.

Stigma causing harm

Stigma harms people who are labeled as mentally ill in several ways. Stereotyping, prejudice, and discrimination can rob people labeled mentally ill of important life opportunities that are essential for achieving their life goals. Studies have shown that public stereotypes and prejudice about mental illness have a deleterious impact on obtaining and keeping good jobs (Baldwin & Johnson, 2004; Farina & Felner, 1973; Link, 1987; Scheid, 2005; Stuart, 2006; Wahl, 1999) and leasing safe housing (Corrigan, Thompson, Lambert, Sangster, Noel, & Campbell, 2003; Farina, Thaw, Lovern, & Mangone, 1974; Ozmen et al. 2004; Wahl, 1999).

Despite substantial advancement in the scientific community's understanding and treatment of mental health problems over the last few decades, stigmatizing public conceptions of mental illness are still very much alive. For example, a central aspect of stigma of mental illness is the attribution of dangerousness (Pescosolido, Monahan, Link, Stueve, & Kikuzawa, 1999; Phelan, Link, Stueve, & Pescosolido, 1996). Link and colleagues (1999) used nationwide survey data to examine contemporary public beliefs pertaining to the perceived dangerousness of, and general interest in interacting with people with mental illness. Although previous empirical studies show only a small actual increase in violence among people with mental illness (Swanson, Holzer, Ganju, & Tsutomu Jono, 1990), the majority of respondents in the survey believed that all diagnosed mental disorders, from major depressive disorder to schizophrenia, substantially increase the risk of violence, reflecting disproportionate public fears. Moreover, the researchers found that the public has a strong desire to maintain social distance from persons with mental illness (Link et al., 1999).

Similar findings were found in studies examining stigma associated with mental illness in children (Pescosolido, 2007). Pescosolido, Fettes, Martin, Monahan, and McLeod (2007) used data from the National Stigma Study for children (NSS-C) to compare perceived dangerousness of children with mental and physical health problems. In their study, a large sample of 1,152 participants were presented with descriptive clinical vignettes describing children with attention-deficit hyperactivity disorder (ADHD), depression, and asthma, and were asked to rate whether they believed these children were likely to be a danger to themselves or others. While only 15% believed children with asthma are potentially dangerous, children with ADHD or depression were perceived as likely to be dangerous to themselves or others (33% and 81%, respectively). Moreover, individuals who labeled a child as "mentally ill" were twice as likely to expect potential violence and five-times more likely to support forced treatment, reflecting the salient public stigma linked with mental illness (Pescosolido et al., 2007)

Stigma also influences the interface between mental illness and the criminal justice system. Police officers, rather than mental health professionals, are first responders to mental health crises, and this is likely one contributor to the increasing prevalence of people with serious mental illness in jail instead of treatment facilities (Watson, Ottati, Lurigio, & Heyrman, 2005). Persons exhibiting signs and symptoms of serious mental illness are more likely than others to be arrested by the police (Teplin, 1984), and people with mental illness tend to spend more time incarcerated than those without mental illness (Hammett, Roberts, & Kennedy, 2000; Steadman, McCarthy, & Morrissey, 1989). Intolerance towards offenders in general has led to harsher laws and also has hampered effective treatment of mentally ill offenders (Jemeka, Trupin, & Chiles, 1989; Lamb & Weinberger, 1998; Metzner & Fellner, 2010).

The negative impact of stigma is also observed in the general healthcare system; people labeled mentally ill are less likely to benefit from the depth and breadth of available physical healthcare services than people without these illnesses. Druss and colleagues (Desai, Rosenheck, Druss, & Perlin, 2002; Druss & Rosenheck, 1997) completed two studies on archival data that suggested people with mental illness receive fewer medical services than those not labeled in this manner. Moreover, studies by this group suggest that individuals with mental illness are less likely to receive the same range of insurance benefits as people without mental illness (Druss, Allen, & Bruce, 1998; Druss & Rosenheck, 1998). An additional study seems to implicate stigma more directly. Druss, Bradford, Rosenheck, Radford, and Krumholz (2000) examined the likelihood of a range of medical procedures after myocardial infarction in a large sample (N = 113,653) of individuals and found that people identified with comorbid psychiatric disorder were significantly less likely to undergo percutaneous transluminal coronary angioplasty, the standard next step in treatment for heart problems.

Controlled social laboratory studies have demonstrated an inverse association between stigmatization and care-seeking. Results of one survey showed members of the general public who blamed individuals for their mental illness and withheld help to them were also less likely to seek mental health services for themselves (Cooper, Corrigan, & Watson, 2003). A second study showed an inverse relationship between stigmatizing attitudes and treatment adherence (Sirey, Bruce, Alexopoulos, Perlick, Friedman, & Meyers, 2001). In this study (N = 134), stigma was measured using the Scale of Perceived Stigma (Link, Cullen, Struening, Shrout, & Dohrenwend, 1989), and scores were associated with whether patients were compliant with their antidepressant medication regimen three months later. Findings from these small samples have been supported by additional population-based studies that frequently incorporate probability samples. One study on a probability sample of approximately 3,000 community residents showed that endorsing negative attitudes about mental illness inhibits personal service utilization in those at risk for psychiatric disorder (Leaf, Bruce, Tischler, & Holzer, 1987). Results from the NCS identified several specific beliefs that might sway people from treatment, including concerns about what others might think and wanting to solve problems independently (Kessler et al., 2001). Evidence suggests similarities in the influence of stigma on care-seeking in younger populations. The National Annenberg Risk Survey of Youth was conducted by telephone in the spring of 2002 with 900 respondents selected via random-digit dialing procedures. Results showed that adolescents who are more likely to endorse the stigma of mental illness are less likely to obtain care when needed (Penn et al., 2005).

An additional interesting finding from the National Annenberg Risk Survey of Youth was that the connection between stigma and treatment-seeking was mediated by perceptions about treatment success (Penn et al., 2005). Views about stigma were less relevant to care-seeking when the adolescent believed treatment was likely to be successful. These results parallel another study done on adults with neurotic disorders; people in this group were less likely to seek treatment when they believed they could not be helped (Meltzer, Bebbington, Brugha, Farrell, Jenkins, & Lewis, 2003).

Stigma as societal phenomena

Thus far, the models we have presented to understand stigma have focused on individual level psychological paradigms. Another approach is to adopt a macrosocial perspective to understand "structural stigma," the policies of private and governmental institutions that intentionally or unintentionally restrict the opportunities of people with mental illness.

"Intentional structural stigma" manifests itself as rules, policies, and procedures of private and public entities in positions of power that consciously and purposefully restrict rights and opportunities of a specific population. Burton (1990) searched the statutes in all 50 states for discriminatory laws using keywords representing mental illness (e.g., mentally ill, mentally incompetent). Ten years later, a similar search of an expanded database was completed (Hemmens, Miller, Burton, & Milner, 2002). The second study sought to determine whether states had passed laws restricting the civil rights of people with mental illness in five areas: voting, holding elective office, serving jury duty, parenting, and remaining married. Both studies showed that approximately one-third of the states restrict the rights of an individual with mental illness to hold elective office, participate in juries, or to vote. Withholding the right to vote is especially harmful given significant debate in the legal community about whether this restriction is even appropriate for convicted felons. Greater limitations were evident in the family domain. Between 42 and 52% of states limited the right of people with mental illness to remain married; more than 40% of states limited the child custody rights of parents with mental illness. Juxtaposing the findings from both studies revealed that over the course of a decade, very little changed in laws restricting civil rights based on mental illness (Corrigan & Lundin, 2001).

To examine current trends in structural stigma in state legislation, Corrigan, Watson, Heyrman, Warpinski, Gracia, Slopen, and Hall (2005b) identified and coded bills introduced in 2002 that directly impacted the liberties, protection from discrimination, and privacy of people with mental illness. Only 42 of the 968 mental health bills surveyed were related to liberties, of which more than 75% contracted liberties, such as permission for involuntary medication and ordering outpatient treatments in some states. About one-quarter of the state bills surveyed related to protection from discrimination. Within this category, bills were about evenly divided between those that expanded protections (e.g., disallowing use of mental health status in child custody) and those that contracted them (e.g., restriction of mental health programs in certain neighborhoods). About 10% of all bills related to privacy and confidentiality issues, with about two-thirds expanding privacy rights (e.g., protections against disclosure of mental health records) and one-third diminishing them (e.g., sharing mental health records for public safety reasons). Interestingly, legislation frequently confused "incompetence" with "mental illness"; for example, several states limited firearm privileges for all people with mental illness, rather than only people who are incompetent as a result of having a mental illness, thereby discriminating against people with mental illness *per se* (Corrigan et al., 2005b).

"Unintentional structural stigma" takes form in institutional policies or principles that result in less opportunity for a stigmatized group relative to the majority, despite an organization's commitment to neutrality (Pincus, 1996; Pincus & Ehrlich, 1999). Link and Phelan (2001), for example, showed that less money is allocated to research and treatment for psychiatric illnesses than other health disorders because illnesses like cancer and cardiovascular disease have dominated the American public health agenda. In addition, many psychiatrists and other mental health professionals choose to opt out of the public service system, which serves people with the most serious psychiatric and substance abuse disorders. Salaries and benefits are better in the private health sector, where providers are more likely to treat less serious illnesses such as adjustment disorders and relational problems. Hence, the quality of services for people with serious mental disorders is often inferior to the quality of services for other conditions.

Problems with mental health insurance parity are another example of unintended structural stigma related to mental illness. The Mental Health Parity Act (MHPA), signed into law in 1997, required that lifetime and annual limits on mental health benefits be set at a similar level as medical and surgical benefits. However, there were notable limitations to the initial version of the act. The MHPA did not require employers to provide mental health coverage. Companies with 50 or fewer employees were exempt. Substance abuse disorders were not covered. Employers who demonstrated that the MHPA would drive up insurance costs by more than 1% could opt out. As is often the case with structural discrimination, this legislation, although intended to be neutral, resulted in less opportunity for members of the targeted group.

The exclusion of substance abuse disorders in the original 1997 legislation was rectified in the Mental Health Parity and Addiction Equity Act of 2008. The new act includes substance abuse disorders and mandates parity for all financial requirements (e.g., deductibles, copayments, coinsurance, and out-of-pocket expenses), treatment limitations (e.g., frequency of treatment, number of visits, days of coverage, or other limits on treatment scope or duration), and out-of-network benefits of group health plans. However, similar to the 1997 provisions, the new law applies only to policies with existing mental health benefits. Group plans are still not required to include mental health coverage. Currently only twelve states mandate that group insurers also cover mental health and substance abuse treatment (Dave & Mukerjee, 2009).

The parity act inadvertently limits availability of financial resources for psychiatric disorders compared with medical illness, resulting in diminished opportunity for people with mental illness (Levinson & Druss, 2000; Mercer, 1998). This disparity does not seem to reflect explicit prejudice – most members of both houses, regardless of political affiliation, support equal care for mental health disorders, as does the American public (Hanson, 1998). Instead, lack of support for many of the provisions stems from financial concerns that are frequently at the root of other forms of structural discrimination.

Minimizing stigma and its impact

We have presented evidence suggesting that stigma associated with mental illness has deleterious effects on the self-esteem, self-efficacy, acquisition of life goals, and availability of resources and opportunities for those with psychiatric problems. Persons with mental illness may choose to avoid labeling by denying their status altogether; by not affiliating with others with mental illness in treatment centers or programs because it may result in subsequent stigmatization; or by neglecting to seek treatment because (due to internalized negative stereotypes) they believe it is futile and they cannot be helped. We now shift our attention to discuss strategies that may assist in preventing the development, maintenance, and negative impact of stigma, with an emphasis on possible implications for treatment-seeking and utilization.

Reducing public stigma, self-stigma, and label avoidance

Programs designed to decrease public stigma, self-stigma, and label avoidance may reduce the attitudes and behaviors that are barriers to care seeking. We have identified four approaches that could diminish stigma experienced by people with mental illness: protest, education, contact, and collaborative care.

Protest

Protest attempts to diminish negative attitudes about mental illness but is somewhat limited in its efficacy in promoting more positive attitudes that are supported by facts. Group protests against inaccurate and hostile representations of mental illness send a clear message that challenges negative views and inaccurate representations of mental illness. Largely anecdotal evidence suggests that protest campaigns have been effective in getting stigmatizing images of mental illness withdrawn (Wahl, 1995). However, controlled studies on changing the stigmatizing attitudes of individuals suggest that protest may also have an unwanted effect, causing "attitude rebound" in the stigmatizing beliefs of the public (Corrigan, Edwards, Green, Diwan, & Penn, 2001a; Macrae, Bodenhausen, Milne, & Jetten, 1994). Instead of decreasing stigma, resistance seems to occur ("don't tell me what to think") and negative attitudes worsen.

Education

Educational programs can provide information that may help the public in making more informed decisions about mental illness. Research on education related to mental illness stigma has suggested that participation in these kinds of programs leads to improved attitudes about people with psychiatric disorders (Corrigan, River, Lundin, Penn, Uphoff-Wasowski, & Campion, 2001b; Holmes, Corrigan, Williams, Canar, & Kubiak, 1999; Keane, 1990; Penn et al., 1994). Having confidence in treatment may diminish the negative effect of stigma on treatment seeking (Meltzer et al., 2003); thus, education programs that present evidence about the success of treatment participation may increase the overall likelihood that people with psychiatric problems will pursue and engage in treatment.

Three groups, in particular, should be the focus of educational efforts: Children, student professionals, and opinion leaders. Schools are natural places to start education for children. Young students are familiar with videotapes and training programs that target racial stereotypes and these methods might also help children develop a more enlightened perspective about mental illness. Parents of school-age children could be invited to special assemblies on mental illness and stigma. These programs are successful when they have the official support of the school board and the principal is present to host the show. School homework could also include anti-stigma exercises, which might be completed with parents. Children struggling with mental problems who undergo anti-stigma education programs will be more likely to explore available resources and less apprehensive about seeking assistance.

The community often turns to mental health professionals for information about psychiatric disability, but survey research has shown that many mental health professionals agree with myths about mental illness (Schulze, 2007). Thus, training programs for psychology interns, psychiatry residents, and social work students are especially warranted. Curricula should focus on attitudes that foster empowerment and undermine any stigmatizing foundation that new students may bring to their training. Moreover, anti-stigma training should not stop when the graduate diploma is earned, and continuing education must address issues of stigma in professionals. Reducing stigmatizing attitudes and corresponding behaviors among professionals will likely impact their interactions with their clients, subsequently reducing self-stigma and hopelessness about treatment.

Perhaps an even more effective way to change attitudes is to target the opinion of leaders in the community, such as mayors, governors, and ministers, who influence the attitudes of large numbers of people. Leaders have a pulpit from which they may change local opinion. Hence, if the leader's views change through contact and education, attitudes of their community may follow.

Contact

Stigma is further diminished when members of the general public have direct contact with people with mental illness who are able to hold jobs or live as good neighbors in the community (Corrigan et al., 2001b; Corrigan, Rowan, Green, Lundin, River, Uphoff-Wasowski, et al., 2002; Pinfold, Toulmin, Thornicroft, Huxley, Farmer, & Graham, 2003; Schulze, Richter-Werling, Matschinger, & Angermeyer, 2003). Research shows that members of the community who meet and interact with people with mental illness as part of an anti-stigma program are less likely to show prejudicial attitudes (Holmes et al., 1999; Penn et al., 1994). Hence, opportunities for the public to meet people with severe mental illness may help discount stigma. In reducing public stigma, self-stigma will also be less likely; reduction in the strength and prevalence of negative stereotypes will subsequently impact their availability for internalization by individuals with mental illness.

Collaborative care

As we discussed earlier, poor treatment adherence is a public health concern that may be exacerbated by stigma. Consumer advocates have argued (Deegan, 1990), and research appears to support the idea (McCubbin & Cohen, 1996; Rappaport, 1987), that many psychosocial and medical treatments disempower people; as a result, people in need decide not to participate fully in services. People with mental illness who self-stigmatize tend to report little personal empowerment in terms of treatment, and thus participation in treatment is diminished. For empowerment to occur, professionals must be able to recognize what adherence means in this context – not blind compliance with what the clinician prescribes, but active participation and engagement in all aspects of care (Drake & Deegan, 2009). Consumer operated self-help, peer support, and peer-delivered services are examples of best practices to this end (Corrigan, 2006; Davidson et al., 1999; Dixon, Dickerson, Bellack, Bennett, Dickinson, Goldberg, et al., 2010).

Psychotherapies that emphasize a collaborative relationship between clinician and client, such as cognitive behavioral treatments (CBT), may be effective in reducing self-stigmatization in people with mental illness. CBT is designed to help people identify and examine the validity of personal beliefs and attitudes (Beck, 1991; Ellis, 1997). In the context of CBT, focusing on reduction of stigma, individuals may learn to identify their own pre-existing biases and negative attitudes towards psychiatric problems and the mentally ill. By changing blaming, over-generalizing, or demonizing stereotypes and attitudes to more realistic beliefs, people with mental illness may become more willing to utilize services that might result in diagnostic labeling, while learning to maintain self-esteem and self-efficacy despite having a mental illness. Family members undergoing family therapy or participating in support groups could also benefit from learning to examine and challenge their beliefs and stigmatizing attitudes, which will likely have a positive impact on those in their lives with mental illness.

Reducing structural stigma

Any effort by the public or private sector to limit civil liberties based on disability due to mental illness must be constrained so as not to curtail those liberties without justifiable reason. We focus our discussion below on four guidelines that are relevant to structural stigma as discussed earlier.

Limiting restriction of rights or opportunities

The government has a public interest and responsibility to make sure that the actions or disabilities of some people do not harm others. Exceptions and limitations to rights are implied in the "undue hardship" clause of the 1990 Americans with Disabilities Act (ADA), which states that reasonable accommodations need not be provided to a person with a disability if the resources needed for the accommodation would do harm given the capabilities of the business. We extend this clause by stating that any rightful opportunity that would be hindered by a psychiatric disability and cause public harm may justifiably be restricted because of that disability. The possible harm assumption, however, suggests that any public rights or privileges that do *not* harm others should *not* be excluded by law or other institutional policy. For example, access to and enjoyment of most public accommodations (e.g., beaches, parks, theaters, hotels, restaurants) should not be restricted by disability or diminished functioning.

Clear definition of the disability on which a person's right is withheld

Disabilities that lead to judgments of incompetence and restriction of rights must be measurable by reliable and valid tools. These measurements need to assess lack of competency due to psychiatric disability in constructs that are based on a comprehensive functional analysis that defines component activities of a right. Therefore, the definition of incompetence related to a specific right or opportunity must extend beyond vague targets, such as psychotic symptoms, to specific skill deficits that comprise the area of concern (e.g., parental rights) and are hindered by disabilities (e.g., inability to regularly serve nutritious meals). Specific laws, rules, or regulations that lack this kind of definition and corresponding assessment strategy may be unnecessarily structurally stigmatizing.

Adequate supportive services must be provided to meet competency criteria

Public and private institutions must provide both environmental and interpersonal supports that help persons with disabilities to function successfully and enjoy the full range of social opportunities. The idea of reasonable accommodations is based on sociopolitical notions that all human competencies (those of people with disabilities and people without disabilities) represent an interaction of the person's ability to complete a task and the resources of the environment in which this task occurs (Hahn, 1984). For example, without making use of many contemporary technological innovations, few office workers, with or without disabilities, could competently carry out their jobs. Similarly, reasonable accommodations are those tools or environmental supports that a person with disabilities needs to perform a job. According to the ADA, one cannot be considered incompetent if these kinds of accommodations are not provided.

Although the ADA framers largely envisioned reasonable accommodations as environmental supports that assist those with ambulatory and sensory disabilities, the Federal Government stated that reasonable accommodations must also be provided to people with psychiatric disabilities (U.S. Equal Employment Opportunity Commission, 1997). The exact nature of these accommodations continues to be negotiated; nevertheless, for people with psychiatric disabilities in the workforce, some examples might include supervision (e.g., having job coaches to provide support and counseling at work), job restructuring (e.g., reallocating marginal job functions), workplace modifications (e.g., providing room dividers or soundproofing to diminish distractions), and sick time (e.g., permitting the use of accrued paid leave or unpaid leave for psychotherapy) (Behnay, Hall, & Keller, 1997).

Future research

Previous research has described why stigma might lead people to avoid labels and underutilize services. Future research needs to build on this literature to develop a more cohesive paradigm for understanding the link between stigma and the utilization of services as well as quality of care available to people with mental illness. We identify a number of specific important domains that require further investigation.

Examination of how varying aspects of individual-level stigmatization interfere with care seeking and their relative impact is necessary. For example, some people with mental illness might not seek treatment in order to avoid the public harm that results from diagnostic labels (public stigma), while others may avoid the label to escape stigma's impact on their sense of self (self-stigma). Research examining the impact of stigma on care seeking also should include awareness as a covariate. Many persons with psychotic disorders are unaware of the nature of their mental illness or its impact on the breadth of life function domains (Amador et al., 1994; Lysaker, Buck, Salvatore, Popoli, & Dimaggio, 2009). As a result, some people with mental illness may not realize they belong to a stigmatized group, and thus they may be relatively immune to individual-level stigma.

To date, research showing that people who endorse some aspect of individual-level stigma are less likely to utilize and engage in treatment has been largely correlational, and researchers should use experimental or multi-panel designs to examine causal relationships between individual-level stigma and utilization and engagement in treatment. For example, the extensive repeated measures design in Experience Sampling Methods (ESM) research allows scientists to examine short-term temporal relationships between variables as they occur in the daily life of people with mental illness (Ben-Zeev, Ellington, Swendsen, & Granholm, 2010; Myin-Germeys, Oorschot, Collip, Lataster, Delespaul, & van Os, 2009). ESM could be used to determine whether increases in individual self-stigmatization at certain measurement points prospectively independently predict treatment avoidance behaviors or poor engagement, increasing confidence in a causal, directional relationship between these variables.

Future research also should incorporate measureable behavioral proxies for care-seeking. Past research has primarily used self-report to assess care-seeking even though it is fundamentally a behavior. Researchers should incorporate measures of actual behavior, including direct observation, clinic logs, or progress reports, to find out whether stigma attitudes impede people from seeking care. Prospective designs, in particular, may be useful in determining how pre-existing attitudes influence care-seeking as the person needs mental health services.

Another important area for further research is the effects of stigma-reduction interventions on utilization of care. Conducting randomized controlled clinical trials of individual and group treatment programs designed to reduce individual public and self-stigma would improve understanding of the relationships between these variables for people with mental illness. Such studies may also help identify practical strategies that reduce stigma while improving patient care and outcomes.

Finally, more research is needed that takes both macro- (e.g., societal, institutional) and micro- (e.g., emotional, behavioral) level variables into consideration when examining stigma. In this chapter, we discussed the impact of structural stigma on the lives of people with mental illness. Structural discrimination involves processes that typically represent collective and macro-level units (e.g., how the insurance programs of the federal government limit mental health benefits); however, the aggregate of individual properties may serve as a proxy for macro-level constructs. For example, an analytic unit representing nation-specific collections of insurers might be represented by the average premiums that individuals pay per year for mental health benefits. Research in this area would require a comprehensive list of aggregate, continuous variables that would represent the extent of structural discrimination.

This macro-to-micro link was an important research paradigm for sociologists in the first half of the 20th century (Blau, 1960; Faris & Dunham, 1939). However, analyses of this nature diminished in the 1970s after a series of critiques concluded that only a small amount of variance in individual-level variables is attributable to macro-level variables (Alexander & Griffin, 1976; Hauser, 1977). Liska (1990) responded to this criticism by arguing that although macro-level variables might account for relatively minor variance in micro-level individual variables (especially compared with other psychological predictors), the social scientist should not overlook the conceptual importance of macro-level variables *per se*. The presence of a mental health parity law is still theoretically important to understanding the impact of individual insurance benefits. Therefore, the interesting research question may not be whether macro-level variables account for more variance than micro-level variables in a group's experience of stigma and willingness to access services, but rather whether macro-level variable A accounts for significantly more variance than macro-level variable B and thereby seems to have a bigger role in the micro (individual) experience of stigma. Future research efforts need to explore the multiple levels of methodological possibilities.

References

Alexander, K. L., & Griffin, L. J. (1976). School district effects on academic achievement: A reconsideration. *American Sociological Review, 52,* 222–237.

Allport, G. (1954). *The nature of prejudice.* Cambridge, MA: Addison-Wesley.

Amador, X. F., Flaum, M., Andreasen, N. C., Strauss, D. H., Yale, S. A., Clark, S. C., & Gorman, J. M. (1994). Awareness of illness in schizophrenia and schizoaffective and mood disorders. *Archives of General Psychiatry, 51,* 826–36.

Baldwin, M. L., & Johnson, W. G. (2004). Labor market discrimination against men with disabilities. *Journal of Human Resources, 29,* 1–19.

Bandura, A. (1977). Self-efficacy: Toward a unifying theory of behavioral change. *Psychological Review, 84,* 191–215.

Bandura, A. (1989). Regulation of cognitive processes through perceived self-efficacy. *Developmental Psychology, 25,* 729–735.

Bebbington, P. (2001). The world health report 2001. *Social Psychiatry and Psychiatric Epidemiology, 36,* 473–474.

Beck, A. T. (1991). Cognitive therapy: A 30-year retrospective. *American Psychologist, 46,* 368–375.

Behney, C., Hall, L., & Keller, J. (1997). *Psychiatric disabilities, employment, and the Americans with Disabilities Act Background Paper.* Washington, DC: U.S. Office of Technology Assessment.

Bellack, A. S., Mueser, K. T., Morrison, R. L., Tierney, A., & Podell, K. (1990). Remediation of cognitive deficits in schizophrenia. *American Journal of Psychiatry, 147,* 650–655.

Ben-Zeev, D., Ellington, K., Swendsen, J., & Granholm, E. (2010). Examining a cognitive model of persecutory ideation in the daily life of people with schizophrenia: A computerized experience sampling study. *Schizophrenia Bulletin.* [ePub ahead of print]. doi:10.1093/schbul/sbq041.

Ben-Zeev, D., Young, M. A., & Corrigan, P. W. (2010). DSM-V and the stigma of mental illness. *Journal of Mental Health, 19*(4):318-327.

Blau, P. M. (1960). Structural effects. *American Sociological Review, 25,* 178–193.

Burton, V. S. (1990). The consequences of official labels: A research note on rights lost by the mentally ill, mentally incompetent, and convicted felons. *Community Mental Health Journal, 26,* 267–276.

Cooper, A., Corrigan, P. W., & Watson, A. C. (2003). Mental illness stigma and care-seeking. *Journal of Nervous and Mental Disease, 191,* 339–341.

Corrigan, P. W. (1998). The impact of stigma on severe mental illness. *Cognitive and Behavioral Practice, 5,* 201–222.

Corrigan, P. W. (2000). Mental health stigma as social attribution: Implications for research methods and attitude change. *Clinical Psychology—Science and Practice, 7,* 48–67.

Corrigan, P. W. (2006). Impact of consumer-operated services on empowerment and recovery of people with psychiatric disabilities. *Psychiatric Services, 57,* 1493–1496.

Corrigan, P. W. (2007). How clinical diagnosis might exacerbate the stigma of mental illness. *Social Work, 52,* 31–39.

Corrigan, P. W., Edwards, A. B., Green, A., Diwan, S. L., & Penn, D. (2001a). Prejudice, social distance, and familiarity with mental illness. *Schizophrenia Bulletin, 27,* 219–226.

Corrigan, P. W., Faber, D., Rashid, F., & Leary, M. (1999). The construct validity of empowerment among consumers of mental health services. *Schizophrenia Research, 38,* 77–84.

Corrigan, P. W., Kerr, A., & Knudsen, L. (2005a). The stigma of mental illness: Explanatory models and methods for change. *Applied and Preventive Psychology, 11,* 179–190.

Corrigan, P. W., Larson, J. E., & Rusch, N. (2009). Self-stigma and the "why try" effect impact on life goals and evidence-based practices. *World Psychiatry, 8,* 75–81.

Corrigan, P. W., & Lundin, R. (2001). *Don't call me nuts! Coping with the stigma of mental illness.* Tinley Park, IL: Recovery Press.

Corrigan, P. W., Markowitz, F. E., & Watson, A. (2004). Structural levels of mental illness stigma and discrimination. *Schizophrenia Bulletin, 30,* 481–491.

Corrigan, P. W., & Matthews, A. K. (2003). Stigma and disclosure: Implications for coming out of the closet. *Journal of Mental Health, 12,* 235–248.

Corrigan, P. W., River, L., Lundin, R. K., Penn, D. L., Uphoff-Wasowski, K., Campion, J., et al. (2001b). Three strategies for changing attributions about severe mental illness. *Schizophrenia Bulletin, 27,* 187–195.

Corrigan, P. W., River, L., Lundin, R. K., Uphoff-Wasowski, K., Campion, J., Mathisen, J., et al. (2000). Stigmatizing attributions about mental illness. *Journal of Community Psychology, 28*, 91–102.

Corrigan, P.W., Rowan, D., Green, A., Lundin, R., River, P., Uphoff-Wasowski, K., et al. (2002). Challenging two mental illness stigmas: Personal responsibility and dangerousness. *Schizophrenia Bulletin, 28*, 293–310.

Corrigan, P. W., Thompson, V., Lambert, D., Sangster, Y., Noel, J. G., & Campbell, J. (2003). Perceptions of discrimination among persons with serious mental illness. *Psychiatric Services, 54*, 1105–1109.

Corrigan, P. W., & Watson, A. C. (2002). The paradox of self-stigma and mental illness. *Clinical Psychology – Science and Practice, 9*, 35–53.

Corrigan, P. W., Watson, A. C., & Barr, L. (2006). The self-stigma of mental illness: Implications for self-esteem and self-efficacy. *Journal of Social & Clinical Psychology, 25*, 875–884.

Corrigan, P. W., Watson, A. C., Heyrman, M. L., Warpinski, A., Gracia, G, Slopen, N., & Hall, L. L. (2005b). Structural stigma in state legislation. *Psychiatric Services, 56*, 557–563.

Cramer, J. A., & Rosenbeck, R. (1998). Compliance with medication regimens for psychiatric and medical disorders. *Psychiatric Services, 49*, 196–210.

Crocker, J., Major, B., & Steele, C. (1998). Social stigma. In D. T. Gilbert, S. Fiske, & G. Lindzey (Eds.), *The handbook of social psychology* (Vol. 2, 4th ed., pp. 504–553). New York: McGraw-Hill.

Dave, D., & Mukerjee, S. (2011). Mental health parity legislation, cost-sharing and substance-abuse treatment admissions. *Health Economics, 20*(2), 161-183. doi: 10.1002/hec.1577.

Davidson, L., Chinman, M., Kloos, B., Weingarten, R., Stayner, D., & Tebes, J. K. (1999). Peer support among individuals with severe mental illness: A review of the evidence. *Clinical Psychology—Science and Practice, 6*, 165–187.

Deegan, P. E. (1990). Spirit breaking: When the helping professions hurt. *Humanistic Psychologist, 18*, 301–313.

Desai, M. M., Rosenheck, R. A., Druss, B. G., & Perlin, J. B. (2002). Mental disorders and quality of care among postacute myocardial infarction outpatients. *Journal of Nervous and Mental Disease, 190*, 51–53.

Devine, P. G. (1995). Prejudice and out-group perception. In A. Tessor (Ed.), *Advanced social psychology* (pp. 467–524). New York: McGraw-Hill.

Dixon, L. B., Dickerson, F., Bellack, A. S., Bennett, M., Dickinson, D., Goldberg, R. W., et al. (2010). The 2009 schizophrenia PORT psychosocial treatment recommendations and summary statements. *Schizophrenia Bulletin, 36*, 48–70.

Drake, R. E., & Deegan, P. E. (2009). Shared decision making is an ethical imperative. *Psychiatric Services, 60*, 1007.

Druss, B. G., Allen, H. M., & Bruce, M. L. (1998). Physical health, depressive symptoms, and managed care enrollment. *American Journal of Psychiatry, 155*, 878–882.

Druss, B. G., Bradford, D. W., Rosenheck, R. A., Radford, M. J., & Krumholz, H. M. (2000). Mental disorders and use of cardiovascular procedures after myocardial infarction. *JAMA, 283*, 506–511.

Druss, B. G., & Rosenheck, R. (1997). Use of medical services by veterans with mental disorders. *Psychosomatics, 38*, 451–458.

Druss, B. G., & Rosenheck, R. (1998). Mental disorders and access to medical care in the United States. *American Journal of Psychiatry, 155*, 1775–1777.

Eagly, A. H., Ashmore, R. D., Makhijani, M. G., & Longo, L. C. (1991). What is beautiful is good, but…: A meta-analytic review of research on the physical attractiveness stereotype. *Psychological Bulletin, 110*, 109–128.

Eagly, A. H., & Chaiken, S. (1993). *The social psychology of attitudes.* Fort Worth, TX: Harcourt Brace Jovanovich.

Ellis, A. (1997). Extending the goals of behavior therapy and of cognitive behavior therapy. *Behavior Therapy, 28*, 333–339.

Farina, A., & Felner, R. D. (1973). Employment interviewer reactions to former mental patients. *Journal of Abnormal Psychology, 82*, 268–272.

Farina, A., Thaw, J., Lovern, J. D., & Mangone, D. (1974). People's reactions to a former mental patient moving to their neighborhood. *Journal of Community Psychology, 2*, 108–112.

Faris, R. E. L., & Dunham, H. W. (1939). *Mental disorders in urban areas: An ecological study of schizophrenia and other psychoses.* Chicago, IL: University of Chicago Press.

Goffman, E. (1963). *Stigma: Notes on management of spoiled identity.* Englewood Cliffs, NJ: Prentice-Hall.

Hammett, T., Roberts C., & Kennedy, S. (2000). Health-related issues in prisoner reentry. *Crime Delinquency, 47*, 390–409.

Hahn, H. (1984). *The issue of equality: European perceptions of employment policy for disabled persons.* New York: World Rehabilitation Fund.

Hanson, K. W. (1998). Public opinion and the mental health parity debate: Lessons from the survey literature. *Psychiatric Services, 49*, 1059–1066.

Hauser, R. M. (1977). *The process of stratification: Trends and analyses.* New York: Academic Press.

Hemmens, C., Miller, M., Burton, V. S., & Milner, S. (2002). The consequences of official labels: An examination of the rights lost by the mentally ill and the mentally incompetent ten years later. *Community Mental Health Journal, 38*, 129–140.

Holmes, E. P., Corrigan, P. W., Williams, P., Canar, J., & Kubiak, M. (1999). Changing public attitudes about schizophrenia. *Schizophrenia Bulletin, 25*, 447–456.

Holmes, E. P., & River, L. P. (1998). Individual strategies for coping with the stigma of severe mental illness. *Cognitive and Behavioral Practice, 5*, 231–239.

Jemeka, R., Trupin, E., & Chiles, J. A. (1989). The mentally ill in prisons: A review. *Hospital and Community Psychiatry, 40*, 481–491.

Julius, R., Novitsky, M., & Dubin, W. (2009). Medication adherence: A review of the literature and implications for clinical practice. *Journal of Psychiatric Practice, 15*, 34–44.

Jussim, L., Nelson, T. E., Manis, M., & Soffin, S. (1995). Prejudice, stereotypes, and labeling effects: Sources of bias in person perception. *Journal of Personality and Social Psychology, 68*, 228–246.

Keane, M. (1990). Contemporary beliefs about mental illness among medical students: Implications for education and practice. *Academic Psychiatry, 14*, 172–177.

Kessler, R. C., Berglund, P. A., Bruce, M. L., Koch, R., Laska, E. M., Leaf, P. J., et al. (2001). The prevalence and correlates of untreated serious mental illness. *Health Services Research, 36*, 987–1007.

Krueger, J. (1996). Personal beliefs and cultural stereotypes about racial characteristics. *Journal of Personality and Social Psychology, 71*, 536–548.

Lamb, H., & Weinberger, L. E. (1998). Persons with severe mental illness in jails and prisons: A review. *Psychiatric Services, 49*, 483–492.

Lauber, C., & Rossler, W. (2007). Stigma towards people with mental illness in developing countries in Asia. *International Review of Psychiatry, 19*, 157–178.

Leaf, P. J., Bruce, M. L., & Tischler, G. L. (1986). The differential effect of attitudes on the use of mental health services. *Social Psychiatry, 21*, 187–192.

Leaf, P. J., Bruce, M. L., Tischler, G. L., & Holzer, C. E. (1987). The relationship between demographic factors and attitudes toward mental health services. *Journal of Community Psychology, 15*, 275–284.

Lehman, A. F., Steinwachs, D. M., Dixon, L. B., Goldman, H. H., Osher, F., Postrado, L., et al. (1998). Translating research into practice: The Schizophrenia Patient Outcomes Research Team (PORT) treatment recommendations. *Schizophrenia Bulletin, 24*, 1–10.

Levinson, C. M., & Druss, B. G. (2000). The evolution of mental health parity in American politics. *Administration and Policy in Mental Health, 28*(2), 139–146.

Link, B. G. (1987). Understanding labeling effects in the area of mental disorders: An assessment of the effects of expectations of rejection. *American Sociological Review, 52*, 96–112.

Link, B. G., Cullen, F. T., Frank, J., & Wozniak, J. F. (1987). The social rejection of former mental patients: Understanding why labels matter. *American Journal of Sociology, 92*, 1461–1500.

Link, B. G., Cullen, F. T., Struening, E. L., Shrout, P. E., & Dohrenwend, B. P. (1989). A modified labeling theory approach to mental disorders: An empirical assessment. *American Sociological Review, 54*, 400–423.

Link, B. G., & Phelan, J. C. (2001). Conceptualizing stigma. *Annual Review of Sociology, 27*, 363–385.

Link, B. G., & Phelan, J. C. (2006). Stigma and its public health implications. *The Lancet, 367*, 528–529.

Link, B. G., Phelan, J. C., Bresnahan, M., Stueve, A., & Pescosolido, B. A. (1999). Public conceptions of mental illness: Labels, causes, dangerousness, and social distance. *American Journal of Public Health, 89*, 1328–1333.

Liska, A. (1990). The significance of aggregate dependent variables and contextual independent variables for linking macro and micro theories. *Social Psychology Quarterly, 53*, 292–301.

Lysaker, P. H., Buck, K. D., Salvatore, G., Popolo, R., & Dimaggio, G. (2009). Lack of awareness of illness in schizophrenia: Conceptualizations, correlates and treatment approaches. *Expert Review of Neurotherapeutics, 9*, 1035–1043.

Macrae, C., Bodenhausen, G. V., Milne, A. B., & Jetten, J. (1994). Out of mind but back in sight: Stereotypes on the rebound. *Journal of Personality and Social Psychology, 67*, 808–817.

Markowitz, F. E. (2001). Modeling processes in recovery from mental illness: Relationships between symptoms, life satisfaction, and self-concept. *Journal of Health and Social Behavior, 42*, 64–79.

McCubbin, M., & Cohen, D. (1996). Extremely unbalanced: Interest divergence and power disparities between clients and psychiatry. *International Journal of Law and Psychiatry, 19*, 1–25.

Meltzer, H., Bebbington, P., Brugha, T., Farrell, M., Jenkins, R., & Lewis, G. (2003). The reluctance to seek treatment for neurotic disorders. *International Review of Psychiatry, 15*, 123–128.

Mercer, W. M. (1998). *Mercer/Foster Higgins national survey of employer-sponsored health plans.* New York: William M. Mercer.

Metzner, J. L., & Fellner, J. (2010). Solitary confinement and mental illness in U.S. prisons: A challenge for medical ethics. *Journal of the American Academy of Psychiatry and the Law, 38,* 104–108.

Mojtabai, R. (2007). Americans' attitudes toward mental health treatment seeking: 1990–2003. *Psychiatric Services, 58,* 642–651.

Moses, T. (2009). Self-labeling and its effects among adolescents diagnosed with mental disorders. *Social Science & Medicine, 68,* 570–578.

Mueser, K. T., Bellack, A. S., Douglas, M. S., & Morrison, R. L. (1991). Prevalence and stability of social skill deficits in schizophrenia. *Schizophrenia Research, 5,* 167–176.

Myin-Germeys, I., Oorschot, M., Collip, D., Lataster, J., Delespaul, P., & van Os, J. (2009). Experience sampling research in psychopathology: Opening the black box of daily life. *Psychological Medicine, 39,* 1533–1547.

Narrow, W., Regier, D., Norquist, G., Rae, D., Kennedy, C., & Arons, B. (2000). Mental health service use by Americans with severe mental illnesses. *Social Psychiatry and Psychiatric Epidemiology, 35,* 147–155.

Ozmen, E., Ogel, K., Aker, T., Sagduyu, A., Tamar, D., & Boratav, C. (2004). Public attitudes to depression in urban Turkey – the influence of perceptions and causal attributions on social distance towards individuals suffering from depression. *Social Psychiatry and Psychiatric Epidemiology, 39,* 1010–1016.

Penn, D. L., Guynan, K., Daily, T., Spaulding, W. D., Garbin, C., & Sullivan, M. (1994). Dispelling the stigma of schizophrenia: What sort of information is best? *Schizophrenia Bulletin, 20,* 567–578.

Penn, D. L., Judge, A., Jamieson, P., Garczynski, J., Hennesy, M., & Romer, D. (2005). Stigma. In D. L. Evans, E. B. Foa, R. E. Gur, H. Hendan, C. P. O'Brien, M. E. P. Seligman, & T. Walsh (Eds.), *Treating and preventing adolescent mental health disorders* (pp. 531–544). Oxford, England: Oxford University Press.

Penn, D. L., & Martin, J. (1998). The stigma of severe mental illness: Some potential solutions for a recalcitrant problem. *Psychiatric Quarterly, 69,* 235–247.

Penn, D. L., Mueser, K. T., & Doonan, R. (1997). Physical attractiveness in schizophrenia: The mediating role of social skill. *Behavior Modification, 21,* 78–85.

Pescosolido, B. A. (2007). Culture, children, and mental health treatment: Special section on the national stigma study-children. *Psychiatric Services, 58,* 611–612.

Pescosolido, B. A., Fettes, D. L., Martin, J. K., Monahan, J., & McLeod, J. D. (2007). Perceived dangerousness of children with mental health problems and support for coerced treatment. *Psychiatric Services, 58,* 619–625.

Pescosolido, B. A., Monahan, J, Link, B. G., Stueve, A., & Kikuzawa, S. (1999) The public's view of the competence, dangerousness, and need for legal coercion of persons with mental health problems. *American Journal of Public Health, 89,* 1339–1345.

Pincus, F. L. (1996). Discrimination comes in many forms: Individual, institutional, and structural. *American Behavioral Scientist, 40,* 186–194.

Pincus, F. L., & Ehrlich, H. J. (Eds.). (1999). *Race and ethnic conflict: Contending views on prejudice, discrimination, and ethnoviolence.* Boulder, CO: Westview Press.

Pinfold, V., Toulmin, H., Thornicroft, G., Huxley, P., Farmer, P., & Graham, T. (2003). Reducing psychiatric stigma and discrimination: Evaluation of educational interventions in UK secondary schools. *British Journal of Psychiatry, 182,* 342–346.

Rappaport, J. (1987). Terms of empowerment/exemplars of prevention: Toward a theory for community psychology. *American Journal of Community Psychology, 15,* 121–148.

Regier, D. A., Narrow, W. E., Rae, D. S., Manderscheid, R. W., Locke, B. Z., & Goodwin, F. K. (1993). The de facto U.S. mental and addictive disorders service system: Epidemiologic Catchment Area prospective 1-year prevalence rates of disorders and services. *Archives of General Psychiatry, 50,* 85–94.

Rosenberg, M. (1965). *Society and the adolescent self image.* Princeton, NJ: Princeton University Press.

Scheff, T. (1974). The labeling theory of mental illness. *American Sociological Review, 39,* 444–452.

Scheid, T. L. (2005). Stigma as a barrier to employment: Mental disability and the Americans with Disabilities Act. *International Journal of Law and Psychiatry, 28,* 670–690.

Schulze, B. (2007). Stigma and mental health professionals: A review of the evidence on an intricate relationship. *International Review of Psychiatry, 19,* 137–155.

Schulze, B., Richter-Werling, M., Matschinger, H., & Angermeyer, M. C. (2003). Crazy? So what! Effects of a school project on students' attitudes towards people with schizophrenia. *Acta Psychiatrica Scandinavica, 107,* 142–150.

Sirey, J. A., Bruce, M. L., Alexopoulos, G. S., Perlick, D. A., Friedman, S. J., & Meyers, B. S. (2001). Stigma as a barrier to recovery: Perceived stigma and patient-rated severity of illness as predictors of antidepressant drug adherence. *Psychiatric Services, 52,* 1615–1620.

Socall, D. W., & Holtgraves, T. (1992). Attitudes toward the mentally ill: The effects of label and beliefs. *Sociological Quarterly, 33,* 435–445.

Steadman, H. J., McCarthy, D. W., & Morrissey, J. P. (1989). *The mentally ill in jail: Planning for essential services.* New York, NY: Guilford Press.

Stuart, H. (2006). Mental illness and employment discrimination. *Current Opinion in Psychiatry, 19,* 522–526.

Swanson, J., Holzer, C., Ganju, V., & Tsutomu Jono, R. (1990). Violence and psychiatric disorder in the community: Evidence from the Epidemiologic Catchment surveys. *Hospital & Community Psychiatry, 41,* 761–770.

Tarrier, N., Yusupoff, L., Kinney, C., McCarthy, E., Gledhill, A., Haddock, G., & Morris, J. (1998). Randomised controlled trial of intensive cognitive behaviour therapy for patients with chronic schizophrenia. *British Medical Journal, 317,* 303–307.

Teplin, L. A. (1984). Criminalizing mental disorder: The comparative arrest rate of the mentally ill. *American Psychologist, 39,* 794–803.

U.S. Equal Employment Opportunity Commission. (1997). *The Americans with Disabilities Act and psychiatric disabilities.* Washington, DC: U.S. EEOC.

Wahl, O. F. (1995). *Media madness: Public images of mental illness.* New Brunswick, NJ: Rutgers University Press.

Wahl, O. F. (1999). Mental health consumers' experience of stigma. *Schizophrenia Bulletin, 25,* 467–478.

Wang, P.S., Demler, O., & Kessler, R.C. (2002). Adequacy of treatment for serious mental illness in the United States. *American Journal of Public Health, 92,* 92–98.

Wang, P. S., Lane, M., Olfson, M., Pincus, H. A., Wells, K. B., & Kessler, R. C. (2005). Twelve-month use of mental health services in the United States: Results from the National Comorbidity Survey Replication. *Archives of General Psychiatry, 62*, 629–640.

Watson, A., Ottati, V., Lurigio, A., & Heyrman, M. (2005). Stigma and the police. In P. Corrigan (Ed.), *On the stigma of mental illness: Practical strategies for research and social change* (pp. 197–218). Washington, D.C.: American Psychological Association.

Weiden, P. J., & Olfson, M. (1995). Cost of relapse in schizophrenia. *Schizophrenia Bulletin, 21*, 419–429.

Willis, A. G., Willis, G. B., Male, A., Henderson, M., & Manderscheid, R. W. (1998). Mental illness and disability in the U.S. adult household population. In R. W. Manderscheid & M. J. Henderson (Eds.), *Mental health, United States, 1998* (pp. 235–246). Washington, DC: U.S. Department of Health and Human Services.

World Health Organization. (2001). *The world health report 2001-Mental health: New understanding, new hope.* Geneva, CH: WHO. Retreived from www.who.int/whr/2001/en/

Part II
Policy

7 Social policy and the American mental health system of care

David Mechanic and Gerald N. Grob

Introduction

Lunacy, insanity, or mental illnesses – whatever the term or diagnostic category used – have seemingly been an omnipresent feature of the human condition. Virtually every society has been forced to confront the presence of persons whose aberrant behavior and condition invariably lead to dependency or community disruption. That persons with severe mental illnesses are generally unable to survive on their own without some form of assistance and support has raised grave problems. What is the responsibility of the family? Can families be required to provide care for dependent members when to do so might destroy their ability to function? Does the community or the state have a moral and legal obligation to provide care and – if possible – treatment? If so, what kinds of arrangements are appropriate? What level of government is best qualified to assume the role of provider and caretaker?

In the United States, a variety of factors have shaped mental health policy, including the changing composition of the population with severe mental disorders; concepts of the etiology and nature of mental illnesses; the organization and ideology of psychiatry; funding mechanisms; and existing popular, political, social, and professional attitudes and values. Equally significant, the structure of the American political system and the division of responsibilities between federal, state, and local governments has played a major role in shaping the mental health system.

The rise of institutional care

The 19th century was notable for the proliferation of institutional solutions and the transfer of functions from families to public or quasi-public structures; thus, the transformation of insanity into a social problem that was seen as requiring institutionalization and the ensuing emphasis on state intervention of this period was by no means unique. In 1820 only one state mental hospital existed, but by the Civil War virtually every state had established one or more institutions. Local communities, however, were deeply involved in institutional care, since they were responsible for paying for the upkeep of their residents in state hospitals. Thus, they had an incentive to retain residents with mental disorders in almshouses, where the cost of care was lower.

For all of the 19th and the first half of the 20th centuries, mental health remained the single largest item in state operating budgets. However, the creation of this vast hospital system led to unanticipated problems. Many patients remained in hospitals for extended periods, increasing inpatient populations and raising new questions. Should states build additional hospitals? Did the presence of long-stay patients undermine therapeutic goals? Should local communities retain persons with severe and persistent mental disorders in almshouses and other welfare institutions? What levels of government – local, state, or national – should bear the largest burden of support?

Toward the close of the 19th century, coalitions that included physicians and social welfare advocates began to lobby for an end to dual responsibility and for the state to be the sole provider for persons with severe mental disorders. New York led the way with the passage of its influential State Care Act in 1890, which mandated that all persons with a severe mental illness were wards of the state. Over time, virtually every state enacted similar legislation, and in the twentieth century state care became the general rule (Grob, 1983).

Although the intent of state assumption of responsibility was to ensure that persons with mental illnesses would receive high-quality care and treatment, local officials saw in the new laws an entrepreneurial opportunity to shift some of their financial obligations onto the state. Traditionally, locally supported and administered almshouses served in part as old-age homes for senile and elderly persons without any financial resources. With economic considerations paramount, and going beyond the intent of the state care acts, local officials redefined senility in psychiatric terms and transferred aged persons from almshouses to state mental hospitals (Grob, 1983). For this and other reasons, between 1890 and 1920, the almshouse populations dropped precipitously. Altered coverage patterns, in turn, transformed the mission of state hospitals by converting them in part into institutions that provided custodial care for large numbers of elderly, incapacitated persons.

Demographic data vividly illustrate this change. Between the 1830s and 1890s, the proportion of long-term or chronic cases in hospitals was relatively low. By 1923, 54% of patients had been hospitalized for five years or more (U.S. Bureau of the Census, 1926). Hospital populations were increasingly heterogeneous, but the aged constituted by far the single largest group. As late as 1958, nearly a third of all state hospital resident patients were over the age of 65 (American Psychiatric Association [APA], 1960).

The rise of community care and treatment

In 1945 there was little evidence that mental health policy would shortly begin to undergo radical changes. At that time, the average daily resident population in public mental hospitals was about 430,000; approximately 85,000 were first-time admissions. Aggregate data, however, conceal as much as they reveal. Hospitals, to be sure, had a high proportion of long-stay patients composed of two groups: persons admitted at a young age, who remained hospitalized for the rest of their lives, and elderly persons who remained until they died. The presence of large numbers of long-stay patients tended to reinforce the belief that hospitals were merely serving a custodial role, though a much larger proportion of patients who were admitted were treated and discharged after relatively brief stays. During the Great Depression of the 1930s and World War II, declining resources led to a neglect of physical facilities and overcrowding, and the loss of professional personnel during the war exacerbated problems.

Few public policies, however long-established or stable, remain immune from broader social, economic, intellectual, and scientific currents. Beginning with World War II, the faith that institutionalization was the proper policy choice slowly began to erode. The change in postwar mental health priorities had diverse roots. The military experiences of World War II allegedly demonstrated that community and outpatient treatment of persons with mental disorders was superior and more efficient. A simultaneous shift in psychiatric thinking fostered receptivity toward a psychodynamic and psychoanalytic model that emphasized life experiences, the important role of socio-environmental factors, and psychotherapy of one form or another. The belief that early identification of individuals at risk and intervention in the community would be effective in preventing subsequent hospitalization became popular. This view was especially encouraged by psychiatrists and other mental health professionals who had a public health orientation; they shared a faith that psychiatry, in collaboration with the social and behavioral sciences, could ameliorate those social and environmental conditions that played an important role in the etiology of mental disorders. The introduction of new psychosocial and biological therapies in the postwar decades – including, but not limited to, psychotropic drugs – held out the promise of a better and more productive life for persons who in the past were committed to mental hospitals. At the same time, psychiatrists began to abandon mental hospital employment for private and community practice. Finally, a series of journalistic and media exposés seemed to buttress the claim that mental hospitals were incarcerating persons and offering little in the way of therapy (Grob, 1991). All of these developments undermined the legitimacy of the traditional institutional policy, and a new paradigm began to emerge, namely, that care and treatment of persons with severe mental disorders should take place in the community.

These developments in conjunction with each other would probably have been enough to promote significant change. Nevertheless, the entry of the federal government into the mental health policy arena proved crucial as it altered the very ways in which policy was conceptualized and implemented. After 1945 the thrust toward medical specialization accelerated; new structural relations were forged among federal agencies; federal funding for biomedical research increased at a rapid pace; and the role of the Public Health Service expanded dramatically. The passage of the Hill-Burton Act in 1946 gave generous subsidies for hospital construction, and third-party medical insurance programs began to grow. The emergence of a health lobby that included members of Congress and influential laypersons hastened the expansion of federal health activities.

The growing role of the federal government in health affairs did not necessarily imply that it would seek to preempt the traditional role of states in providing care and treatment for persons with severe mental disorders. However, the passage of the National Mental Health Act of 1946 (Public Law Chap. 538, 1946) created the National Institute of Mental Health (NIMH), and its first director, Robert H. Felix – who remained the director until 1964 – framed a national agenda that assumed that community care and treatment would replace archaic and obsolete mental hospitals. His interpretation of the legislation precluded support for care and treatment of patients at state mental hospitals. Felix was also able to create a national constituency and to cultivate key congressional legislators.

While Felix was expanding the influence of the NIMH during the 1950s, interest in community alternatives to mental hospitalization was mounting. The development of psychosocial and milieu therapies, as well as the introduction of psychotropic drugs, gave impetus to the belief that early identification and treatment would obviate the need for hospitalization. Support for a community mental health program came from a variety of constituencies. The Council of State Governments and Governors' Conferences in the 1950s endorsed this approach as a means of arresting the seemingly inevitable growth of the institutionalized population and the burden on state finances. Private foundations, such as the Milbank Memorial Fund, as well as leading university departments of psychiatry added to the chorus for change. The growing faith in community mental health services led New York State in 1954, and California in 1957, to enact legislation encouraging communities to expand their mental health services (Council of State Governments, 1950; 1953; Milbank Memorial Fund, 1956; 1957; Grob, 1991).

The Community Mental Health Centers Act of 1963

The major difficulty impeding broad changes in mental health services was that each state had its own policies. Activists, therefore, were faced with the daunting, if not impossible, task of persuading 48 state legislatures to change their mental health policies. That such activists turned to the federal government was not surprising. The New Deal and the experiences of World War II had created a pervasive feeling that the federal government was enlightened, whereas many state governments were tight-fisted and reactionary. The goal of creating new mental health priorities was slowly incorporated into a liberal political coalition dedicated to expanding national authority and diminishing the role of states.

To further their agenda, activists succeeded in creating the Joint Commission on Mental Illness and Health (JCMIH). A private undertaking that received congressional support and financing, the JCMIH worked for nearly six years, published nine studies, and issued its final report, *Action for Mental Health*, in 1961. The report was a sort of smorgasbord of recommendations, including a proposal for the doubling of mental health expenditures in five years and tripling it in ten, of which the largest proportion would be provided by the federal government (Joint Commission on Mental Illness and Health [JCMIH], 1961).

The reception of *Action for Mental Health* was generally favorable, although it had its critics. Due to conflicting political pressure, President John F. Kennedy appointed an inter-agency task force to develop policy recommendations. Since its members were not especially knowledgeable about the subject, they relied on Felix to guide their deliberations. Felix and the NIMH had little use for the recommendations of the JCMIH (which had emphasized the care and treatment of persons with serious disorders), and in its place the NIMH recommended the adoption of a comprehensive community program that envisaged the disappearance of the mental hospital and the development of a broad continuum of mental health services. In place of mental hospitals, they urged the creation of a new institution – a community mental health center (CMHC) (NIMH, 1961; 1962a; 1962b). The presidential task force accepted the NIMH proposals and called for the creation of 500 CMHCs by 1970 and 1,500 by 1980. After complex political maneuvering and with Kennedy's endorsement, Congress enacted legislation that provided a three-year authorization of $150 million for fiscal years 1965–1967 (Public Law 88–164, 1963).

The passage of the CMHC Act of 1963 not only strengthened the policymaking authority of the federal government while diminishing the role of states, it also represented a victory of ideology over reality. A community program model was based on assumptions that patients had a home in the community and a sympathetic family to provide support. In 1960, however, 73% of the hospitalized population was either unmarried, widowed, or divorced. Nor did much of this population have work experience or the economic resources to support community residence, and the legislation also included nothing about the income required to live in the community (Kramer, 1956; 1967; Kramer, Taube, & Starr, 1968; Pollack, Person, Kramer, & Goldstein, 1959). Further, there was no evidence that

CMHCs could provide care and treatment for a severely disabled population in the community. The legislation provided no links between state hospitals and free-standing centers, and state authorities, who continued to run the mental hospitals, were bypassed in favor of a federal-local partnership and their priorities were ignored. The result was that CMHCs had considerable autonomy and freedom from state regulation, which permitted the centers to focus on a set of clients who better fit the orientations of mental health managers and professionals trained in psychodynamic and preventive orientations. The treatment of choice at most centers was individual psychotherapy, an intervention especially adapted to a middle-class, educated clientele with less severe disorders that was congenial to professional staffs composed largely of clinical psychologists and social workers.

Deinstitutionalization

Deinstitutionalization of hospitalized persons with severe mental disorders is often attributed to the introduction of psychotropic drugs in the 1950s, yet this claim is hardly supported by available data. Between 1955 and 1965, state hospital populations fell by only 15%, while in the following decade the decline was 60% (Mechanic & Rochefort, 1992). Indeed, the first wave of deinstitutionalization can be attributed to the enactment of Medicare and Medicaid in 1965, which encouraged the construction of nursing homes by providing a payment source for elderly patients who needed custodial care, or those who needed aftercare following a hospital stay. Although states were responsible for the full costs of patients in state hospitals, they could transfer patients to nursing homes and have the federal government assume from half to three-quarters of the cost. Between 1963 and 1969 the number of persons 65 or older with mental disorders in nursing homes increased from 188,000 to 368,000. Medicaid, according to a General Accounting Office report in 1977, "had become the largest single purchasers of mental health care and the principal federal program funding the long-term care of the mentally disabled" (General Accounting Office, 1977). The shift from mental hospital to nursing facility care was a development more driven by a desire to take advantage of federal resources than by a desire to improve the lot of elderly persons and those with a severe and persistent mental disorder.

A second wave of deinstitutionalization began in the 1970s and included new cohorts of persons with mental illnesses. Between 1946 and 1960 more than 59 million births were recorded. The disproportionately high size of this age cohort meant that the number of persons (most of whom were young) at risk for developing a severe mental illness was relatively high. Persons developing these disorders were often mobile and many abused alcohol and drugs. The availability of a series of federal entitlement programs – including Social Security Disability Insurance (SSDI), Supplementary Security Income for the Aged, the Disabled, and the Blind (SSI),

Medicaid, and food stamps – encouraged states to make admission to mental hospitals more difficult, if only because resources for persons with severe mental disorders in the community were available at lower state expense.

Treatment in the community for clients with multiple needs, as compared with mental hospital care, posed severe challenges. In the community (and particularly in large urban areas) clients were widely dispersed, and their successful management depended on bringing together needed services administered by a variety of bureaucracies, each with its own culture, politics, and preferred client populations. The decentralization of services and lack of integration made it extraordinarily difficult to deal with individuals in the community, and many became part of the street culture. Individuals with a dual diagnosis of serious mental illness and substance abuse presented such serious problems that many mental health professionals refused to deal with them. Moreover, the decline in institutional care created a situation where the "criminalization" of such persons became more common.

When the General Accounting Office prepared a comprehensive report to Congress in 1977, it laid bare the problem of a disorganized and uncoordinated mental health system. Although the report endorsed deinstitutionalization, it was extraordinarily critical of the manner in which it was implemented and lamented that responsibility for the care, support, and treatment of persons with mental disorders was "frequently diffused among several agencies and levels of government." The dramatic growth of federal involvement in mental health had not produced the anticipated benefits, if only because there was little or no coordination between the 135 federal programs administered by eleven major agencies and departments (General Accounting Office, 1977).

Upon taking office in early 1977, Jimmy Carter created a presidential commission to investigate the mental health system. After public hearings and months of deliberations, the commission presented its final report to the president in the spring of 1978. It included more than 100 recommendations that affected not only relations among federal, state, and local governments, but also public and private agencies and such federal programs as Medicare and Medicaid. In many ways the commission's work was influenced by a political climate in which debates were shaped by groups that defined themselves in terms of class, ethnicity, gender, and race. By that time, neither state hospitals nor persons with persistent and serious mental illnesses were at the center of policy debates; the number of competing voices and advocates of other groups had increased substantially. The final report was neither a blueprint for legislative action nor the viewpoints of a particular group, and the diversity of its recommendations could not easily be translated into legislation (President's Commission on Mental Health, 1978; Grob & Goldman, 2006).

For more than two years the administration and Congress struggled in an effort to draft an appropriate piece of legislation. There was an absence of any consensus on mental health policy. Deinstitutionalization – whatever its meaning – was coming under widespread criticism by a variety of interest groups, each with its own agenda. In October, 1980, Congress finally enacted and Carter signed into law the Mental Health Systems Act. While in theory assigning the highest priority to individuals with long-term mental disorders, the legislation also recognized the claims of various other groups whose needs were quite different, including children and adolescents, the elderly, rural residents, and victims of rape. The absence of new resources and vague generalizations about the kinds of services required, however, raised doubts about the legislation's effectiveness. Indeed, in order to make it through Congress, the legislation offered something to everyone and, as a result, lacked focus. Moreover, some provisions – especially those dealing with the prevention of mental illnesses and the promotion of mental health – reflected ideology and were little more than attractive slogans that had no basis in empirical data. Further, the legislation did not offer any guidelines to assist persons with severe mental disorders to negotiate a myriad of programs administered by independent agencies (Foley & Sharfstein, 1983; Grob & Goldman, 2006; Mechanic, 2008; Public Law 96–398, 1980).

Social policy and the American mental health system of care

When President Reagan took office in 1981, the Mental Health Systems Act was repealed. The federal government substantially removed itself from mental health policymaking, and mental health policy debates and policies shifted to states and localities. NIMH considerably narrowed its involvements to research and demonstrations and withdrew from policy formulation. However, earlier trends continued at the local level, and seemingly modest changes in generic federal programs, such as Medicaid, had a dramatic impact.

Deinstitutionalization accelerated in the late 1970s with changes in federal programs, such as SSI, that provided a stronger safety net for surviving in the community. Generic federal programs were enabling, but states in fact reduced inpatient populations at very different rates depending on the size and configuration of their mental health inpatient facilities, the available alternative care arrangements, the power of the hospital bureaucracy to resist downsizing, the vigor of community advocacy for deinstitutionalization, the economic pressures on states to reduce costs, the fiscal arrangements between state and local governments, and the bureaucratic skills and attitudes about shifting costs to the federal government. Between 1955 and 1973 states such as California, Illinois, Massachusetts, Hawaii, and Utah had reduced their mental hospital inpatients by more than two-thirds, while others, such as Texas and South Dakota, by only two-fifths. Nevada reduced its inpatient population by less than 15%, and Delaware by only 17%. As late as 1986, some states had only reduced inpatient populations by about three-fifths (e.g., Wyoming and Delaware), while others had reduced inpatient census by 85% or more (e.g., Illinois, California, Wisconsin, Vermont) (Mechanic & Rochefort, 1992).

In the 1970s and 1980s, care and support for persons with mental illness who were no longer in mental hospitals came from a variety of federal programs that were not designed for persons with mental illnesses in mind. Medicaid became de facto the most important program affecting persons with mental illnesses. Frank and Glied characterized these trends as the "mainstreaming" of mental health services (Frank & Glied, 2006).

The expansion of mental health services

One important influence on mental health service expansion over the decades was the growth in mental health coverage in health insurance. By the turn of the century, 80% of persons with mental illnesses had some form of health insurance (compared with 86% of the population overall) (McAlpine & Mechanic, 2000), and most plans covered at least some mental health services. However, a point of great contention in the mental health community was the greater limitations on mental health than on physical health coverage. Indeed, mental health parity has been a source of continuing struggle over the decades, with incremental improvements over time at both the state and federal levels.

The Wellstone-Domenici Mental Health Parity and Addiction Equity Act was passed in 2008 and went into effect in 2010, representing the largest federal effort to move to full parity. Under this Act, financial requirements and treatment limitations for mental health and substance abuse benefits cannot be more restrictive than those for medical/surgical benefits; this applies to deductibles and other copayments as well as all treatment limitations, including frequency of treatment, number of visits, and days of coverage. Gaps still remain, including exclusions for small employers and no basic requirement that mental health be covered. However, more comprehensive parity laws are in effect in many states (National Alliance on Mental Illness, 2009).

With increased insurance coverage and greater public awareness of mental illnesses and the availability of treatment, use of mental health services became more acceptable over the decades. Two University of Michigan surveys 20 years apart (1957 and 1976) found that despite comparable population levels of well-being, reports of using professional help for psychological problems increased from 14 to 26% (Veroff, Kulka, & Douvan, 1981). Another study comparing help-seeking for mental health problems between 1957 and 1996 found an increase in mental health services use from 1 to 22% (Swindle, Pescosolido, Braboy-Jackson, & Boyer, 1997). The National Comorbidity Survey Replication conducted in 2001 to 2003 found that 18% of adult respondents used a mental health service in the prior year, and 9% used a specialty mental health service (Wang, Lane,

Olfson, Pincus, Wells, & Kessler, 2005). This was a large increase over prior periods using comparable definitions. Persons treated for depression increased from 5.8 million in 1996 to 10.1 million in 2005 (Olfson & Marcus, 2009).

A major change involved the role of the general medical care sector. General physicians have always cared for many patients with psychiatric morbidity and psychological problems, but mental health agencies sought to increase their interest and capacities to recognize psychiatric illness and treat it more effectively. The introduction of new psychiatric drugs, such as the selective serotonin reuptake inhibitors (SSRIs), which general physicians are more comfortable with prescribing than earlier medications, encouraged treatment. Prescription drugs are now the largest influence on growth of mental health cost, and mental disorders are now among the five most costly chronic conditions, with expenditures of $57.5 billion in 2006 (Soni, 2009). Pharmaceutical use increased from 5.6% of all mental health specialty costs in 1971 to 23% in 2003 (Frank & Glied, 2006). Estimated drug spending per capita for mental health care in 2006 was 51% of mental health expenditures, compared with only 26% of per capita costs for general medical services costs (Frank, Goldman, & McGuire, 2009).

Pharmaceutical companies invest large resources in detailing to physicians as well as direct-to-consumer advertising to encourage use (Angell, 2004). Pharmaceutical companies invest heavily in sponsoring continuing medical education, professional meetings, and advocacy groups as a way of encouraging use of new patent-protected medications. These companies fund most of the clinical trials of drugs and often maintain control over their execution and publication. Clinical trials sponsored by these companies report more favorable results than trials supported by other funding (Mechanic, 2008). Selective publication, distortion of research findings, biased interpretation, and other abuses have been commonly noted (Turner, Matthews, Linardatos, Tell, & Rosenthal, 2008). There is now a strong backlash against these practices and new efforts to make transparent and to control the financial relationships between researchers and for-profit entities such as pharmaceutical companies.

With the expansion of diagnostic conceptions over the last 20 years, the medicalization of what many regard as common life problems, and the increased identification of mental health problems in general medical practice, psychiatric drug use also has increased dramatically among the general population. Primary care physicians prescribed almost three-fifths of all psychiatric prescriptions between August 2006 and July 2007 and prescribed more anxiolytics, antidepressants, and stimulants than psychiatrists and addiction specialists (Mark, Levit, & Buck, 2009). Antidepressants were the most common prescription type written in office-based practice, with some 27 million in 2005, more than 10 per 100 persons and almost double the rate of 5.84 per 100 persons in 1996 (Olfson & Marcus, 2009). While depression, bipolar disorder, and anxiety are the most common indications for use of antidepressants, they are also commonly used in non-specific ways for a variety of patient complaints, including sleep disorders, fatigue, adjustment problems, headache, back pain, and the like.

Studies of treatment of depression find that only rarely does it conform to evidence-based practice guidelines, especially in general medical practice, where most such treatment takes place (Wang, Demler, & Kessler, 2002; Kessler, Berglund, Demler, Jin, Koretz, Merikangas, et al., 2003). Despite the widespread use of antidepressants for depression complaints, there is little evidence of efficacy in treating less severe depression (Fournier, DeRubeis, Hollon, Dimidjian, Amsterdam, Shelton, & Fawcett, 2010). Treatment for persons with serious mental illness is even more deficient. Patients rarely receive many of the basic components of good care, such as effective case management, psychosocial rehabilitation, and supported employment (Lehman, 1999). Even basic psychiatric care is often deficient. An assessment of treatment adequacy based on data from the National Comorbidity Study found that only 40% of persons received any treatment in the previous year, 57% from the mental health specialty sector, 20% from the general medical sector, and 23% from both. Of those who received care, only 20% in the general medical sector, 46% in the mental health sector, and 39% with combined care had care that met minimally adequate treatment standards (Wang et al., 2002).

Changing patterns of patient care

With the emptying of large mental hospitals and greater reliance on pharmaceutical treatments, care for most patients now occurs in ambulatory settings with a strong focus on avoiding inpatient admission. Inpatient psychiatric care largely occurs in specialized psychiatric and substance abuse units in non-profit and public general hospitals for acute episodes of serious illness involving either patient or community risk. Typical inpatient stays have fallen to six to eight days, primarily to stabilize symptoms. Many severely ill patients, no longer protected by the custodial services of the mental hospital – housing, nutrition, daily activities, and supervision – have been more likely to get into difficulty, and increasingly use alcohol and drugs, become homeless, and get involved in disorderly conduct and petty crime. These patients are now commonly arrested and jailed. Coordination between inpatient hospital care and community services has been greatly deficient, and the promised coherent network of needed community services has, for the most part, not materialized. In the case of the many persons with serious mental illnesses who are incarcerated, services for appropriate re-entry to the community are highly deficient or not available at all.

In recent decades understanding has grown that serious mental illness is often chronic and requires a long-term treatment orientation with needed integration of services among various bureaucratic domains. Medication monitoring is just one component of an array of functions, including illness and medication education, substance abuse screening and treatment, family involvement, attention to stable housing, linkage to needed social and rehabilitative services, and supported employment. A variety of intensive case management programs have been developed to attempt coordination of these needed services in community settings, but relatively few persons with serious mental illnesses have access to these services. Large-scale efforts to develop more effective mental health authorities or to integrate services at the community level have had limited success (Mechanic, 2008). Patients are often housed in a variety of low-cost sheltered facilities where the level and quality of services are even more deficient than they were in the large mental hospitals condemned in earlier decades.

The rise of managed care

The most important organizational change in recent decades in mental health care has been the growth of managed care. While the backlash against managed care in the general medical sector resulted in substantial weakening of such management strategies (Mechanic, 2004), development of these tools continued in the mental health sector, and now almost all mental health care is managed. The predominant pattern is to carve out the mental health component of insurance coverage and contract with managed care organizations to administer the benefits on either a risk basis or as an administrative intermediary.

In the private insurance sector, utilization review and concurrent review of ongoing treatment were tools introduced in the 1990s and were highly successful in substantially reducing inpatient care, the most expensive component of care. Increasingly, the intensity of treatment was limited by reducing number of visits and length of treatment. Pharmaceuticals became the dominant treatment; the prevalence of psychotherapy was substantially reduced and, when used, was more directive and limited in length, with social workers, psychologists, and nurses often substituted for psychiatrists (Mechanic, 2008).

Over time, managed mental health care was introduced into the Medicaid program. One important advantage of many Medicaid programs compared to private insurance is that they potentially offer a broader range of services needed by people with serious mental illness. The ideal of managed care, relative to fee-for-service, is that managers have flexibility and can arrange the most appropriate and most cost-effective care plan for those with complex needs. In some cases, managed care programs are quite broad and sophisticated, using assertive care management and a range of rehabilitative programs, housing arrangements, and coordination of other needed services. In many other instances, these programs do little more than provide pharmaceutical treatment and medication management. The quality of any managed care approach depends on many specific aspects, and the literature reports quite varied performance (Mechanic, 2008). Management of care tends to spread services more evenly among a population of patients, and questions remain as to whether those with the most severe and persistent conditions receive the intensity and comprehensive care they require (Mechanic & McAlpine, 1999).

In the decades since its passage in 1965, Medicaid has become the mental health program that is most important for persons with severe and persistent mental illnesses, as well as for many less disabled low-income adults and children. Between 1991 and 2001, Medicaid expenditures as a proportion of all public mental health expenditures increased from 33 to 44% (Mark, Coffey, McKusick, Harwood, King, Bouchery, et al., 2005). The President's New Freedom Commission in 2003 reported that 20 to 25% of all mental health services for non-elderly adults are financed exclusively by Medicaid and that between seven and 13% of the Medicaid population uses mental health services (New Freedom Commission on Mental Health, 2003). Nevertheless, federal Medicaid mandated services for mental health are few, and the quality of state programs depends substantially on state agreement to optional service coverage. Thus, there is great variability in quality of care across states.

Mental health expenditures over the past 30 years has been less than 1% of gross national product (GNP) and from 1970 to 2003 grew only at about half the rate of general medical care (Frank et al., 2009). Estimates vary, but mental health clearly has been a decreasing proportion of total health spending; Frank and colleagues (2009) estimate a rate of 5 to 6% in 2006. Among the constraints on mental health expenditures are more forceful managed care and particularly large reductions in inpatient care. As states have faced serious constraints on their Medicaid budgets, they find it easier to limit mental health care than general medical care. With the exception of drugs, expenditures for traditional psychiatric services in a period of growth has at best remained stable or declined (Frank et al., 2009). Since mental health managed care carve outs are not usually responsible for prescription costs, it serves their interests to substitute medication for other mental health traditional services.

New Freedom Commission, recovery, and recent trends

In 2002 President Bush appointed the New Freedom Commission, which was charged with making a comprehensive study of mental health and recommending improvements that would not exceed current levels of expenditures. Six months into its work the Commission issued an interim report once again indicating that the system was fragmented and in disarray. They identified many barriers and gaps in care, and the final report argued for a transformed system with six goals: understanding that

1   mental health was an essential part of health;
2   it should be family and consumer driven;
3   disparities in care should be eliminated;
4   early screening, assessment, and referral should be the norm;
5   research should be accelerated and care excellent; and
6   new technology such as telecare and electronic health records should be used to improve access and coordination of care, particularly in underserved populations and in remote areas (New Freedom Commission on Mental Health, 2003).

Most of these goals are constructive, but the recommendations lacked specificity and the report, like earlier reports, was vague in establishing priorities given the efforts to satisfy various constituencies, particularly in a context of no new resources.

One central concept endorsed by the New Freedom Commission was the idea of "recovery," one of the new buzzwords in mental health services with varying definitions (Davidson, O'Connell, Tondora, Styron, & Kangas, 2006). As in the past, the Commission went beyond the scientific evidence base in its advocacy of prevention and its focus on recovery. The sad fact is that we have a very limited understanding of the major mental illnesses and, at this point, no evidence-based prevention strategy. Nevertheless, if recovery means participating to the fullest extent possible in the community despite one's impairments, we have had an impressive body of evidence for many years indicating that with reasonable treatment and appropriate psychosocial and supportive services many of the secondary disabilities that commonly occur with severe mental illnesses can be prevented or minimized (Wing, 2009). Within this perspective, recovery is consistent with broader social and legal trends in our society seeking to maximize integration and participation of persons with disabilities in the community. It is also consistent with the important 1999 Supreme Court *Olmstead* decision that institutionalizing persons capable of receiving care in the community constitutes discrimination under the Americans with Disabilities Act.

The New Freedom Commission gained no more than an immediate media flurry and has received little public attention. Many of the subsequent developments and activity are at the state level, but states face continuing fiscal problems and focus more on constraining costs than on expansion. For example, passage of Proposition 63 in California, imposing a 1% mental health tax on adjusted gross incomes exceeding $1 million, generated billions of dollars for restructuring services (Scheffler & Adams, 2005), but subsequently, California's enormous budget deficits have led to suspension and reduction of other important health and welfare programs. It remains unclear whether supplemental funds from Proposition 63 have been fully protected as planned and what progress has been made with such large added mental health investments. Studies underway will eventually inform us of these and other related issues.

The Obama domestic focus has been on health reform and economic recovery, and mental health per se has not been salient. Nevertheless, some early extensions of the State Children's Health Insurance Program (SCHIP) and Medicaid and many proposals for further expansions of insurance coverage and generic health programs have important implications for future mental health services. Still, the most significant transformation in mental health policy over recent decades is the extent to which mental health has increasingly been incorporated into the larger health domain and the dependence of this sector on important federal programs that affect the health and welfare of the population as a whole.

Upstream determinants

Decades of research show that prevention of low-weight births and provision of appropriate care and socialization, good nutrition, effective schooling, parental caring and emotional support, avoidance of abuse and neglect, and many other aspects of development contribute constructively to reducing future behavioral problems and dysfunctions. Economic security, preventing privation and providing opportunities for the future are also formative of healthy adulthoods. Preventing noxious behavior – particularly abuse of substances – and promoting a healthy lifestyle regimen are also important. However, we still lack understanding of the specific causal pathways of these influences and how to prevent serious mental illnesses (Mrazek & Haggerty, 1994).

For those with the most severe and persistently disabling disorders, the system, if one can call it that, remains in tatters. Far too many persons with mental illnesses are incarcerated rather than in treatment, care for those with serious chronic disorders is too often fragmented and uncoordinated, and people with these disabilities develop many secondary problems that are preventable. Translation of much of what we have learned to clinical practice has been exceedingly slow. As in earlier decades there is an unwillingness to acknowledge how little we really know with any confidence and too many claims and treatments that cannot be sustained by any reliable evidence. Mental health services have become too much of a business, the power of the pharmaceutical industry and its corruptions too pervasive, and too many psychiatric researchers have compromised ties with the industry. There is an emerging determination among medical leaders and medical schools to diminish these arrangements and create an environment where training, research, and service can be less guided by proprietary interests and better guided by the welfare of patients.

Future opportunities, risks, and prospects

The treatment of serious mental illness traditionally has been uncomfortably situated between the medical, social welfare, and, increasingly, the criminal justice sectors. With more attention to biological issues, research in the neurosciences, and medications and other medical treatments, psychiatry has moved closer to other medical concerns and general physicians now receive more training and exposure to psychiatric morbidity than in the past. However, the driving factor in the changes we have observed has been the integration of mental health coverage within health and social insurance programs that finance and shape medical practice, access to care, and predominant treatment approaches. Whether a particular treatment modality or type of clinician will prosper or be neglected depends very much on whether public and private plans provide coverage and adequate reimbursement. About half of all formal care for persons with mild and moderate mental health conditions is managed by the general medical sector within the context of everyday medical care. Those more seriously and chronically ill are more likely to make contact with the mental health specialty sector in a range of venues such as community mental health centers, emergency departments, hospital outpatient and inpatient psychiatric units, and mental health services associated with jails and prisons.

The future of mental health services depends a great deal on the outcomes of health reform deliberations. To the extent that uninsured persons with serious mental illness gain access to insurance with mental health coverage, both access to care and attention from service providers will increase. Nevertheless, we know that progress is not linear and policy moves by starts and stops. With future predicted budget deficits and the need to constrain health care growth well into future decades, it is by no means assured that mental health advocates will be able to promote their priorities successfully. This is a particularly difficult challenge for the mental health sector, which depends more completely than the physical health sector on state and federal governments for the broad range of services that support functioning, prevent secondary disabilities, and allow a minimal decent quality of life. In the absence of support for expanded medical and social rehabilitative services, more responsibility will default to the criminal justice arena.

For those who are less seriously ill, the general medical sector will continue as the first, and for many, the exclusive formal treatment of their psychiatric complaints. The long-term trend of lesser tolerance of everyday emotional problems and psychosocial stressors and continuing commercial promotion of drugs and psychiatric treatments encourages both a redefinition of normal distress in medical and psychiatric terms and increased help-seeking and treatment (most likely by pharmaceuticals). As with other drugs, some psychiatric pharmaceuticals for the less serious but prevalent disorders are likely to become available without prescriptions. Likely, stigma in seeking treatment for mild and moderate disorders among otherwise reasonably functioning individuals will continue to abate, but overcoming stigma associated with severe and disabling illnesses, such as schizophrenia, will continue as a serious challenge.

As we look to the future, uncertainty abounds. Much depends not only on developing scientific knowledge and new treatment discoveries, but also on trends in the economy and the fiscal pressures faced by varying levels of government, employers, and households. Additionally, we cannot forecast the uncertainties of environmental disasters, unpredictable catastrophes, wars, and other calamities that impact large populations. Finally, whatever our state of knowledge, it is difficult to foresee political developments or government and public priorities or how they might shape future patterns of financing and care. We know from the past that policy typically is built on prior trends, institutions, infrastructures, and cultural conceptions, and rarely is discontinuous with the past. Our understanding of the problems and barriers that characterize current mental health and mental health policy give us the opportunity to rethink and reorder priorities so we are better prepared not only to improve current services but also to shape constructive responses to whatever comes.

References

American Psychiatric Association. (1960). *Report on patients over 65 in public mental hospitals.* Washington, DC: American Psychiatric Association.

Angell, M. (2004). *The truth about the drug companies: How they deceive us and what to do about it.* New York: Random House.

Council of State Governments. (1950). *The mental health programs of the forty-eight states: A report to the governors' conference.* Chicago, IL: Council of State Governments.

Council of State Governments. (1953). *Training and research in state mental health programs: A report to the governors' conference.* Chicago, IL: Council of State Governments.

Davidson, L., O'Connell, M., Tondora, J., Styron, T., & Kangas, K. (2006). The top ten concerns about recovery encountered in mental health system transformation. *Psychiatric Services, 57,* 640–645.

Foley, H. A., & Sharfstein, S. S. (1983). *Madness and government: Who cares for the mentally ill?* Washington, DC: American Psychiatric Press.

Fournier, J. C., DeRubeis, R. J., Hollon, S. D., Dimidjian, S., Amsterdam, J. D., Shelton, R.C., & Fawcett, J. (2010). Antidepressant drug effects and depression severity: A patient-level meta-analysis. *Journal of the American Medical Association, 303,* 47–53.

Frank, R. G., & Glied, S. A. (2006). *Better but not well: Mental health policy in the United States since 1950.* Baltimore, MD: Johns Hopkins University Press.

Frank, R. G., Goldman, H. H., & McGuire, T. G. (2009). Trends in mental health cost growth: An expanded role for management? *Health Affairs, 28,* 649–659.

General Accounting Office. (1977). *Returning the mentally disabled to the community: Government needs to do more.* (HRD-76-152). Washington, DC: U.S. General Accounting Office.

Grob, G. N. (1983). *Mental illness and American society 1875–1940.* Princeton, NJ: Princeton University Press.

Grob, G. N. (1991). *From asylum to community: Mental health policy in modern America.* Princeton, NJ: Princeton University Press.

Grob, G. N., & Goldman, H. H. (2006). *The dilemma of federal mental health policy: Radical reform or incremental change*. New Brunswick, NJ: Rutgers University Press.

Joint Commission on Mental Illness and Health. (1961). *Action for mental health: Final report of the Joint Commission on Mental Illness and Health 1961*. New York: Basic Books.

Kessler, R. C., Berglund, P., Demler, O., Jin, R., Koretz, D., Merikangas, K.R., et al. (2003). The epidemiology of major depressive disorder: Results from the national comorbidity survey replication (NCS-R). *Journal of the American Medical Association, 289*, 3095–3105.

Kramer, M. (1956). *Facts needed to assess public health and social problems in the widespread use of the tranquilizing drugs*. (Public Health Service, Publication 486*)*. Washington, DC: U.S. Government Printing Office.

Kramer, M. (1967). *Some implications of trends in the usage of psychiatric facilities for community mental health programs and related research*. (Public Health Service, Publication 1434). Washington, DC: U.S. Government Printing Office.

Kramer, M., Taube, C., & Starr, S. (1968). Patterns of use in psychiatric facilities by the aged: Current status, trends, and implications. *Psychiatric Research Reports, 23*, 89–150.

Lehman, A. F. (1999). Quality of care in mental health: The case of schizophrenia. *Health Affairs, 18*, 52–65.

McAlpine, D. D., & Mechanic, D. (2000). Utilization of specialty mental health care among persons with severe mental illness: The roles of demographics, need, insurance and risk. *Health Services Research, 35*(1, Part II), 277–292.

Mark, T. L., Coffey, R. M., McKusick, D. R., Harwood, H., King, E., Bouchery, E., et al. (2005). *National expenditures for mental health services and substance abuse treatment, 1991–2001* (SAMHSA Publication No. SMA 05-3999). Rockville, MD: Substance Abuse and Mental Health Services Administration.

Mark, T. L., Levit, K. R., & Buck, J. A. (2009). Datapoints: Psychotropic drug prescriptions by medical specialty. *Psychiatric Services, 60*, 1167.

Mechanic, D. (2004). The rise and fall of managed care. *Journal of Health and Social Behavior, 45*(Extra Issue), 76–86.

Mechanic, D. (2008). *Mental health and social policy: Beyond managed care* (5th ed.). Boston: Allyn and Bacon.

Mechanic, D., & Rochefort, D. A. (1992). A policy of inclusion for the mentally ill. *Health Affairs, 11*, 128–150.

Mechanic, D., & McAlpine, D. D. (1999). Mission unfulfilled: Potholes on the road to mental health parity. *Health Affairs, 18*, 7–21.

Milbank Memorial Fund. (1956). *The elements of a community mental health program. Papers presented at the 1955 annual conference of the Milbank Memorial Fund*. New York: Milbank Memorial Fund.

Milbank Memorial Fund. (1957). *Programs for community mental health. Papers presented at the 1956 annual conference of the Milbank Memorial Fund*. New York: Milbank Memorial Fund.

Mrazek, P. J., & Haggerty, R. J. (Eds.). (1994). *Reducing risks for mental disorders: Frontiers for preventive intervention research*. Institute of Medicine Committee on Prevention of Mental Disorders, Washington, DC: National Academy Press.

National Alliance on Mental Illness. (2009). *State Mental Health Parity Laws*.

Retrieved from www.nami.org/Template.cfm?Section=Parity1&Template=/Content-Management/ContentDisplay.cfm&ContentID=45313.

National Institute of Mental Health. (1961). *National Institute of Mental Health Position Paper on Report of the Joint Commission on Mental Illness and Health. National Institute of Mental Health Records 1965–1967, Box 1, Record Group 511.2.* Washington, DC: National Archives.

National Institute of Mental Health. (1962a). *Preliminary Draft Report of NIMH Task Force on Implementation of Recommendations of the Report of the Joint Commission on Mental Illness and Health. National Institute of Mental Health Records 1965–1967, Box 1, Record Group 511.2.* Washington, DC: National Archives.

National Institute of Mental Health. (1962b). *A Proposal for a Comprehensive Mental Health Program to Implement the Findings of the Joint Commission on Mental Illness and Health. National Institute of Mental Health Records 1965–1967, Box 1, Record Group 511.2.* Washington, DC: National Archives.

New Freedom Commission on Mental Health. (2003). *Achieving the promise: Transforming mental health care in America: Final Report* (DHHS Publication No. SMA-03–3832). Rockville, MD: DHHS.

Olfson, M., & Marcus, S. C. (2009). National patterns in antidepressant medication treatment. *Archives of General Psychiatry, 66,* 848–856.

Pollack, E. S., Person, P. H., Jr., Kramer, M., & Goldstein, H. (1959). *Patterns of retention, release, and death of first admission to state mental hospitals* (Public Health Service, Publication 672). Washington, DC: U.S. Government Printing Office.

President's Commission on Mental Health. (1978). *Report to the President from the President's Commission on Mental Health,* 4 volumes. Washington, DC: Government Printing Office.

Public Law Chap. 538. (1946). *U.S. Statutes at Large, 60,* 421–426.

Public Law 88–164. (1963). *U.S. Statutes at Large, 77,* 282–299.

Public Law 96–398. (1980). *U.S. Statutes at Large, 94,* 1564–1613.

Scheffler, R. M., & Adams, N. (2005). Millionaires and mental health: Proposition 63 in California. *Health Affairs Web Exclusive,* W5–212–224. Retrieved from http://content.healthaffairs.org/cgi/reprint/hlthaff.w5.212v1.

Soni, A. (2009). *The five most costly conditions, 1996 and 2006: Estimates for the U.S. civilian non-institutionalized population.* (Statistical Brief #248, Agency for Healthcare Research and Quality). Retrieved from www.meps.ahrq.gov/mepsweb/data_files/publications/st248/stat248.pdf.

Swindle, R., Pescosolido, B. A., Braboy-Jackson, P., & Boyer, C. A. (1997). *Confronting mental health problems: How Americans experienced and coped with mental health problems in three decades.* Paper presented at the annual meeting of the American Sociological Association. Toronto, Canada.

Turner, E. H., Matthews, A. M., Linardatos, E., Tell, R. A., & Rosenthal, R. (2008). Selective publication of antidepressant trials and its influence on apparent efficacy. *New England Journal of Medicine, 358,* 252–260.

U.S. Bureau of the Census. (1926). *Patients in hospitals for mental disease 1923.* Washington, DC: Government Printing Office.

Veroff, J., Kulka, R. A., & Douvan, E. (1981). *Mental health in America: Patterns of help-seeking from 1957 to 1976.* New York: Basic Books.

Wang, P. S., Demler, O., & Kessler, R. C. (2002). Adequacy of treatment for serious mental illness in the United States. *American Journal of Public Health,* 92, 92–98.

Wang, P. S., Lane, M., Olfson, M., Pincus, H. A., Wells, K. B., & Kessler, R. C. (2005). Twelve-month use of mental health services in the United States: Results from the national comorbidity survey replication. *Archives of General Psychiatry, 62*, 629–640.

Wing, J. K. (2009). *Reasoning about madness* (reissued, with a new introduction by David Mechanic). New Brunswick, NJ: Transaction Publishers.

8 Legislating social policy
Mental illness, the community, and the law

John Petrila, Jeffrey Swanson

Introduction

Most people with mental illnesses reside in the community. Evidence-based treatments now enable many with even the most serious mental illnesses to have sustained community tenure. Recovery from mental illness, rather than symptom reduction, has become the primary focus of treatment, and there is an emerging emphasis on person-centered care. However, care is often inadequate and unavailable. Even when services exist, many people have difficulty obtaining access because of poverty and lack of health insurance (Cunningham, McKenzie, & Taylor, 2006), and the great majority of people who obtain services do not receive evidence-based care (Drake, Bond, & Essock, 2009). Thus, the question of how to create and assure access to adequate treatment capacity is a significant challenge for public policy.

Despite some advances in the public's understanding of mental illness, the public's fear of "the mentally ill" as dangerous remains entrenched (Pescosolido, Monahan, Link, Stueve, & Kikuzawa, 1999) and in fact may have hardened over the years in response to incidents like the killings at Virginia Tech in 2007 (Bonnie, Reinhard, Hamilton, & McGarvey, 2009). As a result, policymakers concerned with public safety have extended the use of coercion to the community; protection of the public, rather than access to care, often dominates policy discussions.

Resolving the issues of access to quality care, public safety, and the use of coercion plays out in an environment in which mental health systems have dramatically eroded and fragmented in many communities. The assessment and treatment of mental illnesses now occurs in multiple settings, such as the school, justice, and social welfare systems. For example, it is estimated that more than two million people booked into U.S. jails in a year may have a serious mental illness (Steadman, Osher, Robbins, Case, & Samuels, 2009), and in many communities, judges have assumed mental health policymaking roles (Petrila & Redlich, 2008). The complex role of law as a social policy tool to address all of these challenges is the subject of this chapter.

The role of law

The law plays an integral role in shaping the environment in which community services are delivered. Indeed, the law has helped shape mental health policy in the U.S. for more than 50 years, beginning with legal challenges to a state hospital-dominated service system. Today, however, the core question is how to provide access to community care for those with serious mental illnesses in a fragmented, disconnected service system. Creation of sufficient treatment capacity is crucial, and yet the availability of services alone does not assure their use. In the context of community-based management of mental illness and disability, treatment non-adherence and discontinuity are critical problems that contribute to poor long-term outcomes in the affected populations and may in some cases increase risk to public safety. Accordingly, new tools of "leverage" are being used in the legal and social welfare systems in an effort to engage people in treatment; the underlying assumption is that treatment over time will reduce rehospitalization, involvement in the criminal justice system, and risk to the public. These tools of leverage include outpatient civil commitment, mental health courts and jail diversion programs, specialty probation, subsidized housing programs, representative payeeship for disability benefits, and psychiatric advance directives (Monahan, Redlich, Swanson, Robbins, Appelbaum, Petrila, et al., 2005). In each case, decision-makers attempt to use "the law" in some way to affect treatment outcomes while preserving public safety. These laws may work on a number of levels: by modifying social environments that affect the quality of life of people with mental illness; by motivating institutions, organizations, and systems that provide direct services to people with mental illnesses; and by constraining the individual behavior of people with mental illnesses.

Some of these tools are overtly coercive, while others seek to maximize individual autonomy and choice. Due to public perceptions regarding the dangerousness of people with mental illnesses, most policymakers assume that social control must be available to mental health clinicians acting in concert with legal authorities. At the same time, with the ascendant belief that patient-centered care is essential to recovery, most consumers (as well as policymakers and treatment providers) now assume that patient autonomy is a critical value. The inherent tension between these twin concerns – the individual's freedom and right to self-determination versus the exigencies of social control to manage public risk – creates a challenge for constructing social policy regarding the treatment of persons with mental illness at the population level, as well as for making clinical decisions at the individual level.

This chapter explores the use of several of these legal tools, including outpatient civil commitment, leveraging of disability entitlements to ensure treatment adherence, firearm restrictions applied to people with mental illness, psychiatric advance directives, the Americans with Disabilities Act, and the "criminalization" of mental illness. In doing so, we touch on other areas where the law has attempted to address questions of treatment non-adherence and discontinuity in care. We consider areas where federal and state legislatures have created social policy through statutory change, and we also look at the attempt of a system concerned primarily with public safety (the criminal justice system) to identify people with mental illnesses and divert them into treatment.

The role of research in community care and law

In each area discussed below, we also discuss recent research that sheds light on the comparative success of these legal efforts in developing social policies for people with mental illnesses in community settings. Research has influenced mental health policy at various times, particularly regarding the relationship, if any, between mental illness and violence. Social scientists have held competing views regarding this relationship. On the one hand, the tradition of social-psychiatric epidemiology has addressed the problem within a public health framework, using survey research tools and clinical assessment to identify risk and protective factors for violence (e.g., Swanson, Holzer, Ganju, & Jono, 1990; Steadman, Mulvey, Monahan, Robbins, Appelbaum, Grisso, et al., 1998; Monahan et al., 2005; Catalano & McConnell, 1996). This line of scientific work has been driven largely by an applied policy-research agenda of protecting the public; the goal has been to understand violence and mental illness for the purpose of improving risk assessment and risk management. On the other hand, the tradition of the sociology of deviance and social control has studied public perceptions of the link between mental illness and violence to understand how society labels, represents, and responds to deviance; the nature and function of social stigma; and how perceptions of dangerousness may produce social discrimination (Goffman, 1963; Link & Phelan, 2001; Corrigan, Watson, Byrne, & Davis, 2005; Pescosolido, Olafsdottir, & McLeod, 2007) For this tradition, the applied research agenda has been driven largely by a reform concern for the civil rights, autonomy, and well-being of individuals diagnosed with mental illness, rather than a focus on protecting the public from such persons. Each of these perspectives and the tension between them has shaped the development of legal principles applied to people with mental illnesses. Patients' violence risk is not the only issue of concern to mental health law and policy, of course; systemic factors and the behavior of other parties (such as the police, or probation officers) are also the province of law and policy, and research has begun to examine how these variables may affect outcomes such as public safety and access to care for people with mental illness.

We begin this discussion by briefly describing legal challenges to the state hospital system and to medically oriented civil commitment statutes. These challenges resulted in the establishment of a legal framework for the use of coercion that still influences legislative and judicial thinking.

Setting the stage: state hospitals, the U.S. Constitution, and civil commitment law

The first broad application of law to the treatment of people with mental illnesses emerged in response to abuses in state psychiatric facilities. The policy of using separate asylums to treat mental illness rested on the benevolent philosophy of "moral treatment" and assumed that "insanity" could best be treated in small asylums in pastoral settings, with good hygiene and diet, occupational activities, medical care, and religious practice (Tuke, 2009/1813). However, by the middle of the 20th century, the census of state hospitals had exploded, and in 1955, state psychiatric hospitals housed 558,922 individuals in a nation of 166 million people (Appelbaum, 1994). Some of these institutions were virtual cities. For example, Pilgrim Psychiatric Center, the largest, housed 13,875 patients at its peak. As they grew in size, many of these institutions became unsafe, understaffed, and overcrowded. Overdrugging was routine, with dangerous side effects, and people could spend decades confined, lost to the outside world.

People often came to these institutions through involuntary civil commitment. States historically have had broad authority to use civil commitment, and in the 1960s, most state statutes used a medical model of commitment. Individuals could be committed indefinitely on the certification of a physician that the person had a mental illness; independent review of the need for continuing confinement was virtually non-existent, and people could be (and sometimes were) confined for life.

By the late 1960s, civil rights lawyers took note of conditions in state hospitals and began challenging both the medically-oriented civil commitment statutes that provided a gate into these institutions and the often dangerous conditions in which people were confined. Scores of lawsuits were brought, asserting that states were violating fundamental constitutional rights to liberty and due process. Courts were sympathetic to these challenges and found that states routinely violated the constitutional rights of people with mental illnesses. In response, courts ordered states to improve conditions in state institutions and in some cases assumed control over the administration of those facilities. In addition, and most important here, states were directed to revise their civil commitment laws (*Lessard vs. Schmidt*, 1971, is the seminal case on this issue). People subject to commitment were given several rights usually associated with criminal proceedings, including the right to counsel, the right to present evidence, and the right to an impartial decision-maker, typically a judge. This marked a significant shift from the more medically oriented commitment laws of the era. In addition, states were ordered to revise the substantive criteria for commitment contained in statute. A finding of mental illness was no longer legally sufficient to commit someone. Rather, the person also had to be a danger to his or her self or others due to mental illness. As a result of these decisions, most states rewrote their civil commitment laws. A legal framework based on individual constitutional rights, rather than medical paternalism, became the statutory norm.

Mandated community treatment: Deinstitutionalization and the emergence of oupatient civil commitment

These rulings were one of many factors that contributed to the continuous depopulation of state hospitals from the mid-1950s onward. New psychotropic medications, changes in financing rules that permitted reimbursement for various types of community care, and changing treatment philosophies also were important drivers of deinstitutionalization (Gelman, 1997; Mechanic & Rochefort, 1990). The decline in state hospital census over 50 years was dramatic. In 2003, even with the rate of deinstitutionalization slowing (Salzter, Kaplan, & Atay, 2006), state hospitals held fewer than 50,000 people – down from over a half million in the mid 1950s (Manderscheid, Atay, & Crider, 2009).

While deinstitutionalization became the centerpiece of mental health policy, it was almost immediately judged a failure, largely because of inadequate community treatment resources (General Accounting Office, 1977; President's Commission on Mental Health, 1978). Over time, advocates for people with mental illnesses brought lawsuits designed to create legal entitlements to community care and housing, but those efforts were largely unsuccessful as courts ruled that neither federal nor state law mandated states to create such services (Klapper, 1993).

As deinstitutionalization proceeded apace, homelessness increased dramatically and became much more visible in every major urban area in the U.S. A complex problem, with many social and economic causes, homelessness emerged as a dominant public concern in the 1980s. Two widespread assumptions about the problem led to important consequences for mental health policy and law. First, many policymakers assumed that deinstitutionalization caused homelessness and thus concluded that most people who were homeless were also mentally ill. Second, based on the first assumption, many believed that the increase in homelessness necessarily would result in an increase in random acts of violence against the public and the degradation of urban environments. As a result, some argued that expanding the reach of civil commitment laws to community settings was an appropriate policy response to these issues (Torrey, 1997; Torrey & Zdanowicz, 2001).

Visible homelessness and the perceived dangerousness of people with mental illness, coupled with the increasingly costly problem of revolving-door admissions of "noncompliant" patients to state psychiatric and community hospitals, helped to fuel a movement to adopt outpatient commitment laws throughout the U.S. While outpatient commitment statutes vary, they all permit courts to order certain people who are diagnosed with mental illness and reside in the community to comply with court-imposed treatment conditions. Statutorily specified findings are necessary before a person can be committed to outpatient care. For example, many statutes require that the person be unwilling to seek treatment voluntarily, that the person have a history of "failed" treatment, and that resources are available to provide the necessary treatment. If the person fails to adhere to treatment, he or she may be removed to an inpatient facility for further assessment.

Courts have ruled that these statutes meet federal and state constitutional standards (see, for example, *In re K.L.*, 2004, upholding New York's statute, popularly called Kendra's Law). Such decisions are striking because they shift the legal framework for civil commitment back in the direction of more medically oriented criteria. For example, the New York Court of Appeals in *In re K.L.* (2004) explicitly endorsed state intervention to guard against prospective relapse, writing:

> The state's interest in immediately removing from the streets noncompliant patients previously found to be, as a result of their noncompliance, at risk of a relapse or deterioration likely to result in serious harm to themselves or others is quite strong. The state has a further interest in warding off the longer periods of hospitalization that, as the Legislature has found, tend to accompany relapse or deterioration.
>
> (p. 487)

Single jurisdiction studies of outpatient civil commitment, also known as assisted outpatient treatment (AOT), have examined the impact of this legal intervention on rehospitalization and involvement with the criminal justice system. In North Carolina, research found that extended involuntary outpatient commitment (six months or more) combined with intensive mental health services in the community reduced hospitalizations (Swartz, Swanson, Wagner, Burns, Hiday, & Borum, 1999), violent behavior (Swanson, Swartz, Borum, Hiday, Wagner, & Burns, 2000), arrests (Swanson, Borum, Swartz, Hiday, Wagner, & Burns, 2001), and criminal victimization (Hiday, Swanson, Swartz, Wagner, & Borum, 2002); improved treatment adherence (Swartz, Swanson, Wagner, Burns, & Hiday, 2001); and improved subjective quality of life for people with serious mental disorders (Swanson, Swartz, Elbogen, Wagner, & Burns, 2003). The most important finding was that neither treatment nor a court order alone had these effects, but both treatment and judicial involvement were essential. A more recent study of Kendra's Law (New York's AOT law) resulted in similar findings on hospitalization and re-arrest and also found that people on AOT had increased levels of services such as intensive case management and appropriate medication (Swartz, Swanson, Steadman, Robbins, & Monahan, 2009).

While research suggests that outpatient commitment can be effective, implementation often has been difficult. A multi-state study found that outpatient commitment is used principally by inpatient facilities discharging people to the community (Ridgely, Borum, & Petrila, 2001; see also Christy, Petrila, McCranie, & Lotts, 2009). The Ridgely, et al. study also identified numerous barriers to implementation, including a lack of treatment resources, insufficient housing, transportation problems, and disinterest on the part of law enforcement and treatment providers in engaging in a time-consuming court process. As a result of these and related issues, outpatient commitment use is inconsistent in the U.S. While used extensively in New York, a state that appropriated substantial resources for implementation, it is seldom used in Florida and California, two of the four largest states in the country (Petrila & Christy, 2008; Appelbaum, 2003).

Community tenure: Money and housing mandates

Outpatient commitment has drawn the most attention in the debate regarding the use of coercion in community settings. However, clinicians, judges, family, and other decision-makers sometimes use leverage in other areas to ensure adherence to treatment. For example, in a study of 1,011 psychiatric outpatients in public mental health outpatient programs in five sites throughout the U.S., Monahan and colleagues found that between 23 and 40% of participants across the sites reported that access to housing had been made contingent on treatment compliance (Monahan et al., 2005). This meant that of all forms of leverage studied, housing was the most commonly utilized. The use of leverage was more likely to occur in "special" housing, available only to people with mental illnesses and designed explicitly to provide treatment with housing (Robbins, Petrila, LeMelle, & Monahan, 2006). However, residents in special housing and in housing-first programs (that is, housing for people with mental illnesses where treatment participation is not mandatory) reported no significant differences in overall satisfaction with their residence (Robbins, Callahan, & Monahan, 2009).

In addition, approximately 7 to 19% of respondents in the five-site study reported that they had an experience in which access to money was made contingent on treatment compliance. The law provides a number of formal mechanisms for transferring control of money from a person who lacks capacity to another decision-maker. Two examples include guardianship and the establishment of a representative payee. A representative payee may be appointed when an individual becomes incapable of managing Social Security or Supplemental Security Income (SSI) payments (for a description, see www.ssa.gov/payee). Family members and clinicians often become representative payees, and in a study of 50 dyads of consumers with psychiatric disabilities and family members acting as representative payees, Elbogen, Ferron, Swartz, Wilder, Swanson, and Wagner (2007) found that the majority of consumers and family members believed that the arrangement led to enhanced living stability. However, 36% of consumers and 50% of payees reported conflicts over money, and many payees lacked basic money management knowledge and skills. Another study of 205 adult patients in a large urban community mental health center found that 53% of patients had a money manager or payee, and

79% of this group had a clinician as a payee. A large percentage (40%) of those with a clinician payee reported that they believed that the payee had conditioned access to and use of money on treatment adherence; the authors concluded that when a clinician acted as payee, it appeared to increase the risk of conflict in the therapeutic relationship because of the clinician's use of money as a source of leverage (Angell, Martinez, Mahoney, & Corrigan, 2007).

In summary, the law provides a number of ways for judges, clinicians, and family members to condition access to a presumably desired good (freedom, housing, money) on a person's compliance with community-based treatment. Available research suggests that outpatient commitment, perhaps the most formally coercive of these tools, can increase participation in community-based treatment, as well as reduce hospitalizations and arrests in some circumstances, but a variety of problems create barriers to implementing outpatient commitment statutes. Research on leveraged housing suggests that individuals in special housing for people with mental illnesses are more likely to perceive themselves as coerced (though overall satisfaction with housing is not reduced), while representative payee relationships may give rise to conflict within families and may contaminate the therapeutic relationship when a clinician acts as payee. In the criminal justice system, coercion is an even more explicit part of the lives of people with mental illnesses, a topic discussed in the next section.

Mandated treatment: The criminal justice system

As a result of federal and state legislative policies, the U.S. has the highest rate of incarceration in the world. In 1972, 160 of every 100,000 people in the U.S. were incarcerated. By 1997, 645 of every 100,000 people were confined, and by 2007, that number had increased to 775 per 100,000 – a rate five to seven times that in other Western countries (Kennedy, 2003; Tonry, 2008).

As arrest and incarceration rates have risen sharply, the number of people with serious mental illnesses in the criminal justice system has increased dramatically as well. In a recent study of a sample of 822 inmates in two Maryland and three New York jails, use of the Structured Clinical Interview for *Diagnostic and Statistical Manual of Mental Disorders, Fourth Edition* (DSM-IV) (SCID) showed that 14.5% of male and 31% of female inmates had a current serious mental illness (Steadman et al., 2009). Assuming similar prevalence among all arrestees, Steadman and colleagues infer that more than two million people with serious mental illnesses are booked into U.S. jails in a given year. Overall prevalence of mental illness and substance abuse disorders among people in correctional facilities approaches 80% and may be even higher for juveniles (Teplin, Abram, McClellan, & Dulcan, 2002).

While federal and state correctional policies have been responsible for increasing the size of the population under control of the justice system, local jurisdictions have increasingly developed their own strategies to address the needs of large numbers of justice-involved people with mental illnesses. There has been a particular emphasis on diverting people from the criminal justice system into treatment, though the point at which diversion occurs and the amount of continuing control exercised over the person varies. In some cases, diversion occurs prior to booking the person for an offense. The goal of pre-booking diversion is to provide access to appropriate care without formal involvement of the criminal justice system (Hartford, Carey, & Mendonca, 2006). Insofar as these strategies often depend on police officers identifying people who might be appropriate for diversion, changing police practice has been a particular focus. A notable example is Crisis Intervention Training (CIT). Developed in Memphis, this training rests on a standardized 40-hour curriculum for police officers. The curriculum instructs officers about mental illness, local treatment resources, and techniques for identifying and apprehending people with mental illnesses in ways that minimize the prospect of violence and enhance opportunities to access the treatment system (National Alliance for the Mentally Ill, 2010). CIT has become very popular, and there is evidence that it can be effective in diverting people with serious mental illnesses into treatment when they might otherwise have been arrested (Teller, Munetz, Gill, & Ritter, 2006).

While CIT attempts to change the behavior of police officers, diversion strategies used after the person is arrested often involve judges as decision-makers. As a result, the courts have become the locus of considerable innovation. Therapeutic courts, including drug courts and mental health courts, have multiplied over the past two decades. The first drug court was created in Dade County, Florida, in 1989, in response to the "war on drugs" that drove many new first-time offenders into the criminal justice system. Designed to divert non-violent defendants with substance abuse-related charges into judicially supervised treatment, drug courts have now become a familiar part of the judicial landscape, with 2,140 courts in operation and another 284 in development or planning (Office of National Drug Control Policy, 2009). Mental health courts emerged a decade later and today there are more than 250 mental health courts, and the number is growing (Raines & Laws, 2009). While participation in treatment is voluntary, courts retain the option to sanction a person for non-adherence to treatment and other conditions imposed by the court. In this respect, therapeutic courts represent another effort to blend respect for the person's autonomy (through voluntary agreement to enter the court) with the use of leverage (the court's use of jail and other sanctions) to achieve the twin goals of access to care and protection of public safety.

There is evidence that therapeutic courts can be effective for at least some individuals. Drug courts in particular appear to reduce recidivism rates (United States Government Accountability Office, 2005), and while the evidence on mental health courts is sketchier, single-site studies suggest that mental health courts may increase access to services while reducing time to arrest and time spent in jail (Cosden, Ellen, Schnell, Yasmeen, & Wolfe, 2003; Poythress, Petrila, McGaha, & Boothroyd, 2002; Redlich, 2005; Ridgely, Engberg, Greenberg, Turner, DeMartini, & Dembosky, 2007).

Other people enter treatment after conviction for a crime, as a condition of sentencing. Probation and parole officers exercise social control, and today there are more than five million people in the U.S. on probation or parole (Pew Center on the States, 2009), many with serious mental illnesses. Just as the growing number of people with serious mental illnesses in the criminal justice system has caused changes in police and judicial behavior, a number of jurisdictions in the U.S. have adopted specialty probation programs for probationers with mental illnesses. The touchstone of such programs is specialized training and a reduced caseload for the specialty probation officer, who then monitors compliance with both the ordinary conditions of probation and special conditions regarding mental health treatment.

Do these interventions work, and if so, how? What is the mechanism by which specialty probation can improve mental health and/or criminal justice outcomes for mentally ill offenders on probation? According to Skeem, Eno Louden, Polasheck, & Cap (2007); Skeem & Manchak (2008); and Skeem, Eno Louden, Manchak, Vidal, & Haddad (2009), there are significant differences between regular and specialty mental health probation in the manner in which violations are handled (traditional probation officers are more likely to report violations than specialty officers), as well as the characteristics of the relationship between the officer and probationer. Specifically, the investigators found evidence that the quality of the relationship between specialty officers and probationers was the key mechanism that resulted in improved compliance with the conditions of probation as well as the reduction in violations for those on specialty probation. As with outpatient commitment and therapeutic courts, specialty probation may be effective in increasing access to care; in addition, probation officers with specialized mental health caseloads appear to achieve better mental health and criminal justice outcomes for probationers.

In each of the examples provided above, police, judges, and probation officers adopt roles that are at least in part explicitly therapeutic. Skeem's work suggests that the relationship between the legal decision maker and person with mental illness is critical to attaining the policy goals of access to care with reduced public risk. Exploring this in more detail, in the context of probation as well as judge- and police-based interventions is an important research question for the future.

Laws restricting access to firearms for people with mental illness

Federal and state laws restricting access to firearms for people with a history of involuntary commitment or other mental health adjudication provide another timely example of legislating social policy and the need to balance protection of individual rights with risk to public safety. Individuals with a history of involuntary psychiatric hospitalization have been legally disqualified from purchasing firearms for over 40 years, since the enactment of the Omnibus Crime Control and Safe Streets Act and the Gun Control Act in 1968. However, it was not until 1998, with the implementation of the National Instant Criminal Background Check System (NICS), mandated by the 1993 Brady Handgun Violence Prevention Act, that a potentially effective and comprehensive method emerged for enforcing restrictions on gun purchases from federally licensed dealers by persons with disqualifying conditions. In January 2008, in the wake of the shootings at Virginia Tech, the Brady Handgun Violence Prevention Act was amended by the National Instant Criminal Background Check System Improvement Act (NICSIA) to essentially require states to report to the federal registry all persons legally barred from possessing or purchasing a handgun, including those with disqualifying mental health records. The NICSIA also requires states to create relief-from-disabilities programs, providing people with mental illness who are excluded from firearms purchase the opportunity to apply for relief from that exclusion (Appelbaum & Swanson, 2010).

Without denying that gun violence is a major public health problem in the U.S. – firearms kill some 50,000 people annually (Centers for Disease Control and Prevention (CDC), 2010a, 2010b) – there are, nevertheless, serious questions about whether current gun restrictions as they apply to persons with mental illness constitute a rational policy. Epidemiological evidence suggests that only 3 to 5% of violent acts may be attributable to mental illness and most do not involve guns (Swanson, 1994). Whether the categories of persons with mental illness affected by the laws actually pose a significantly higher risk of gun violence is unknown. Criminogenic risk factors affect people with and without mental illness alike, and gun restrictions already apply to those with felony convictions. Do laws that base gun restrictions specifically on mental health history confer additional public safety benefit, i.e., beyond the effect of restrictions based on criminal history? Does the social and legal presumption of increased risk of gun violence in people with mental illness bear unintended consequences – perhaps unnecessarily infringing on the civil liberties of some people with mental illness, reinforcing the negative stereotype of dangerousness that perpetuates stigma and discrimination, increasing reliance on involuntary commitment, and incurring public costs in collecting, managing, and reporting disqualifying mental health records? Solid research is needed to examine whether these policies are achieving their intended social benefit in protecting the public or whether they might be doing more harm than good.

Expanding autonomy: Psychiatric advance directives

In contrast to coercion and leverage, psychiatric advance directives (PADs) are an effort to expand patient choice. The introduction of PADs is regarded as one of the more significant developments in U.S. mental health law and policy in recent years (Appelbaum, 1991; 2004; Srebnik & Lafond 1999; Winick, 1996; Swanson, Swartz, Elbogen, Van Dorn, Wagner, McCauley, & Kim, 2006). Thomas Szasz in 1982 proposed the "psychiatric will" as a way to legally protect patients against unwanted mental health intervention; the origin of PADs thus resonates with the civil rights focus of the constitutional era of mental health law. However, PADs also have origins in medical advance directives, powers of attorney for healthcare, and "living wills" for end-of-life care.

While most states prior to the 1990s had statutory provisions for medical advance directives, interest in and use of these instruments increased dramatically following the U.S. Supreme Court's decision in *Cruzan* v. *Director, Missouri Dept. of Health* (1990), which dictated that "clear and convincing evidence" was needed of patients' wishes in order to withdraw life-sustaining treatment. Soon thereafter, Congress enacted the federal Patient Self-Determination Act (PSDA) (Omnibus Budget Reconciliation Act, 1990) to promote the use of written advance directives (ADs). The PSDA requires healthcare facilities receiving federal funds to ask patients upon admission whether they have executed an AD and to inform patients of their rights to prepare one (Greco, Schulman, Lavizzo-Mourey, & Hansen-Flaschen, 1991).

In the wake of the PSDA, mental health consumer advocates appropriated ADs and applied these instruments to the context of decisional incapacity associated with psychiatric crises. Persons with serious mental illnesses were seen to be particularly vulnerable to loss of autonomy and at risk of receiving unwanted interventions during times of mental health crisis and thus seemed to be a logical target population for this legal intervention (Kapp, 1994; Hoge, 1994; Backlar, 1995). However, while medical ADs applied mainly to end-of-life care, PADs were designed to promote recovery. In contrast to the singular event of death, the episodic nature of incapacity in severe mental illness may provide the affected person with valuable experience regarding what to expect and how best to manage future psychiatric crises (Backlar, 1997, Halpern & Szmukler, 1997).

Twenty-six states have enacted specific PAD statutes. Clearly, expansion of PAD legislation and policy in the U.S. was driven in part by mental health consumer advocacy organizations' resistance to legal coercion in mental health care (California Protection and Advocacy, Inc., 2001). Concern over the expansion of coercion or "leverage" in community-based care (Monahan et al., 2005) led to a broadened view of PADs' potential role as an antidote or remedy for coercion – an alternative vehicle for "self-directed care" (Srebnik & La Fond, 1999; Srebnik, Russo, Sage, Peto, & Zick, 2003). Specifically, advocates hoped that PADs would give persons with severe mental illness greater control over their own treatment, decreasing the need for involuntary interventions (Appelbaum, 1991; 2004; Winick, 1996).

A study funded by the MacArthur Network on Mandated Community Treatment in five U.S. cities (combined N = 1,011) found a large latent demand for these legal instruments (Swanson, Swartz, Ferron, Elbogen, & Van Dorn, 2006). The study reported that PADs were completed by only 4 to 13% of mental health consumers sampled from public-sector outpatient treatment, yet large majorities – 66 to 77% – indicated that they would want to complete PADs if given the opportunity and necessary assistance.

Despite this apparent interest on the part of consumers, the expected widespread use of PADs has yet to materialize, due to skepticism and lack of familiarity with PADs by clinicians, slow progress in implementing and integrating them into routine care, and lack of resources to assist consumers in preparing PADs (Van Dorn, Swartz, Elbogen, Swanson, Kim, Ferron, et al., 2006). These barriers are not insurmountable: A large, longitudinal implementation trial in North Carolina found that a formal, structured intervention to facilitate PADs can help consumers with serious mental illness understand and complete legal PADs, and completed facilitated PADs tend to contain treatment instructions that comport with clinical standards of care as well as consumers' personal goals for treatment (Swanson et al., 2006; Elbogen, Ferron, Swartz, Wilder, Swanson, & Wagner, 2007).

Evidence to date suggests that PADs, if widely implemented, could improve the health of the population with mental illness (Swanson, Swartz, Elbogen, Van Dorn, Wagner, Moser, et al., 2008.) However, far more needs to be learned about how best to facilitate PAD completion, especially within fiscally constrained mental health care systems. Information is lacking in how to overcome barriers to PADs at the clinician level as well as the consumer level. Research is needed to better identify the populations that could most benefit from PADs and under what conditions. Also needed is research regarding the mechanisms – the pathways of effect – by which PADs may benefit consumers, and whether subgroups of interest, such as those under mandated community treatment, may benefit differentially.

Expanded opportunities and access to care: Americans with Disabilities Act

The 1990 Americans with Disabilities Act (ADA) is another important example of the use of law to pursue a broad social policy that may improve the lives of people with mental illness. The ADA was intended to eliminate disability as a basis of discrimination in employment and access to public services – a goal that makes the ADA the most important civil rights legislation since the original civil rights bills passed in the 1960s. At the time of passage, Congress estimated that approximately 43 million Americans had a physical or mental disability covered by the ADA (Melton, Petrila, Poythress, & Slobogin, 2007). Two applications of the legislation to people with mental illnesses in community settings are relevant here: The first is in the context of employment, and the second is in the pursuit of a legal remedy for attaining access to services. Each is discussed below.

If a person has a mental disability, as defined by the ADA, and can perform the essential functions of the job, the ADA requires that the employer make reasonable accommodation if necessary to enable the person to overcome the effects of the disability. Mental disability is one of the leading causes of complaints under the ADA, and given the stigma associated with mental illness, a reasonable empirical question is whether claims based on mental impairment are treated similarly to claims based on physical impairments. A study by Swanson, Burris, Moss, Ullman, and Ranney (2006) addressed this latter question by comparing characteristics, perceptions, legal processes, and outcomes in litigation for persons with psychiatric and non-psychiatric disabilities who filed employment discrimination lawsuits under Title I of the ADA from 1993 to 2001. The study found that people with psychiatric disability fared significantly worse in employment discrimination lawsuits than their counterparts with non-psychiatric disabilities, controlling for other significant predictors of litigation outcome. Plaintiffs with mental impairments were also significantly less satisfied with the overall process of filing a discrimination claim and filing a lawsuit under the ADA. The study did not show *why* these differences exist, but the findings are important in the context of larger public attitudes about mental illnesses.

While employees with mental disabilities appear to fare less well than those with physical disabilities in pursuing ADA claims, all employees were affected by a series of decisions by the U.S. Supreme Court that narrowed the application of the ADA and made it increasingly difficult for employees to prevail. Those decisions interpreted the ADA in a way that constricted the group of people who might be found to have a disability and thereby receive the protection of the Act. In response, Congress in 2008 enacted legislation designed to restore the ADA to its original intent (Petrila, 2009). These amendments may stimulate an increase in ADA claims for both physical and mental disabilities. Whether the seeming disparities in outcomes between the two types of claims persist is a subject for further research.

The ADA has also been the basis of litigation designed to assure access to community services for people who are confined despite the judgment of their treatment providers that they are appropriate for treatment in community settings. In *Olmstead* v. *L.C.* (1999), the U.S. Supreme Court held that such confinement can constitute illegal segregation under the ADA. In its decision, the Court's majority was forthright in its description of the harm caused by inappropriate institutional confinement. While *Olmstead* also created defenses for state government that has slowed broad application of the Court's ruling, newly decided cases may presage the development of a right to community-based care that goes beyond what the federal courts historically have been willing to countenance. Thus, *Olmstead* merits discussion.

In *Olmstead,* two residents of a Georgia psychiatric facility brought a lawsuit arguing that their continued confinement violated the ADA because treatment staff had determined that community placement was appropriate and yet they had not been placed. The U.S. Supreme Court, in a six to three decision, agreed. Justice Ginsburg, for the majority, wrote that under the ADA:

> states are required to place persons with mental disabilities in community settings rather than in institutions when the State's treatment professionals have determined that community placement is appropriate, the transfer from institutional care to a less restrictive setting is not opposed by the affected individual, and the placement can be reasonably accommodated, taking into account the resources available to the State and the needs of others with mental disabilities.
>
> (p. 607)

In supporting its conclusion, the Court described the impact of forced institutionalization of people who could live in community settings:

> First, institutional placement of persons who can handle and benefit from community settings perpetuates unwarranted assumptions that persons so isolated are incapable or unworthy of participating in community life ... Second, confinement in an institution severely diminishes the everyday life activities of individuals, including family relations, social contacts, work options, economic independence, educational advancement, and cultural enrichment ... In order to receive needed medical services, persons with mental disabilities must, because of those disabilities, relinquish participation in community life they could enjoy given reasonable accommodations, while persons without mental disabilities can receive the medical services they need without similar sacrifice.
>
> (p. 600)

The Court provided states with a defense to claims that the ADA required community placement in individual cases, noting that the State's obligation was not boundless, that the ADA required the State to make only reasonable modifications, and that the State was not required to make modifications that fundamentally altered its services and programs. In its most important language regarding state duties, the Court wrote:

If, for example, the State were to demonstrate that it had a comprehensive, effectively working plan for placing qualified persons with mental disabilities in less restrictive settings, and a waiting list that moved at a reasonable pace not controlled by the State's endeavors to keep its institutions fully populated, the reasonable modifications standard would be met.

(pp. 605–606)

After the Court's decision, when confronted with similar claims the lower federal courts read *Olmstead* fairly narrowly, holding, for example, that the ADA did not obligate a state to create new resources or, in the context of Medicaid, to offer services not already offered under the State's Medicaid plan (Smith & Calandrillo, 2001). Courts did order community placement for individuals confined to nursing homes, facilities for people with mental retardation and developmental disabilities, and psychiatric facilities, but typically ruled in favor of states that appeared to be making active efforts to effectuate change even when individuals were on waiting lists for services for years (Rosenbaum & Teitelbaum, 2004).

However, in September, 2009, a federal judge in New York put aside this judicial reticence and issued the most expansive ruling ever made in a case involving access to community services for people with mental illnesses. In *Disability Advocates* v. *Paterson* (2009), Judge Garaufis ruled that the state had discriminated against more than 4,300 individuals living in large, private group homes licensed by the state when it did not provide them with the opportunity to move into apartments and homes of their own, with appropriate social services and mental health treatment. The court described the adult homes as institutions that segregate residents from the community and impede interactions with people without disabilities. The homes in question are very large; the court noted that there were 28 adult homes with more than 120 beds per home at issue in the case. After a lengthy recitation of facts supporting its conclusion that confinement to adult homes in the circumstances of the case constituted illegal segregation, the court turned to the State's defense that it would have to fundamentally alter its program and services to accommodate the needs of the plaintiffs. The court rejected these arguments, finding that New York did not have an *Olmstead* plan in place. While the court acknowledged that the State would have to develop additional supported housing to place the 4,300 individuals living in the affected adult homes, the court also found that this would not require additional spending by the State.

The court directed the parties to propose remedies to implement its order. On March 1, 2010, the court rejected the State's proposal to develop 1,000 alternative placements over six years, a proposal the U.S. Department of Justice characterized as "unreasonable and inadequate." Instead, the court directed the State to develop placements for all of the individuals in the relevant adult homes (www.bazelon.org/In-Court/Current-Cases/Disability-Advocates-Inc.-v.-Paterson.aspx). At the time of writing, the State had appealed the district court's decision to a federal court of appeals, and one may reasonably anticipate that the case will go to the U.S. Supreme Court. Judge Garaufis has ordered relief that goes far beyond any *Olmstead* related decision, and so his order may not stand. However, if it does, it will transform the ADA into a system-changing tool for people in various residential settings seeking access to more "normalized" services and residences.

Conclusion

As this chapter illustrates, law has affected mental health policy in a number of ways. While the law can construct social policies designed to accomplish certain aims, the implementation of those policies comes down to multiple decisions by patients, treatment providers, and other officials in systems where the assessment and treatment of mental illness have become important tasks, largely by default.

A fundamental issue in creating community care systems is assuring universal and voluntary access to care, a task the law has approached with only limited success. Paradoxically, perhaps, law has been much better at codifying standards for using coercion and other forms of leverage in efforts to induce treatment adherence. Part of policymakers' long-standing willingness to permit coercion of people with mental illness is based on the public perception that mental illness poses a threat to public safety. However, coercion can only do so much. Its efficacy is limited by many things, including the lack of treatment resources that in some cases give rise to its use.

Providing adequate public resources to ensure access to evidence-based mental health treatment for all those in need is a worthy aspiration but one that has eluded policymakers even in less challenging economic environments than the present. However, even if adequate resources were suddenly to appear, there will always be individuals who do not want treatment, who discontinue treatment prematurely, and who pose a risk to themselves or others. Clearly, more efficacious and tolerable pharmacotherapies are needed, along with psychosocial interventions that will effectively engage people with psychiatric disorders and disabilities in meaningful recovery on their own terms. At the same time, an important research task for the future is to better understand why people decline or discontinue treatment for serious mental illnesses and the strategies that clinicians and other decision-makers can use to induce people to accept treatment. On occasion, that may include the use of various forms of leverage or coercion. Gaining better understanding of these issues empirically in turn will inform policymakers interested in broader questions of creating treatment capacity that maximizes the number of people willing to use it, without coercion.

Acknowledgments

This chapter is part of a larger work commissioned as part of the *Theory, Practice and Evidence Series* of the Public Health Law Research Program, a national program of the Robert Wood Johnson Foundation.

References

Angell, B., Martinez, N. I., Mahoney, C. A., & Corrigan, P. W. (2007). Payeeship, financial leverage, and the client-provider relationship. *Psychiatric Services, 58*, 365–372.

Appelbaum, P. S. (1991). Advance directives for mental health treatment. *Hospital and Community Psychiatry, 42*, 983–984.

Appelbaum, P. S. (2004). Psychiatric advance directives and the treatment of committed patients. *Psychiatric Services, 55*, 751–752,763.

Appelbaum, P. S. (1994). *Almost a Revolution: Mental Health Law and the Limits of Change*. London: Oxford.

Appelbaum, P. S. (2003). Ambivalence codified: California's new outpatient commitment statute. *Psychiatric Services, 54*, 26–28.

Appelbaum, P. S., & Swanson, J. W. (2010). Gun laws and mental illness: How sensible are the current restrictions? *Psychiatric Services, 61*, 652–654.

Backlar, P. (1995). The longing for order: Oregon's Medical Advance Directive for Mental Health Treatment. *Community Mental Health Journal, 31*,103–108.

Backlar, P. (1997). Anticipatory planning for psychiatric treatment is not quite the same as planning for end-of-life care. *Community Mental Health Journal, 33*, 261–268.

Bonnie, R., Reinhard, J. S., Hamilton, P., & McGarvey, E. L. (2009). Mental health system transformation after the Virginia Tech tragedy. *Health Affairs, 28*, 793–804.

California Protection and Advocacy, Inc. (2001). *Advance Health Care Directives*. Sacramento: California Protection and Advocacy, Inc.

Catalano R. A., & McConnell W. (1996). A time-series test of the quarantine theory of involuntary commitment. *Journal of Health and Social Behavior, 37*, 381–387.

Centers for Disease Control and Prevention. (2010a). *WISQARS Leading Causes of Death Reports, 1999–2006*. Atlanta, GA: Centers for Disease Control and Prevention, National Center for Injury Prevention and Control. Retrieved from webappa.cdc.gov/sasweb/ncipc/leadcaus10.html.

Centers for Disease Control and Prevention. (2010b). *WISQARS Injury Mortality Reports, 1999–2006*. Atlanta, GA: Centers for Disease Control, National Center for Injury Prevention and Control. Retrieved from webappa.cdc.gov/sasweb/ncipc/mortrate10_sy.html.

Christy, A., Petrila, J., McCranie, M., & Lotts, V. (2009). Involuntary outpatient commitment in Florida: Case information and provider experience and opinions. *International Journal of Forensic Mental Health Services, 8*, 122–130.

Corrigan P. W., Watson A. C., Byrne P., & Davis K. E. (2005). Mental illness stigma: Problem of public health or social justice? *Social Work, 50*, 363–368.

Cosden, M., Ellens, J., Schnell, J., Yasmeen, Y., & Wolfe, M. (2003). Evaluation of a mental health treatment court with assertive community treatment. *Behavioral Sciences & the Law, 21*, 415–427.

Cruzan v. *Director* v. *Missouri Department of Health.* (1990). (497 U.S. 261).

Cunningham, P., McKenzie, K., & Taylor, E. F. (2006). The struggle to provide community-based care to low-income people with serious mental illnesses. *Health Affairs*, 694–705.

Drake, R. E., Bond, G. R., & Essock, S. M. (2009). Implementing evidence-based practices for people with schizophrenia. *Schizophrenia Bulletin, 35*, 704–713.

Eastern District of New York. (2009). *Disability Advocates* v. *Paterson* (03-CV-3209 [NGG]).

Elbogen, R. B., Ferron, J. C., Swartz, M. S., Wilder, C. M., Swanson, J. W., & Wagner, H. R. (2007). Characteristics of representative payeeship involving families of beneficiaries with psychiatric disabilities. *Psychiatric Services, 58*, 1433–1440.

Gelman, S. (1997). The law and psychiatry wars: 1960–1980. *California Western Law Review, 34*, 153–175.

General Accounting Office. (1977). *Returning the mentally disabled to the community: Government needs to do more.* Washington, DC: United States Government Printing Office.

Goffman E (1963). Stigma: Notes on the management of a spoiled identity. New York: Simon & Schuster.

Greco, P. J., Schulman, K. A., Lavizzo-Mourey, R., & Hansen-Flaschen, J. (1991). The Patient Self-Determination Act and the future of advance directives. *Annals of Internal Medicine, 115*, 639–643.

Halpern, A., & Szmukler, G. (1997). Psychiatric advance directives: Reconciling autonomy and non-consensual treatment. *Psychiatric Bulletin, 21*, 323–327.

Hartford, K., Carey, R., & Mendonca, J. (2006). Pre-arrest diversion of people with mental illness: Literature review and international survey. *Behavioral Sciences & the Law, 24*, 845–856.

Hiday, V. A., Swanson, J. W., Swartz, M. S., Wagner, H. R., & Borum, W. R. (2002). The impact of outpatient commitment on victimization of persons with severe mental illness. *American Journal of Psychiatry, 159*, 1403–1411.

Hoge, S. (1994). The Patient Self-Determination Act and psychiatric care. *Bulletin of the American Academy of Psychiatry & the Law, 22*, 577–586.

In re K.L. 806 N.E. 2d 480 (NY 2004). (2004).

Kapp, M. (1994). Implications of the Patient Self-Determination Act for psychiatric practice. *Hospital and Community Psychiatry, 45*, 355–358.

Kennedy, J. E. (2003). The new data: Over-representation of minorities in the criminal justice system: Drug wars in black and white. *Law & Contemporary Problems, 66*, 153–179.

Klapper, A. B. (1993). Finding a right in state constitutions for community treatment of the mentally ill. *University of Pennsylvania Law Review, 142*, 739–835.

Lessard v. *Schmidt*, 349 F. Supp. 1078 (1972).

Link B. G., & Phelan, J. (2001). Conceptualizing stigma. *Annual Review of Sociology, 27*, 363–385.

Manderscheid, R. W., Atay, J. E., & Crider, R. A. (2009). Changing trends in state psychiatric hospital use from 2002 to 2005. *Psychiatric Services, 60*, 29–34.

Mechanic, D., & Rochefort, D. A. (1990). Deinstitutionalization: An appraisal of reform. *Annual Review of Sociology, 16*, 301–327.

Melton, G. B., Petrila, J., Poythress, N. G., & Slobogin, C. (2007). *Psychological evaluations for the courts: A handbook for mental health professionals and lawyers* (3rd ed.). New York: Guilford.

Monahan, J., Redlich, A., Swanson, J., Robbins, P., Appelbaum, P., Petrila, J., et al. (2005). Use of leverage to improve adherence to psychiatric treatment in the community. *Psychiatric Services, 56*, 37–44.

National Alliance for the Mentally Ill. (2010). *Crisis Intervention Team Resource Center*. Retrieved from www.nami.org/template.cfm?section=CIT2.

Office of National Drug Control Policy. (2009). Drug courts. Retrieved from www.whitehousedrugpolicy.gov/enforce/drugcourt.html.

Olmstead v. *L.C.* (527 U.S. 581). (1999).

Pescosolido, B. A., Monahan, J., Link, B. G., Stueve, A., & Kikuzawa, S. (1999). The public's view of the competence, dangerousness, and need for legal coercion of persons with mental health problems. *American Journal of Public Health, 89*, 1339–1345.

Pescosolido, B. A., Olafsdottir, S., & McLeod, J. D. (2007). The construction of fear: Americans' preferences for social distances from children and adolescents with mental health problems. *JourSSnal of Health and Social Behavior, 48*, 50–67.

Petrila, J. (2009). Congress restores the Americans with Disabilities Act to its original intent. *Psychiatric Services, 60*, 878–879.

Petrila, J., & Christy, A. (2008). Florida's outpatient commitment law: A lesson in failed reform? *Psychiatric Services, 59*, 21–23.

Petrila, J., & Redlich, A. (2008). Mental illness and the courts: Some reflections on judges as innovators. *Court Review, 43*, 154–164.

PEW Center on the States. (2009). 1 in 31: The long reach of American Corrections. Retrieved from www.pewcenteronthestates.org/uploadedFiles/PSPP_1in31_report_FINAL_WEB_3-26-09.pdf.

Poythress, N., Petrila, J., McGaha, A., & Boothroyd, R. (2002). Perceived coercion and procedural justice in the Broward County Mental Health Court. *International Journal of Law and Psychiatry, 25*, 517–533.

President's Commission on Mental Health. (1978). *Report to the President from the President's Commission on Mental Health, Volume 1*. Washington DC: United States Government Printing Office.

Raines, J. B., & Laws, G. T. (2009). Mental health court survey. *Criminal Law Bulletin, 45*, 4.

Redlich, A. (2005). Voluntary, but knowing and intelligent: Comprehension in mental health courts. *Psychology, Public Policy, and the Law, 11*, 605–619.

Ridgely, M. S., Borum, R., & Petrila, J. (2001). *The Effectiveness of Involuntary Outpatient Treatment: Empirical Evidence and the Experience of Eight States*. Santa Monica: RAND.

Ridgely, M. S., Engberg, J., Greenberg, M. D., Turner, S., DeMartini, C., & Dembosky, J. W. (2007). *Justice, treatment, and cost: An evaluation of the fiscal impact of Allegheny County Mental Health Court*. Santa Monica: RAND.

Robbins, P. C., Callahan, L., & Monahan, J. (2009). Perceived coercion to treatment and housing satisfaction in housing-first and supportive housing programs. *Psychiatric Services, 60*, 1251–1253.

Robbins, P. C., Petrila, J., LeMelle, S., & Monahan, J. (2006). The use of housing as leverage to increase adherence to psychiatric treatment in the community. *Adminstration and Policy in Mental Health and Mental Health Services Research, 33*, 222–236.

Rosenbaum, S., & Teitelbaum, J. (2004). *Olmstead at Five: Assessing the Impact*. Kaiser Commission on Medicaid and the Uninsured. Retrieved from www.kff.org/medicaid/upload/Olmstead-at-Five-Assessing-the-Impact.pdf/.

Salzter, M. S., Kaplan, K., & Atay, J. (2006). State psychiatric hospital census after the 1999 Olmstead decision: Evidence of decelerating deinstitutionalization. *Psychiatric Services, 57*, 1501–1504.

Skeem, J., Eno Louden, J., Manchak, S., Vidal, S., & Haddad, E. (2009). Social networks and social control of probationers with co-occurring mental and substance abuse problems. *Law and Human Behavior, 33*, 122–135.

Skeem, J., & Manchak, S. (2008). Back to the future: From Klockars' model of effective supervision to evidence-based practice in probation. *International Journal of Offender Rehabilitation, 47*, 220–247.

Skeem, J., Eno Louden, J., Polasheck, & Cap, J. (2007). Relationship quality in mandated treatment: Blending care with control. *Psychological Assessment, 19*, 397–410.

Smith, J. D. E., & Calandrillo, S. P. (2001). Forward to fundamental alteration: Addressing ADA Title II integration lawsuits after *Olmstead* v. *L.C. Harvard Journal of Law and Public Policy, 24*, 695.

Srebnik, D., & LaFond, J. (1999). Advance directives for mental health services: current perspectives and future directions. *Psychiatric Services, 50*, 919–925.

Srebnik, D., Russo, J., Sage, J., Peto, T., & Zick, E. (2003). Interest in psychiatric advance directives among high users of crisis services and hospitalization. *Psychiatric Services, 54*, 981–986.

Steadman, H. J., Mulvey, E. P., Monahan, J., Robbins, P. C., Appelbaum, P. S., Grisso, T., Roth, L. H., & Silver, E. (1998). Violence by People Discharged From Acute Psychiatric Inpatient Facilities and by Others in the Same Neighborhoods. *Archive of General Psychiatry, 55*, 393–401.

Steadman, H. J., Osher, F., Robbins, P., Case, B., & Samuels, S. (2009). Prevalence of serious mental illnesses among jail inmates. *Psychiatric Services, 60*, 761–765.

Swanson, J. W. (1994). Mental disorder, substance abuse, and community violence: An epidemiological approach. In Monahan J and Steadman H (Eds.), *Violence and Mental Disorder* (pp. 101–136). Chicago, IL: University of Chicago Press.

Swanson, J. W, Borum, W. R, Swartz, M. S, Hiday, V. A, Wagner H. R, & Burns, B. J (2001). Can involuntary outpatient commitment reduce arrests among persons with severe mental illness? *Criminal Justice and Behavior, 28*, 156–189.

Swanson, J., Burris, S., Moss, K., Ullman, M. A., & Ranney, L. M. (2007). Justice Disparities: Does the ADA enforcement system treat persons with psychiatric disabilities fairly? *Maryland Law Review, 7*, 94–139.

Swanson, J., Holzer, C., Ganju, V., & Jono, R. (1990). Violence and psychiatric disorder in the community: evidence from the Epidemiologic Catchment Area Surveys. *Hospital and Community Psychiatry.* 41, 761–770.

Swanson, J. W., Swartz, M. S., Borum, R. B., Hiday, V. A., Wagner, H. R., & Burns, B. J. (2000). Involuntary out-patient commitment and reduction of violent behaviour in persons with severe mental illness. *British Journal of Psychiatry, 176*, 324–331.

Swanson, J. W., Swartz, M., Elbogen, E., Van Dorn, R., Wagner, H., McCauley, B., & Kim, M. (2006). Facilitated psychiatric advance directives: A randomized trial of an intervention to foster advance treatment planning among persons with severe mental illness. *American Journal of Psychiatry, 163*, 1943–1951.

Swanson, J. W., Swartz, M. S., Elbogen, E. B., Van Dorn, R. A., Wagner, H. R., Moser, L. A., Wilder, C., & Gilbert, A. R. (2008). Psychiatric advance directives and reduction of coercive crisis interventions. *Journal of Mental Health, 17*, 255–267.

Swanson, J. W, Swartz, M. S., Elbogen, E., Wagner, H. R, & Burns, B. J. (2003). Effects of involuntary outpatient commitment on subjective quality of life in persons with severe mental illness. *Behavioral Sciences and the Law, 21,* 473–491.

Swanson, J. W., Swartz, M. S., Ferron, J., Elbogen, E. B., & Van Dorn, R. A. (2006). Psychiatric advance directives among public mental health consumers in five United States cities: Prevalence, demand, and correlates. *Journal of American Academy of Psychiatry and the Law, 34,* 43–57.

Swartz, M., Swanson, J., Steadman, H., Robbins, P., & Monahan, J. (2009). *New York State Assisted Outpatient Treatment Program Evaluation.* Duke University School of Medicine. Durham, North Carolina.

Swartz, M., Swanson, J., Wagner, H. R., Burns, B., & Hiday, V. (2001). Effects of involuntary outpatient commitment and depot antipsychotics on treatment adherence in persons with severe mental illness. *Journal of Nervous and Mental Disease, 189,* 583–592.

Swartz, M. S., Swanson, J. W., Wagner, H. R., Burns, B. J., Hiday, V. A., & Borum, W. R. (1999). Can involuntary outpatient commitment reduce hospital recidivism? Findings from a randomized trial in severely mentally ill individuals. *American Journal of Psychiatry, 156,* 1968–1975.

Szasz, T. (1982). The psychiatric will: A new mechanism for protecting persons against "psychosis" and psychiatry. *American Psychologist, 37,* 762–770.

Teller, J. L., Munetz, M. R., Gill, K. M., & Ritter, C. (2006). Crisis intervention team training for police officers responding to mental disturbance calls. *Psychiatric Services, 57,* 232–237.

Teplin, L. A., Abram, K. M., McClelland, G. M., & Dulcan, M. K. (2002). Psychiatric disorders in youth in juvenile detention. *Archives of General Psychiatry, 59,* 1133–1143.

Tonry, M. (2008). Crime and human rights—how political paranoia, protestant fundamentalisms, and constitutional obsolescence combined to devastate black America: The American society of criminology 2007 presidential address. *Criminology, 46,* 1–33.

Torrey, E. F. (1997). *Out of the shadows: Confronting America's mental illness crisis.* New York: John Wiley.

Torrey, E. F., & Zdanowicz, J. D. (2001). Outpatient commitment: What, why, and for whom. *Psychiatric Services, 52,* 337–341.

Tuke, S. (2009/1813). *Description of the retreat: An Institution near York, for insane persons of the Society of Friends.* Charleston, SC: BiblioLife.

Van Dorn, R. A., Swartz, M. S., Elbogen, E. B., Swanson, J. W., Kim, M., Ferron, J., et al. (2006). Clinicians' attitudes regarding barriers to the implementation of Psychiatric Advance Directives. *Administration and Policy in Mental Health and Mental Health Services, 33,* 449–60.

United States Government Accountability Office (2005). *Adult Drug Courts: Evidence Indicates Reduced Recidivism Reductions and Mixed Results for Other Outcomes.* Washington DC: GAO-05-219.

Winick, B. J. (1996). Advance directive instruments for those with mental illness. *University of Miami Law Review, 51,* 57–95.

9 Community rights, recovery, and advocacy

David Roe and Kim T. Mueser

Introduction

For over 20 years, the vision of recovery from severe mental illnesses (SMI) such as schizophrenia and severe mood disorders, was the focus of only those on the margin of the mental health field. However, recently this vision has taken center stage in major policy documents and initiatives in the U.S. and throughout the world. In this chapter we discuss the concept of recovery for people with SMI. We begin by briefly reviewing major developments in medicine, social values, research, and policy that led to community support systems and the practice of psychiatric rehabilitation for persons with SMI. We then discuss the concept of recovery, including its many different definitions and meanings to different stakeholder groups, such as people with SMI and their families, clinicians, policymakers, and researchers. Finally, we look at recovery-oriented services, including the challenges and opportunities it generates for policymakers and the key issues and research agendas it poses for public mental health in the 21st century.

From early deterioration to psychiatric rehabilitation: Advancements in conceptualizing severe mental illness

Towards the end of the 19th century, Kraepelin (1899; 1904), the German psychiatrist who pioneered the classification of psychiatric disorders, described a disease he called *dementia praecox* (which means "early deterioration"). He characterized it as having an early onset, usually after adolescence or during early adulthood, and resulting in a downward and deteriorating course of mental and psychosocial functioning. Although his observations were based primarily on long-term residents of institutions, his core conjecture – that *dementia praecox*, later referred to as schizophrenia by Bleuler (1950), invariably leads to progressive deterioration – still reigns dominant today in the mental health field and in general society. This leads to frequent pessimistic pronouncements about the lifelong prospects of persons with SMI. As schizophrenia and SMI are often equated, the public perception continues to be that people with SMI cannot improve or recover and have little hope for a future other than one of dependence on others and often on institutions. However, in the latter half of the 20th century, a number of developments contributed to a more optimistic view of people with SMI and their prospects for improving their lives.

One important development was pharmaceutical advancements, such as the discovery of chlorpromazine and other antipsychotic medications and the development of antidepressants and mood stabilizers. These medications were found to be effective in decreasing symptoms, thereby increasing the feasibility of community living for many people with SMI. A second development was the trend away from institutional care and towards community care, based on economic concerns regarding the soaring costs of institutional care (Johnson, 1990).

As deinstitutionalization of people with SMI grew in the 1960s and 1970s, and increasing numbers of persons with SMI were never institutionalized in the first place, research teams throughout the world began to critically examine the assumption that schizophrenia always had a progressive deteriorating course by conducting a series of rigorous longitudinal studies (Harding, Zubin, & Strauss, 1987). Contrary to expectations, the long-term outcome of schizophrenia was found to be heterogeneous, with 46 to 68% achieving significant improvement and often even full recovery over time (Ciompi, Harding, & Lehtinen, 2010). More recently, a large-scale, multicultural outcome study conducted as part of the International Study of Schizophrenia concluded that the global outcome of schizophrenia was favorable for over half of the people followed up over two to three decades after the initial onset of their disorder (Harrison, Hopper, Craig, Laska, Siegel, Wanderling, et al., 2001).

In addition to research on the long-term outcome of schizophrenia, the pessimistic outlook about the course of SMI was challenged by the people who had experienced psychiatric symptoms and had been diagnosed with a SMI. These people used different terms to describe themselves, including mental health "consumers," "service users," "ex-patients," and "survivors." We will refer to them here as consumers. Despite grim predictions, which were often accompanied by discouraging messages and barriers to fair opportunities (Deegan, 1990), individuals with SMI often protested against these pronouncements. They defied expectations by demonstrating that they were capable of earning socially valued roles and developing personally meaningful lives, often in spite of continuing to experience some symptoms of their psychiatric disorder.

Nonetheless, the actual consequences of deinstitutionalization made it clear that medications alone were not sufficient to address the needs of people with SMI. During the 1960s, a growing number of people were being released without serious consideration of their needs, which often led to devastating results (Bachrach, 1981). In response, efforts were made to address the housing needs of consumers who had been recently discharged from hospitals through development of a variety of continuum housing models. In these models, residents were expected to gradually move to less restrictive settings with fewer or no staff based on improvements in their level of functioning.

Other initial efforts revolved around community-based care. In 1963 the Community Mental Health Centers Act authorized the creation of a network of community mental health centers (CMHCs) (U.S. Congress, 1963). These centers, which were intended to address the overall mental health needs of all community members, included outpatient care, emergency services, partial hospitalization, and consultation and education (Bloom, 1984). Although the number of CMHCs grew over the years, they did not serve the SMI population as fully as was hoped. Possible reasons included staff who lacked sufficient training to treat people with SMI and preferred instead to provide insight-oriented therapy to the "worried well" and the mistaken assumption that people discharged from the hospital would actively seek and use CMHC services (Torrey, 2006). Additionally, partial hospitalization (also known as day treatment) was developed as a less restrictive and less expensive alternative to hospitals, with the goal to deliver comprehensive, multidisciplinary services to people with SMI. While these programs were less restrictive than institutions, they did not prove especially effective in helping people move out of treatment settings and achieve valued social roles in the community (Corrigan, Mueser, Bond, Drake, & Solomon, 2008; Schene, 2004).

Over time, it became increasingly clear that the services developed following deinstitutionalization fell short of meeting the psychosocial needs of many people with SMI. While the vast majority of people with SMI were discharged from mental hospitals, most did not have the skills to develop the opportunities and supports necessary to meet their basic needs for friends, work, and a decent place to live. Lacking these basic building blocks on which the lives of most people are based, along with various levels and periods of symptoms, made individuals with SMI vulnerable to frequent relapses and rehospitalizations. Indeed, more than half of the people who were discharged from psychiatric state hospitals returned within two years (Weiden & Olfson, 1993), and similarly, many individuals experienced multiple hospitalizations for briefer periods of time, while never sustaining stable housing in the community – a phenomenon that became known as the "revolving door."

Efforts to better meet the needs of people being discharged from psychiatric hospitals led to the development of the community support program (CSP) approach (Turner & TenHoor, 1978), which emphasized a continuous system of care and included identified core service agencies responsible for addressing the comprehensive needs of consumers. In line with this trend, during the 1980s, "protected" approaches (such as day treatment programs and group homes) began to be replaced by "supported" approaches. The supported approach aims to provide consumers with access to settings of their choice and then with whatever supports were necessary for pursuing their goals within these settings. Notable examples of supported services include the areas of housing, employment, and education. These services emphasize empowering consumers to choose and attain their housing, employment, and educational goals in integrated community settings and provide help in the form of giving practical assistance, teaching requisite skills, and collaborating with natural supports such as family members, friends, landlords, teachers, and employers (Anthony, 1993).

While these important mental health system changes were rapidly occurring, psychiatric rehabilitation was being developed at various psychosocial rehabilitation centers, notably those at University of California at Los Angeles Psychiatric Rehabilitation Program, the Center for Psychiatric Rehabilitation at Boston University, and Western Pennsylvania Psychiatric Institute and Clinic. Social skills training (SST) programs for persons with SMI were developed, implemented, and investigated, revealing positive results. SST is aimed at helping consumers learn and use the skills needed to pursue their goals in natural settings (Corrigan et al., 2008). In parallel, important developments were taking place at the Fountain House in New York City, which later became known as a "clubhouse" (Corrigan et al., 2008; Pratt, Gill, Barrett, & Roberts, 2007). Emphasis on a sense of belonging and being productive was translated into voluntary membership and transitional work placements. The number of clubhouses across the U.S. and around the world grew rapidly, but perhaps even more important is that many of the core values of psychiatric rehabilitation, especially consumers taking a more active role in setting and pursuing their own goals, can be traced back to the clubhouse movement.

The development of psychiatric rehabilitation fit in well with new values and legislation. For example, since the passage of the American Rehabilitation Act of 1973, the independent living movement established that society has an obligation to promote the independence and self-sufficiency of people with disabilities. Fulfilling this obligation involves identifying the special needs of people with various disabilities and providing them with appropriate accommodations and compensatory strategies to maximize their access to the resources needed to lead the life they want in their community of choice. The growing mental health consumer movement justifiably began to demand that, just as wheelchairs and Braille signs increased community access and opportunity for those with physical disabilities, strategies for increasing community integration and participation for people with psychiatric disabilities were needed.

Indeed, psychiatric rehabilitation refers to adapting and applying rehabilitation principles and practices used with a variety of disabilities to help improve the quality of life and community participation of people with SMI. Since the 1980s, the concept has been increasingly applied and integrated into the mainstream of community mental health. While different definitions of psychiatric rehabilitation slightly vary with regard to their emphasis, it is define by the United States Psychiatric Rehabilitation Association (USPRA) as follows:

> Psychiatric rehabilitation promotes recovery, full community integration and improved quality of life for persons who have been diagnosed with any mental health condition that seriously impairs their ability to lead meaningful lives. Psychiatric rehabilitation services are collaborative, person directed and individualized. These services are an essential element of the health care and human services spectrum, and should be evidence-based. They focus on helping individuals develop skills and access resources needed to increase their capacity to be successful and satisfied in the living, working, learning, and social environments of their choice.
>
> (InterComunity, Inc, 2010)

Recovery in the context of mental health

The combination of more progressive legislation, greater opportunities in the community, and better treatment and rehabilitation services contributed to the development and strengthening of the consumer movement. A growing number of consumers became advocates and leaders, striving to reform mental health policy and practice and adapting the slogan "nothing about us without us," reflecting their demand for growing involvement in shaping mental health services. For example, Patricia Deegan (1988), a psychologist and pioneer activist who was diagnosed with schizophrenia, contributed importantly to the shift from rehabilitation to a recovery model, pointing out that

> Persons with a disability do not "get rehabilitated" in the sense that cars "get" tuned up or televisions "get" repaired. They are not passive recipients of rehabilitation services. Rather, they experience themselves as recovering a new sense of self and of purpose within and beyond the limits of the disability.
>
> (p. 11)

William Anthony, the director of the Center for Psychiatric Rehabilitation at Boston University, who led the development of one of the first psychiatric rehabilitation models, expanded his view of the concept of psychiatric rehabilitation and issued a call for recovery to become the "guiding vision" of mental health services (Anthony, 1993). According to Anthony (1993), recovery is

> A deeply personal, unique process of changing one's attitudes, values, feelings, goals, skills and/or roles. It is a way of living a satisfying,

hopeful and contributing life, even with limitations caused by the illness. Recovery involves the development of new meaning and purpose in one's life as one grows beyond the catastrophic effects of mental illness.

(p. 15)

Introducing the concept of recovery to psychiatric rehabilitation and mental healthcare had an inspiring and influential effect on practitioners and consumers, promoting hope throughout the field. Perhaps its major contribution has been in drawing attention to the fact that many people with SMI can live personally meaningful lives as integral members of their communities, despite and beyond the limits of their psychiatric disorder. While the vision of recovery has been widely embraced of late by state and federal authorities in the U.S. (Department of Health and Human Services (DHHS), 2003), recovery is still an evolving concept, the definitions and dimensions of which require further development (Liberman & Kopelowicz, 2005; Noordsy et al., 2002; Roe, Rudnick, & Gill, 2007).

The different definitions of recovery can be generally organized into two types, which Davidson and Roe (2005) referred to as "recovery from" versus "recovery in" and Slade (2009) referred to as "clinical recovery" versus "personal recovery". The first, "recovery from" or "clinical recovery", refers to the more scientific-professional view of recovery as an outcome based on whether operationally defined criteria are met. The latter "recovery in" or "personal recovery" allude to the more consumer experience-based approach that views recovery as an ongoing process of identity change, including a broadening of self-concept (Silverstein & Bellack, 2008). The next section elaborates on these two central definitions of recovery.

"Recovery from" or "clinical recovery"

Generally speaking, the scientific community continues to view recovery as an outcome defined by emphasis on reduction of clinical symptoms (e.g., psychosis, negative symptoms, cognitive disorganization, depression and anxiety) and improved everyday functioning (role and social functioning, self-care and independent living skills). This form of "recovery from" or "clinical recovery" involves the amelioration of symptoms and the person's returning to a healthier state following onset of the illness. This definition is based on explicit criteria of levels of signs, symptoms, and impairments associated with the illness and identification of a point at which "recovery from" or "clinical recovery" can be considered to have occurred. Thus, such a definition has many advantages from clinical and research perspectives, as it is a clear, reliable, and relatively easy to define measure. A consensus definition of "clinical remission" recently has been proposed (Andreasen, Carpenter, Kane, Lasser, Marder, & Weinberger, 2005) and has included definitions for remission of clinical symptoms, which are part of the active phase·of illness criteria. Remission, according to these criteria, is defined as the absence (i.e., no greater than mild level) of the central symptoms: positive, negative, or disorganized symptoms of the illness. The temporal duration of remission was defined as a six-month period.

In addition to attempts to define symptom remission, efforts also have been directed to develop a remission criterion for functional disability (Harvey & Bellack, 2009). Such attempts have focused on role function-ing, which includes major social roles that involve some form of produc-tive activity that are impaired by SMI. The first domain is work and school, the second is residential (which includes self-care and community living), and the third is social-leisure functioning. Each functional domain includes multiple levels of achievement on two criteria: level and breadth of accomplishment (Harvey & Bellack, 2009). For example, the first criterion includes an assessment of accomplishment within each domain scored across a continuum where one end is "Not actively working toward change/functional improvement" and whose anchors include "making attempts", "making progress", "partial success", and finally, "full success." The second criterion refers to the breadth of accomplish-ment as reflected in the number of domains in which the various levels·of accomplishment were made.

Together, these efforts towards establishing operational criteria to assess the degree of "recovery from" mental illness across key domains such as severity of symptoms and level of functioning signify important progress. Widely agreed upon and used criteria can improve research efforts to investigate the prevalence, course, and determinants of recovery from mental illness.

Being "in recovery" and "personal recovery"

While few would argue the importance of defining and studying the intens-ity of symptoms and level of functioning, these efforts clearly fall short of representing a broader picture of what one would hope for in life. Focus-ing on the person rather than the disorder (Strauss, 1989) shifts attention to one's well-being, fullness of life, and self-directed efforts to find meaning, reconstruct a sense of self, and achieve some recognition by others as a person (Barham & Hayward, 1990). These more subjective aspects of a person are better captured in the concept "in recovery" (Davidson & Roe, 2005) or "personal recovery" (Slade, 2009). This form of recovery does not reflect the clinical or scientific reality emphasized in the outcome-oriented definition of "recovery from" but rather a personal, experiential one.

"Being in recovery" or "personal recovery" is about reclaiming autonomy and self-determination without first having to clinically recover from the illness. In this respect, someone with SMI can be "in recovery" depending on how he or she defines what recovery means to him or her. A person with paraplegia, for example, does not have to regain his or her mobility in order to have a satisfying and personally meaningful life in the community (Davidson & Roe, 2005). Similarly, being "in recovery" refers to the process of pursuing one's personal hopes and aspirations, with dignity and autonomy, despite the person's presumed vulnerability to relapse. Thus "recovery in" does not require a cure, remission of one's psychiatric disorder, or a return to a pre-existing state of health. Instead, it involves a redefinition of one's illness as only one aspect of a multidimensional sense of self and connotes the process of trying to identify, choose, and pursue personally meaningful aspirations, which are not dependent upon symptom remission (Davidson & Roe, 2005).

One of the most widely used definitions of recovery was offered by the Substance Abuse and Mental Health Services Administration (SAMHSA, 2005). Based upon a meeting attended by panelists from multiple backgrounds, a list of fundamental components of recovery was generated: being self-directed, individualized, empowered, holistic, non-linear, strengths-based, and having peer support, respect, responsibility, and hope. Taken together, these components offer a view of recovery as experienced by the consumer, driven by hope, and tailored to his or her needs. An overlapping list of key elements of recovery was offered by Davidson, Tondora, Lawless, O'Connell, and Rowe (2005), who proposed that recovery is comprised of the following elements: renewing hope and commitment, redefining self, incorporating illness as only a minor part of a newly emerging sense of self, being involved in meaningful activities, overcoming stigma, assuming control, becoming empowered, managing symptoms, and being supported by others. While these elements parallel the SAMHSA components, they also emphasize that people must develop their own understanding of their illness and recovery process, as well as ways of dealing with aspects that may persist over time. This conceptualization stresses how subjective changes in the way people understand and experience themselves as individual human beings may be an essential element of recovery.

Some have suggested that medical versus personal and subjective conceptualizations of recovery should be viewed as complementary rather than incompatible (Silverstein & Bellack, 2008). Each definition contributes to portraying and understanding key aspects of living with SMI, helps to evaluate where a person is along the multidimensional course of illness and recovery, and guides the tailoring of individualized care. From the perspective of scientists, policymakers, and clinicians, it would be problematic to ignore symptoms and level of functional disability, as the need for treatment and access to supplementary resources for managing a disability presumably needs to be based on at least some objective criteria. Of equal importance, however, are dimensions that have been emphasized primarily by the consumer movement, such as feeling hopeful, valued, and having a sense of meaning in life (Slade, 2009).

Recovery-oriented services

As the vision of recovery becomes more widespread and influencial, there have been growing international efforts to go beyond traditional clinical practices that stress symptom remission and functional improvement and to focus on supporting the broader range of recovery outcomes desired by consumers. The landmark 1999 publication of the U.S. Surgeon General's *Report on Mental Health* was an important step, with its assertion that all mental health services be consumer- and family-oriented and have as their overarching aim the promotion of recovery (DHHS, 1999). Specifically, the report stated that

> all services for those with a mental disorder should be consumer oriented and focused on promoting recovery. That is, the goal of services must not be limited to symptom reduction but should strive for restoration of a meaningful and productive live.
>
> (p. 455)

Expanding on this position, the subsequent report from the President's New Freedom Commission on Mental Health, entitled *Achieving the Promise: Transforming Mental Health Care in America* (DHHS, 2003), pushed even further the need for fundamental reform of the mental health system. Furthermore, the *Federal Action Agenda* for implementing the New Freedom Commission stressed the need for profound and revolutionary change at its very core (DHHS, 2005). Frese, Knight, and Saks (2009) note that with the report of the President's New Freedom Commission in 2003, a clinical emphasis on recovery became not only possible but also expected.

But just what is a "recovery oriented system" or "recovery oriented services"? One definition comes from Davidson et al. (2009):

> To offer people with serious mental illness a range of effective and culturally responsive interventions from which they may choose those services and supports they find useful in promoting or protecting their own recovery. In addition to diagnosis and reducing symptoms and deficits, a recovery-oriented system of care also identifies and builds on each individual's assets and areas of health and competence to support that person in achieving a sense of mastery over his or her condition while regaining a meaningful, conductive sense of membership in the broader community.
>
> (p. 89)

Defining what is meant by "recovery-oriented services" is necessary, for otherwise, how would anyone know whether the services are recovery-oriented? As part of this effort, Davidson and colleagues (2009) published a practical guide to recovery-oriented practice in which they presented eight recovery practice standards to help guide practitioners in their provision of services:

1   Primacy of participation – giving the primacy to the participation of people in recovery and their loved ones in all aspects and phases of care delivery.
2   Promoting access and engagement – recovery-oriented programs promote access to swift and easy to receive, barrier-free services, which engage the person and not the disability.
3   Ensuring continuity of care – treatment, rehabilitation, and support need to be carefully designed as a system of care that ensures continuity of services by constant healing relationships.
4   Employing strengths-based assessment – providers assess the strengths a person possesses in order to help them meet their own needs.
5   Offering individualized recovery planning – the multidisciplinary recovery plan needs to be individualized and developed in full collaboration with the person receiving services.
6   Functioning as a recovery guide – professionals supply the people receiving services with tools they can use during their whole recovery process.
7   Conducting community mapping, development, and inclusion – community resources and capacities are mapped out to identify possible places where people with disabilities will be welcomed and valued.
8   Identifying and addressing barriers to recovery – the health care provider supplies people with the tools and strategies needed to identify the barriers to their own recovery, both in the mental health care system and also within the broader community.

These guidelines are aimed at helping practitioners and agencies in providing recovery-oriented care and thus offer an initial roadmap to ways of promoting and sustaining such care.

Challenges to the concept of recovery

While the concept of recovery, and particularly the notion of "being in recovery" or "personal recovery", has generated much hope and positive change, it also faces some challenges. In order to convey hope and depathologize illness, one could argue that everyone with a psychiatric disability is in recovery. This, however, runs the risk of making recovery not amenable to scientific study (Roe et al., 2007). If everyone is "in recovery," and there is no variability in degree of recovery, exploring correlates or predictors of recovery is not possible. Thus, to help policymakers and systems planners develop more recovery-oriented services, it is essential to invest in further defining and operationalizing the concept so that it can be more reliably measured.

As Silverstein and Bellack (2008) point out, it is important to study what promotes recovery. Beyond the important humanitarian goal of training practitioners to provide services that are consistent with recovery values (such as self-determination, hope, independence), evaluating the effectiveness of practices that are thought to promote recovery is crucial. Thus, studying the impact of shared decision-making, consumer-run services, psychiatric advanced directives, and other practices that are considered "recovery-oriented," can make important contributions to the currently modest body of knowledge on the relationship between recovery-oriented practice and evidence-based practice, two important approaches that we believe are compatible (Bond, Salyers, Rollins, Rapp, & Zipple, 2004).

One potentially useful direction for work in this area is to recognize that new conceptualizations of recovery have both subjective and objective qualities and that they need to be studied together in order to get a full picture. Such attempts should include efforts to capture individual's preferences, values, and experiences, while not losing sight of the more objective and functional aspects of recovery, such as community integration, effective role functioning, and involvement in rewarding social relationships.

Conclusion

Introducing the concept of recovery to the field of mental health has had inspiring and influential effects on the lives of many consumers and their family members and has influenced the thinking and work of service providers and policy-makers. This exciting development poses an enormous challenge for 21st century public mental health policymakers and systems planners. As evident from this chapter, efforts to implement a recovery-oriented perspective that will yield a more consumer-based mental health system have just begun. The pressing need to investigate these efforts, while taking into consideration the complexity and many meanings of "recovery", is beginning to manifest itself in the mental health research agendas.

References

Andreasen, N., Carpenter, W. T., Kane, J., Lasser, R., Marder, S., & Weinberger, D. A. (2005). Remission in schizophrenia: Proposed criteria and rationale for consensus. *American Journal of Psychiatry, 162,* 441–449.

Anthony, W. A. (1993). Recovery from mental illness: The guiding vision of the mental health service system in the 1990s. *Psychosocial Rehabilitation Journal, 16,* 11–23.

Bachrach, L. L. (1981). Continuity of care for chronic mental patients: A conceptual analysis. *American Journal of Psychiatry, 33,* 189–197.

Barham, P., & Hayward, R. (1990). Schizophrenia as a life process. In R. P. Bentall (Ed.), *Reconstructing Schizophrenia* (pp. 61–85). London, UK: Routledge.

Bleuler E. (1950). *Dementia Praecox or the Group of Schizophrenias*. (J. Zinkin, Trans.) New York, NY: International University Press.

Bloom, B. L. (1984). *Community mental health: A general introduction*. Monterey, CA: Brooks/Cole.

Bond, G. R., Salyers, M. P., Rollins, A. L., Rapp, C. A., & Zipple, A. M. (2004). How evidence-based practices contribute to community integration. *Community Mental Health Journal, 40*, 569–588.

Ciompi, L., Harding, C. M., & Lehtinen, K. (2010). Deep Concern. *Schizophrenia Bulletin, 36*, 437–439.

Corrigan, P. W., Mueser, K. T., Bond, G. R., Drake, R. E., & Solomon, P. (2008). *Principles and practice of psychiatric rehabilitation*. New York: Guilford Press.

Davidson, L., & Roe, D. (2005). Recovery from versus recovery in serious mental illness: One strategy for lessening confusion plaguing recovery. *Journal of Mental Health, 16*, 1–12.

Davidson, L., Tondora, J., Lawless, M. S., O'Connell, M., & Rowe, M. A. (2009). *Practical guide to recovery-oriented practice tools for transforming mental health care*. Oxford, UK: Oxford University Press.

Deegan, P. E. (1988). Recovery: The lived experience of rehabilitation. *Psychosocial Rehabilitation Journal, 11*, 11–19.

Deegan, P. E. (1990). Spirit breaking: When the helping professionals hurt. *The Humanistic Psychologist, 18*, 301–313.

Department of Health and Human Services. (1999). *Mental Health: A Report of the Surgeon General*. Retrieved from http://mentalhealth.samhsa.gov/cmhs/surgeongeneral/larrysgr2.asp

Department of Health and Human Services. (2003). *Achieving the promise: Transforming mental health care in America. President's New Freedom Commission on Mental Health. Final Report*. Rockville, MD: Substance Abuse and Mental Health Services Administration, U.S. Department of Health and Human Services.

Department of Health and Human Services. (2005). *Transforming mental health care in America: Federal action agenda, first steps*. Rockville, MD: Substance Abuse and Mental Health Services Administration, U.S. Department of Health and Human Services.

Frese III, F. J., Knight, E. L., & Saks, E. (2009). Recovery from schizophrenia: With views of psychiatrists, psychologists, and others diagnosed with this disorder. *Schizophrenia Bulletin, 35*, 370–380.

Harding, C. M., Zubin, J., & Strauss, J. S. (1987). Chronicity in schizophrenia: Fact, partial fact, or artifact? *Hospital and Community Psychiatry, 38*, 477–486.

Harrison, G., Hopper, K., Craig, T., Laska, E., Siegel, C., Wanderling, J., et al. (2001). Recovery from psychotic illness: A 15- and 25-year international follow-up study. *British Journal of Psychiatry, 178*, 506–517.

Harvey, P. D., & Bellack, A. S. (2009). Toward a terminology for functional recovery in schizophrenia: Is functional remission a viable concept? *Schizophrenia Bulletin, 35*, 300–306.

Hughes, R. (1994). Psychiatric Rehabilitation: An essential health service for people with serious and persistent mental illness. In Publications Committee of IAPSRS (ed.), *IAPSRS, An Introduction to Psychiatric Rehabilitation (pp. 172–176)*. Columbia, MD: Author.

InterCommunity, Inc. (2010). Retrieved from https://www.netforumondemand. com/eWeb/DynamicPage.aspx?Site=USPRA&WebCode=about://www.icmhg. org/about %20us.html.

Johnson, A. B. (1990). *Out of bedlam: The truth about deinstitutionalization*. New York: Basic Books.

Kraepelin, E. (1899). Zur diagnose und prognose der dementia praecox [On the diagnosis and prognosis of dementia praecox]. *Allgemeine Z Psychiatr Psychisch-Gerichtliche Med, 56*, 254–263.

Kraepelin, E. (1904). *Psychiatrie. Ein Lehrbuch für Studierende und Ärzte* [Psychiatry. A Manual for Students and Physicians] (7th ed.). Leipzig, Germany: Barth.

Liberman, R. P., & Kopelowicz, A. (2005). Recovery from schizophrenia: A criterion-based definition. In R. O. Ralph & P. Corrigan (Eds.), *Recovery in mental illness: Broadening our understanding of wellness* (pp. 101–129). Washington, D.C.: American Psychological Association.

Noordsy, D. L., Torrey, W. C., Mueser, K. T., Mead, S., O'Keefe, C. O., & Fox, L. (2002). Recovery from severe mental illness: An interpersonal and functional outcome definition. *International Review of Psychiatry, 14*, 318–326.

Pratt, C. W., Gill, K. J., Barrett, N. M., & Roberts, M. M. (2007). *Psychiatric rehabilitation* (2nd ed.). San Diego, CA: Academic Press.

Roe, D., Rudnick, A., & Gill, K. J. (2007). The concept of 'being in recovery': Commentary. *Psychiatric Rehabilitation Journal, 30*, 171–173.

Schene, A. H. (2004). The effectiveness of psychiatric partial hospitalization and day care. *Current Opinion in Psychiatry, 17*, 303–309.

Silverstein, S. M., & Bellack, A. S. (2008). Scientific agenda for the concept of recovery as it applies to schizophrenia. *Clinical Psychology Review, 28*, 1108–1124.

Slade, M. (2009). *Personal recovery and mental illness: A guide for mental health professionals*. Cambridge: Cambridge University Press.

Strauss, J. S., (1989). Subjective experience in schizophrenia: Towards a new dynamic psychiatry. *Schizophrenia Bulletin, 15*, 179–187.

Substance Abuse and Mental Health Services Administration. (2005). *National Consensus Conference on Mental Health Recovery and Systems Transformation*. Rockville, MD: Department of Health and Human Services.

Torrey, E. F. (2006). *Surviving schizophrenia: A manual for families, consumers, and providers* (5th ed.). New York: Harper-Collins.

Turner, J. E., & TenHoor, W. J. (1978). The NIMH Community Support Program: Pilot approach to a needed social reform. *Schizophrenia Bulletin, 4*, 319–348.

United States Congress. (1963). *Mental Retardation Facilities and Community Mental Health Centers Construction Act of 1963* (P. L. 88–164). Washington, DC.

Weiden, P. J., & Olfson, M. (1993). The cost of relapse in schizophrenia. *Schizophrenia Bulletin, 21*, 419–428.

10 "No health without mental health"

The global effort to improve population mental health

Mark Tomlinson, Leslie Swartz, and Karen Daniels

Introduction

Mental disorders are a major contributor to the burden of disease in all regions of the world, with about 14% of the global burden attributable to neuropsychiatric disorders (Prince, Patel, Saxena, Mai, Maselko, Phillips, & Rahman, 2007). Even in sub-Saharan Africa, where communicable diseases are common, mental disorders account for nearly 10% of the total burden of disease (Lopez, Mathers, Ezzati, Jamison, & Murray, 2006). The health systems in many low- and middle-income countries (LMICs) face a scarcity of financial resources and qualified staff – a situation that is often compounded by a lack of commitment from public health policymakers and inefficient use of resources (Rahman, 2005). As a result, at least 40 to 70% of individuals never receive any kind of care (Rahman, 2005). In this chapter, we first briefly outline the context of mental health in LMICs, with a particular focus on the Millennium Development Goals (MDGs), and discuss the issue of mental health and poverty. We then present a description and analysis of a number of promising interventions implemented in LMICs that are providing important data in terms of delivery and potential scale-up of mental health interventions. Finally, we discuss the concept of task shifting and present a case for family-based interventions as key efforts to improve population mental health.

Context of mental health in low- and middle-income countries

Of all mental conditions, depression is the most common. In the World Health Organization World Mental Health survey, lifetime prevalence of any mood disorder ranged from 3.3% in Nigeria to 21.4% in the U.S., while projected lifetime risk for any mood disorder ranged from 7.3% in China to 31.4% in the U.S. (Kessler, Angermeyer, Anthony, De Graaf, Demyttenaere, Gasquet, et al., 2007). Depression is often comorbid with other health conditions, such as diabetes, which in South Africa affects 2.6

million people and was the sixth leading cause of natural death in 2005 (Statistics South Africa, 2007). Mental disorders are also among the most costly health conditions in terms of projected health care expenditures (Stein & Seedat, 2007). The poorest countries spend the lowest percentages of their overall health budgets on mental healthcare compared to other countries (Shah & Beinecke, 2009). Two-thirds of the world's population live in countries that spend less than 1% of their health budget on mental health (Shah & Beinecke, 2009). In 40% of LMICs, mental healthcare is funded directly by individuals in the form of out-of-pocket expenses (Shah & Beinecke, 2009). Where funding does exist in these countries, it is significantly supplemented by donor funds and managed by nongovernmental organizations (NGOs) that, unfortunately, do not have a good track record in terms of prioritizing mental health (Shah & Beinecke, 2009).

In addition to financial constraints, there are also substantial workforce issues facing LMICs in terms of meeting the mental health needs of their population. In sub-Saharan Africa there are 0.05 psychiatrists per 100,000 people, which translates to about one psychiatrist for every two million people, compared to Europe where the figure is one psychiatrist for every 11,000 people (Shah & Beinecke, 2009).

The Global Forum for Health Research has long highlighted the major imbalance between the magnitude of mental health problems (especially in LMICs) and the resources devoted to addressing them. This is the so-called "10/90 gap" – only 10% of global spending on health research is directed towards the primary problems affecting the poorest 90% of the world's population (Global Forum for Health Research, 2000). This gap stunts the development of evidence-based health policies and practice in LMIC and limits progress in medicine and public health (Saxena, Paraje, Sharan, Karam, & Sadana, 2006). The impact of the gap is particularly evident in the field of mental health, in which the evidence base depends mainly on European and North American cultural norms and data (Chisholm, Flisher, Lund, Patel, Saxena, Thornicroft, & Tomlinson, 2007; Razzouk, Sharan, Gallo, Gureje, Lamberte, Mari, et al., 2010; Sharan, Gallo, Gureje, Lamberte, Mari, Mazzotti, et al., 2009). Up to 94% of the published literature in high-impact psychiatric journals is from North America, Europe, and Australia/New Zealand (Patel & Sumathipala, 2001), with as little as 3% originating from LMICs (Patel & Sumathipala, 2001; Tomlinson & Swartz, 2003). Africa in particular continues to lag behind in terms of research relative to the rest of the world (Adams, King, & Hook, 2010).

The Millennium Development Goals

The Millennium Development Goals (MDGs) are a set of targets that aim to eradicate extreme poverty; to reduce child mortality; to improve maternal health; to combat HIV/AIDS, malaria, and other diseases; to ensure environmental sustainability; and to develop a global partnership for development. The MDGs were ratified by most nations of the world in 2000 and set specific targets for poverty reduction, eradication of hunger, and improved health and maternal health by 2015 (United Nations Development Programme, 2010). For many countries and donor agencies, addressing the MDGs has become the central platform of their health agenda. While this is laudable, the MDGs almost entirely ignore noncommunicable disorders, such as mental disorders, which Zolnierek (2008) argues is indicative of the lower prioritization of mental health in comparison to illnesses such as HIV and malaria.

Miranda and Patel (2005) make a compelling case for how mental disorders, though not explicitly included in the MDGs, are linked to many of the priority areas and are thus a key consideration in any strategy to improve population health. With regard to the first goal of eradicating extreme poverty and hunger, they argue that mental disorders impoverish people because of the increased healthcare costs as well as associated unemployment or lost employment. Mental health is also linked to maternal and child morbidity and mortality. Rahman, Iqbal, Bunn, Lovel, and Harrington (2004) found that in rural Pakistan, infants of mothers depressed in the prenatal or postpartum periods showed growth retardation at several time points in the first year of life. In addition, chronic depression carried a greater risk for poor outcome than did episodic depression, while maternal mental state was associated with risk of diarrhea in infants. Estimates based on these data suggest that the incidence of infant stunting in rural Pakistan would be reduced by 30% if maternal depression was eliminated (Rahman, 2005). There is an increased risk of poor fetal growth, premature birth, and low birth weight among antenatally depressed women (Hedegaard, Henricksen, Sabroe, & Secher, 1993; Hoffman & Hatch, 2000), and depression is associated with riskier lifestyles such as poor diet and smoking (Milberger, Biederman, Faraone, Chen, & Jones, 1996). Rahman (2005) makes the important point that in LMICs, environments are hostile, and caregivers need to be vigilant about potential dangers to their infants and children. In India and China, suicide is the leading cause of death in women during the reproductive years (Aaron, Joseph, Abraham, Muliyil, George, Prasad, et al., 2004; Phillips, Li, & Zhang, 2002), with depression implicated in these suicides. Preventing or treating depression would therefore make a substantial contribution to improving maternal health.

Miranda and Patel (2005) point out that, in addition to ignoring noncommunicable diseases, the MDGs also do not address health systems strengthening. This, combined with their focus on specific targets, may marginalize mental healthcare delivery, which requires multicomponent interventions within a strong health system (Miranda & Patel, 2005). Finally, the MDGs have been criticized for dependence on indicators, which can skew understanding of progress from an equity point of view. The most vulnerable in society often fare poorly – something that is masked when progress is described only in terms of national averages (Miranda & Patel, 2005). This phenomenon is of particular concern in the case of mental health, given the low priority of mental health on the health agenda of most countries and because of the stigma associated with mental illness.

Mental health and poverty

In the 50 years since the end of World War II, countries outside of North America and Western Europe have seen breathtaking improvements in healthcare and living conditions (Desjarlais, Eisenberg, Good, & Kleinman, 1995). These improvements include increased life expectancy, the eradication of smallpox, lower infant mortality rates, better access to safe water, the availability of healthcare services, and higher levels of literacy in LMICs.

These improvements are misleading, however, as, due to population growth, the actual number of people living in poverty has hardly changed. In 2005, 1.4 billion people in LMICs were living in extreme poverty (less than $1.25 a day) (United Nations, 2009). The worst "performer" has been sub-Saharan Africa, where almost 50% of the population live in extreme poverty (United Nations Population Fund, 2008). Of the 559 million children under five years old in LMICs, 219 million (39%) can be considered disadvantaged (stunted or living in absolute poverty) (Grantham-McGregor, Cheung, Cueto, Glewwe, Richter, & Strupp, 2007).

The most widely used definition of poverty makes a distinction between absolute poverty and relative poverty. Absolute poverty is defined as the severe deprivation of human needs, such as food, safe water, and basic shelter (United Nations, 1995). This form of poverty is characteristic of many LMICs and it often includes a lack of education and access to services. Relative poverty, on the other hand, refers to income in relation to the average of that particular country. Relative poverty is no less detrimental than absolute poverty, and research has shown that morbidity is more closely related to relative income within countries than to differences in absolute income, and countries with lower levels of relative deprivation tend to have lower mortality rates (Wilkinson, 1997).

Interventions to improve population mental health in low- and middle-income countries

Saraceno, Van Ommeren, Batniji, Cohen, Gureje, Mahoney, et al. (2007) have outlined five barriers to the improvement of mental health services in LMICs:

1 Lack of funding for services.
2 Concentration of available resources in urban areas and scarcity in rural areas.

3   Dearth of adequately trained and supervised mental health workers.
4   Lack of public health skills and experience in mental health leadership.
5   The complexities of trying to integrate mental health care into primary health care services.

Shah and Beinecke (2009) summarize these barriers into three integrated themes – scarcity, inequity, and inefficiency. Despite this, in the context of the relative neglect of mental health, pervasive poverty, and weak health systems, a number of interventions have been implemented and tested, providing an evidence base on improving population mental health. In the next section we focus on selected examples of such interventions, chosen because each adopts a somewhat different approach and focus, and each highlights particular limitations characteristic of implementation in LMICs.

Interpersonal group therapy (Uganda)

While there is good evidence for the efficacy of antidepressants in reducing symptoms of depression – in high-income countries as well as LMICs – the use of antidepressants is not possible in many African countries due to the high cost, infrastructure issues (supply problems), and human resource problems, such as the number of primary care doctors (Bolton, Bass, Neugebauer, Verdeli, Clougherty, Wickramaratne, et al., 2003). In this context, Bolton and colleagues (2003) developed a group intervention using interpersonal psychotherapy (IPT) in rural Uganda. While IPT was developed for individual treatment for depression, there are considerable data documenting its applicability to other mood and non-mood disorders. In IPT, four areas of interpersonal experience form the focus of treatment – bereavement, interpersonal conflict, changes in life circumstances, and personal problems in initiating and maintaining relationships.

The IPT intervention was tested in a cluster randomized controlled trial consisting of weeks of group meetings, each lasting an hour and a half. Group leaders (therapists) received two weeks of intensive training in IPT. The Uganda study demonstrated a reduction in depression-like illness and depression symptoms, as well as associated dysfunction. Recovery in the intervention group at the end of treatment was 93.5%, compared to 45.3% in the comparison group; this difference narrowed slightly at six months (88.3% versus 45.1%) (Bolton et al., 2003). Patel and Thornicroft (2009) argue that the study suggests that providing group treatment in a rural setting using local community workers to deliver the interventions is an effective method for reducing costs of treatment.

Limitations

Despite the efficacy of the Uganda intervention, there are few studies that demonstrate the feasibility of large-scale delivery of group interventions in rural settings in LMICs. This limits our ability to draw firm conclusions about this form of intervention (Wiley-Exley, 2007). In addition, while group interventions also have been successful in neonatal interventions in Nepal (Manandhar, Shrestha, Mesko, Morrison, Tumbahangphe, et al., 2004), there remain questions about the suitability of group interventions in many LMICs, particularly because of the stigma of mental disorder and traditions in which it is considered inappropriate to discuss personal details with people outside the family. Finally, 16 sessions of an hour and a half each represents a considerable time investment from the health system and therefore has scalability questions in most LMICs.

Cognitive therapy-based intervention using community health workers (Pakistan)

Rahman and colleagues (2004) have conducted seminal work in rural Pakistan, describing the epidemiology of depression in the region and the consequent development issues and poor growth of infants. Following this work, they implemented a cognitive behavioral intervention in which local health workers, known as Lady Health Workers, delivered a mental health intervention component (Rahman, Malik, Sikander, Roberts, & Creed, 2008). Rahman and colleagues argue that one of the difficulties with implementing cognitive behavior therapy (or even interpersonal therapy) is the lack of adequately trained mental health professionals in most LMICs. In Pakistan, Lady Health Workers are women who have completed secondary school and are trained to deliver preventive maternal, neonatal, and child healthcare and education in the community. There are approximately 96,000 Lady Health Workers who provide services to about 80% of the rural population of Pakistan (100 households per village per worker).

The Pakistan study was a cluster randomized controlled trial conducted in rural Rawalpindi, Pakistan. Participants were women in their third trimester of pregnancy who were depressed. Lady Health Workers were trained to deliver the intervention, while in control clusters Lady Health Workers who had not been trained in mental health made an equal number of visits to depressed women. The intervention consisted of four weekly sessions in the last month of pregnancy, three sessions in the first month after birth, and then monthly sessions for nine months. In light of the association in South Asia between maternal depression and infant growth, the primary outcomes of the study were infant weight and height at six and 12 months. Unexpectedly, the intervention had no impact on infant growth but did halve the rate of prenatal depression in the intervention group. In addition, women receiving the intervention had better overall functioning and less disability up to a year later. Other health benefits included fewer episodes of diarhhea and higher levels of immunization in the intervention group.

The intervention is a pivotal one in that it is not dependant for its delivery on a new or separate mental health workforce. The addition of the integrated cognitive therapy approach had a direct impact on immunization rates and infant health, which are direct indicators of Lady Health Worker performance. Rahman and colleagues argue that evidence of this sort is crucial in order to convince LMICs policymakers of the importance of integrating interventions such as these into the existing health system.

Limitations

One of the limitations in generalizing the Pakistan findings to other LMICs is the lack of similar existing cadres of functioning community health workers such as the Lady Health Workers. Most LMICs do not have such an extensive workforce, and when they do there are significant problems with management, care delivery, and supervision (Daniels, Nor, Jackson, Ekstrom, & Doherty, 2010).

Treating depression in primary care (Chile)

Araya and colleagues (2003) implemented an intervention in Chilean primary healthcare clinics to treat depression among poor women. According to the researchers, the treatment of depression is a complex sequence of management decisions with more than one therapeutic component, and they therefore argue for what they call a sequential multicomponent program (stepped care model). In this model, patients with mild depression receive low-intensity treatment, while those with severe and chronic depression receive additional intensive treatment, including medication.

The intervention was a randomized controlled trial that took place in three primary health clinics that are the main source of care for poor people. Women with depression were allocated to stepped care or usual care. The stepped care was led by a non-medical health worker and included a psycho-educational group intervention with drug treatment for severe depression. Doctors were involved only in the prescription of medication. The study showed a large and significant difference in favor of the stepped care program compared with usual care on all outcomes, and this remained the case at a six-month follow-up.

Limitations

Araya and colleagues (2003) do note several considerations for broader implementation. The psychological intervention included nine group sessions, which may not be feasible in other LMICs. In addition, the primary healthcare system of most LMICs is not as well-resourced or high-functioning as Chile's. Finally, one of the challenges of targeted programs is the incentive for resources to be shifted to cover other priority diseases. (Araya et al., 2003)

Improving the mother–infant relationship using community health workers (South Africa)

There have been several trials in wealthier countries of early interventions aimed at improving maternal sensitivity and reducing infant attachment insecurity, and although these studies have not involved populations with maternal psychiatric disorder, they have produced encouraging findings (Cooper, Landman, Tomlinson, Molteno, Swartz, & Murray, 2002). Based on this research, Cooper and colleagues (2002) carried out a pilot intervention to determine whether a mother–infant intervention delivered in a peri-urban settlement in South Africa would similarly be of benefit. In a small case series, women who received home visits from trained mothers from the community were found at six months postpartum to be more sensitive in engagement with their infants and to express more positive affect than those that did not receive the intervention. Both these factors have been associated with longer-term positive outcomes for infants.

Based on these encouraging preliminary findings, the same team completed a randomized controlled trial in Khayelitsha, a peri-urban settlement of around half a million people on the outskirts of Cape Town, South Africa. The program incorporated key principles developed by the World Health Organization for promoting healthy psychosocial development (World Health Organization [WHO], 1995). The aim of the intervention was to encourage the mother to have sensitive, responsive interactions with her infant. A major aspect was the use of particular items from the Neonatal Behavioural Assessment Schedule (NBAS) (Brazelton & Nugent, 1995) to sensitize the mother to her infant's individual capacities and needs.

The intervention was delivered by women residing in Khayelitsha. The women had no formal specialist qualifications, although all were mothers. They received training in basic parenting and counseling skills, as well as in the specific mother-infant intervention, and they received weekly group supervision throughout the study by an experienced community clinical psychologist. The intervention was delivered in participants' homes in hour-long sessions. The women in the index group were visited twice antenatally, twice in the first postpartum week, weekly for the next seven weeks, biweekly for a further month, and then monthly for two months (i.e., 15 sessions in total, ending at five months postpartum). Those in the control group received the normal service provided by the local infant clinic, which involved visits from community health workers who made assessments of maternal and infant physical and medical progress.

Compared with women who received no specific help or support, women in Khayelitsha who received a home-based intervention interacted with their infants with greater sensitivity and with less intrusiveness, both shortly after completion of the intervention (six months postpartum) and at a longer term follow-up (12 months postpartum). At 18 months postpartum, infants whose mothers had received the intervention were more likely to be rated as securely attached to their mothers than were infants of control group mothers.

The findings of this study show that early intervention in LMICs can benefit the mother–infant relationship. The intervention was delivered by women from the local community who had no formal training, apart from that received from the study team for delivery of the intervention. This indicates that the intervention is potentially sustainable and that it could be broadly implemented in developing countries with relatively limited resources. In addition, the community health workers had a focused task (rather than responsibility for comprehensive community health), were given appropriate support and supervision, and had strong community support, all of which are regarded as essential for effective community health worker programs (Haines, Sanders, Lehmann, Rowe, Lawn, & Jan, 2007).

Limitations

The Khayelitsha mother infant intervention is a relatively intensive intervention (15 one-hour sessions) and one that is not integrated with primary healthcare services. There remain some questions about possible scale-up (in South Africa), as well as in other LMICS.

The MANAS project: Improving the outcomes of primary care attenders (India)

Patel and colleagues (2010) conducted a cluster randomized controlled trial of an intervention in Goa, India, (based on the successful Chilean trial (Araya et al., 2003) described above) using a collaborative stepped care intervention approach. The bulk of the work in this intervention is undertaken by trained health counselors and health assistants. Health assistants screen for depression and refer to primary care physicians. Psycho-education and all non-drug treatments, including adherence management, are provided by health counselors. Where needed, primary care physicians prescribe and monitor antidepressants. A visiting psychiatrist consults on cases that do not respond to lower levels of care and for patients who express suicidal ideation. The trial provided modest evidence for a beneficial effect of the intervention on recovery from common mental disorder (Patel et al., 2010).

Lessons learned

When we consider the studies discussed above, it is clear that there is now compelling evidence that it is possible to implement efficacious mental health interventions in low-income countries and contexts. Carefully designed and well-supervised community- or primary care-based mental health programs can work even with the front-line care delivered by people with minimal training.

While this is good news, questions remain regarding how to translate the promising findings from well-designed and evaluated interventions into existing healthcare systems. Patel and colleagues (2008) highlight the following obstacles to implementing effective programs in developing countries:

1   Low recognition of common mental disorders by primary care physicians, partly because of somatic presentation.
2   Inadequate use of evidence-based medicines (including antidepressants) and widespread use of medicine for which there is no evidence of efficacy.
3   Lack of personnel resources for non-drug (psychosocial) interventions.
4   Severe shortage of skilled mental health practitioners.
5   Low adherence to treatment regimens.
6   Health system challenges in integrating mental health care into primary health care (summarized from Patel et al., 2008).

Thus, even with encouraging results from the studies above, global mental health challenges are formidable. Key to questions of scale-up and effectiveness of interventions in the real world is the question of who in the long term should be providing interventions, especially in the context of limited skills of healthcare workers and enormous existing workloads. Every intervention discussed above depends in some way on what has been termed "task shifting", and it is to this issue that we now turn.

Task shifting in mental health

The WHO has estimated that 57 countries face health worker shortages; 36 of these countries are in sub-Saharan Africa (WHO, 2006). In recent years this crisis has been exacerbated by the stress that HIV care needs put on already overstretched health systems (Lehmann, Van Damme, Barten, & Sanders, 2009; Zachariah, Ford, Philips, Lynch, Massaquoi, Janssens, & Harries, 2009). However, HIV is not the sole cause of health worker shortages. Other factors include migration, poor staff morale, and lack of appropriate incentives (Zachariah et al., 2009). The workforce problem unfortunately is not only limited to shortages but also manifests as inequitable healthcare staff distribution both within countries and between countries, skewing benefits toward both wealthy countries and wealthy urban areas within poor countries (Coovadia, Jewkes, Barron, Sanders, & McIntyre, 2009; Patel, 2009; Zachariah et al., 2009).

A response to this human resource crisis has been the call for task-shifting in healthcare services, especially since the release of the 2006 *World Health Report* (WHO, 2006). When task shifting occurs, medical and health service tasks that previously were performed by higher level cadres are shifted or delegated to lower level cadres (Zachariah et al., 2009). In South Africa, for example, this delegation of tasks occurs at two levels (Lehmann, 2009). The first level is within the health system in the delegation of prescribing and diagnosing tasks from doctors to nurses and more recently the delegation of tasks to mid-level workers. At the second level, tasks are delegated outside of the formal health system to trained lay community members, such as community health workers and caregivers. These tasks usually involve health promotion or treatment support, but research is underway to assess an increase in the range of community health worker responsibilities to more clinical tasks, such as immunization and HIV testing. Task shifting may occur when lower level cadres are required to perform a function if they can produce the same quality as higher level cadres, which is more efficient and cost-effective service delivery. In another scenario, there may simply not be sufficient higher level cadre resources to meet healthcare needs, forcing lower level cadres to take on the tasks.

In discussing the mental health and development agenda in sub-Saharan Africa, Jenkins, Baingana, Belkin, Borowitz, Daly, and Francis (2010) argue that "there is the erroneous presumption that mental health services can only be delivered by specialists." The oldest explanations for the failure of community health worker interventions throughout the world have been the inadequacy of the supervision and the lack of support from formal health care staff (Daniels et al., 2010). The lack of support sometimes has been linked to higher-level health workers feeling threatened if tasks they have done are reallocated to more junior staff or community health workers. The issue requires a sensitive re-examination of the appropriate scope of practice for different levels of providers in constrained circumstances (Lehmann, 2009). Effective supervision remains crucial in this discussion, with the provision of skilled and sophisticated supervision becoming more central to the tasks of higher-level personnel (Ofosu-Amaah, 1983).

As Lehmann (2009) has argued, task shifting is not simply an emergency response, since lower-level cadres may be as good as, or better than, those originally trained for the task. According to Lehmann (2008), task shifting is in line with growing evidence that health worker cadres (other than medical doctors) can deliver aspects of care at primary and community levels as well as, or perhaps better than, medical doctors. At the same time, while task shifting holds significant promise for improving population level mental health across LMICs, it should not be seen as a panacea for the human resources challenges faced by LMICs (Philips, Zachariah, & Venis, 2008).

It stands to reason that if tasks are to be shifted, it should be easier if the new tasks integrate well with and add to existing roles undertaken by health workers. Further, new roles that succeed likely will be ones which hold demonstrable advantages to existing roles. Discussing development issues more broadly, Max-Neef (1989) suggests that, in order to address human needs, policy planners must search for what he terms "synergistic satisfiers" – interventions that simultaneously address a number of human needs. For example, breastfeeding has benefits both for the nutritional status and for the growth of infants under conditions of poverty, and it also contributes to improved relationships between mothers and children. At this stage, we are not aware of empirical data comparing task shifting that aligns and improves existing tasks with task shifting that does not. In the following section, however, we discuss an approach that has the arguable advantage of aligning new roles to existing goals.

Family-centered interventions

Claeson and Waldman (2000) have convincingly argued that significant gains in child survival and improvements in child health will depend to an increasing degree on what happens in the household in combination with a responsive and supportive health system. They further contend that focus should be on the promotion of a limited number of household behaviors that have a direct link to childhood illness. Traditionally, a narrow disease-focused model has dominated health interventions. For example, the primary aim of most interventions that target pregnant, HIV-positive women is to prevent transmission of infection from mother to child. Once transmission has been prevented the program is considered successful and usually ends. A broader family-based approach to wellness would reduce the potential for the broader implications of any health condition to be overlooked. Applied to the example above, this approach would thus extend the benefits of the prevention of mother to child HIV transmission.

A focus on the family in no way excludes consideration of the health system or disease-specific strategies. What it does do, however, is include in program design an understanding of how any health issue is firmly embedded within a familial context. In the case infant feeding, for example, the family-based approach acknowledges that simply providing information about exclusive and appropriate feeding, and even garnering maternal buy-in to these concepts, is simply the first step in a complex chain of familial negotiations that will have to take place for the knowledge to become translated into practice.

Interventions must address the environmental barriers to implementation. Siblings constitute an important aspect of the family environment that is seldom considered. Positive sibling relationships can be protective for children exposed to stressors, especially in homes characterized by parental conflict (Gass, Jenkins, & Dunn, 2007; Jenkins & Smith, 1990). Thus, those designing interventions should consider strategies for strengthening relationships between siblings to reduce the effects of any adverse experiences (Gass et al., 2007). With the increasing occurrence of child-headed households, implementing preventive family-based interventions that target siblings from the outset is vital.

In the case of treating depression, given the lack of access to mental health care and psychotropic medication due to weak health systems in many LMICs, an important consideration is the role of alternative care-givers (Murray, Halligan, & Cooper, 2010. There is evidence that infants of depressed mothers respond positively during interactions with their non-depressed fathers (Hossain, Field, Gonzalez, Malphurs, & Delvalle, 1994) as well as other caregivers, such as child-minders or day care nurses (Pelaez-Nogueras, Field, Cigales, Gonzalez, & Clasky, 1994). Interestingly, Cohn, Campbell, Matias, and Hopkins (1990) found a positive benefit for the mother-infant relationship when the depressed mother was not based at home full-time. Alternative care has also been shown to reduce behavio-ral problems in children aged two and three years among depressed mothers (Lee, Halpern, Hertz-Picciotto, Martin, & Suchindran, 2006). These data are highly pertinent for other mental health concerns in that they illustrate how the functioning of other family members is central in beneficial child outcome (even in the context of maternal depression).

Rotheram-Borus, Swendeman, and Chovnick (2009) have argued that a paradigm shift is needed as lack of skilled staff, poorly developed health systems, and financial constraints all make the continued focus on categor-ical (disease specific) funding ineffective (Rotheram-Borus et al., 2009). They argue categorically funded, vertically integrated interventions (for depression, for instance) are highly stigmatized and will not have the capacity to address the health needs of Africa. Unless packages of care for depression or other mental disorders (Patel & Thornicroft, 2009) are integ-rated into family-based community intervention models, they are unlikely to be successfully implemented at scale. The evidence from research in the area of parental depression offers insights into how a shift from viewing depression as the primary focus, together with a family-based approach, allows us to see with greater clarity the extent to which health conditions are embedded in contexts characterized by interpersonal violence, poor child attendance at school, absent parents, chaotic family routines, inter-generational transmission of trauma, mental illness, youth violence and risk taking, and disempowerment of women.

Mental illness is a highly stigmatized condition, while the family is a valued social unit. Furthermore, mental disorders have repercussions for family members that go beyond the individual and their illness. Therefore, a family-focused wellness perspective is likely to be a more acceptable vehicle of intervention than a focus on any single condition or disease entity. Models of intervention focusing on early parenting, familial cohe-sion, illness detection, appropriate health-seeking behavior, cognitive-behavioral strategies of behavior change, linking people to poverty alleviation programs, and comprehensive strategies that begin early in life and continue over time are urgently needed.

Many of these components are characteristic of many successful intervention programs in the domain of youth violence (Tremblay, 2006), but the broader diffusion of these successful programs has not happened in any significant way (Rotheram-Borus et al., 2009). There are many reasons for this, not least of which is the continuing search for the "magic bullet" for single disease entities. Another reason for poor diffusion is that delivering efficacious treatments under ideal conditions is quite different from implementation at scale in community settings. Interventions are embedded within the "messiness" of family life, which includes the chaos of families without meaningful routines and multiple familial actors that all contribute to the problem as well as its solution. Behavioral change can only be sustained when it is supported by the routines and personal relationships that characterize daily family life (Rotheram-Borus et al., 2009), which is simply not possible in individual-focused, disease-targeted interventions.

While family-level interventions offer the potential for significant gains, their implementation will face many of the same barriers that individual-focused interventions do. Scaling up family-based interventions will require linkages to existing service delivery systems, including integration with the healthcare system. In addition, such interventions will require a trained, well-managed, and adequately supported workforce in order to deliver the interventions. As noted earlier, in the context of the significant human resource crisis that characterizes many LMICs (Coovadia et al., 2009), community health workers are increasingly being used to deliver interventions. There are, however, significant barriers to the effective deployment of community health workers, such as training, monitoring, and supervision.

Significant strides have recently been made in terms of understanding how best to improve global mental health. We know from a number of studies across three continents that it is possible to design and implement interventions that are efficacious and relatively low-cost. However, further exploration of how to take the lessons from these successes and translate them into larger-scale, sustainable health system innovations is sorely needed. Given the resource constraints and the stress under which health systems operate, this scale-up is an enormously complex challenge.

Much more needs to be done to explore the mundane but crucial questions about how health systems, comprising both professionally trained and lay workers, can include mental health work to improve not only mental health outcomes but other outcomes as well. In this regard we have suggested three interlocking principles, the utility of which needs to be more fully explored: First, align mental health interventions with existing goals of healthcare so as not to add to the burden of healthcare personnel; second, focus on broader packages of care that have multiple benefits rather than targeting individual illnesses separately; and third, reconsider the unit of intervention for all this work. That is, family-focused care may both strengthen the area within which most health issues are experienced and managed (the family) and also help overcome the huge barrier of stigma that bedevils illness-focused mental healthcare. Rigorous work on a large scale to explore and address these issues will assist the field in understanding whether these are useful pointers towards improved global mental health or whether other approaches should be taken.

References

Aaron, R., Joseph, A., Abraham, S., Muliyil, J., George, K., Prasad, J., et al. (2004). Suicides in young people in rural southern India. *Lancet, 363*, 1117–1118.

Adams, J., King, C., & Hook, D. (2010). *Global research report: Africa.* London, UK: Thomson Reuters.

Araya, R., Rojas, G., Fritsch, R., Gaete, J., Rojas, M., Simon, G., & Peters, T. J. (2003). Treating depression in primary care in low-income women in Santiago, Chile: A randomised controlled trial. *Lancet, 361*, 995–1000.

Bolton, P., Bass, J., Neugebauer, R., Verdeli, H., Clougherty, K. F., Wickramaratne, P., et al. (2003). Group interpersonal psychotherapy for depression in rural Uganda: A randomized controlled trial. *JAMA, 289*, 3117–3124.

Brazelton, T. B., & Nugent, J. K. (1995). *Neonatal behavioral assessment scale. Clinics in developmental medicine.* London: McKeith Press.

Chisholm, D., Flisher, A., Lund, C., Patel, V., Saxena, S., Thornicroft, G., & Tomlinson, M. (2007). Scale up services for mental disorders: A call for action. *Lancet, 370*, 1241–1252.

Claeson, M., & Waldman, R. J. (2000). The evolution of child health programmes in developing countries: From targeting diseases to targeting people. *Bulletin of the World Health Organization, 78*, 1234–1245.

Cohn, J. F., Campbell, S. B., Matias, R., & Hopkins, J. (1990). Face-to-face interactions of postpartum depressed and nondepressed mother-infant pairs at 2 months. *Developmental Psychology, 26*, 15–23.

Cooper, P., Landman, M., Tomlinson, M., Molteno, C., Swartz, L., & Murray, L. (2002). The impact of a mother-infant intervention in an indigent peri-urban South African context: Pilot study. *British Journal of Psychiatry, 180*, 76–81.

Coovadia, H., Jewkes, R., Barron, P., Sanders, D., & McIntyre, D. (2009). The health and health system of South Africa: Historical roots of current public health challenges. *Lancet, 374*, 817–834.

Daniels, K., Nor, B., Jackson, D., Ekstrom, E. C., & Doherty, T. (2010). Supervision of community peer counselors for infant feeding in South Africa: An exploratory qualitative study. *Human Resources for Health, 8*, 6.

Desjarlais, R., Eisenberg, L., Good, B & Kleinman, A. (1995). *World mental health: Problems and priorities in low-income countries.* New York: Oxford University Press .

Gass, K., Jenkins, J., & Dunn, J. (2007). Are sibling relationships protective? A longitudinal study. *Journal of Child Psychology and Psychiatry, 48*, 167–175.

Global Forum for Health Research. (2000). *10/90 report on health research 2000* (2nd annual report). Geneva: Global Forum for Health Research.

Grantham-McGregor, S., Cheung, Y. B., Cueto, S., Glewwe, P., Richter, L., & Strupp, B. (2007). Developmental potential in the first 5 years for children in developing countries. *Lancet, 369*, 60–70.

Haines, A., Sanders, D., Lehmann, U., Rowe, A. K., Lawn, J. E., Jan, S., et al. (2007). Achieving child survival goals: Potential contribution of community health workers. *Lancet, 369,* 2121–2131.

Hedegaard, M., Henriksen, T. B., Sabroe, S., & Secher, N. J. (1993). Psychological distress in pregnancy and preterm delivery. *BMJ, 307,* 377–378.

Hoffman, S., & Hatch, M. C. (2000). Depressive symptomatology during pregnancy: evidence for an association with decreased fetal growth in pregnancies of lower social class women. *Health Psychology, 19,* 535–543.

Hossain, Z., Field, T., Gonzalez, J., Malphurs, J., & Del Valle, C. (1994). Infants of "depressed" mothers interact better with their non-depressed fathers. *Infant Mental Health Journal, 15,* 348–357.

Jenkins, J. M., & Smith, M. A. (1990). Factors protecting children living in disharmonious homes: Maternal reports. *Journal of the American Academy of Child and Adolescent Psychiatry, 29,* 60–69.

Jenkins, R., Baingana, F., Belkin, G., Borowitz, M., Daly, A., Francis, P., et al. (2010). Mental health and the development agenda in sub-Saharan Africa. *Psychiatric Services, 61,* 229–234.

Kessler, R. C., Angermeyer, M., Anthony, J. C., De Graaf, R., Demyttenaere, K., Gasquet, I., et al. (2007). Lifetime prevalence and age-of-onset distributions of mental disorders in the world health organization's world mental health survey initiative. *World Psychiatry, 6,* 168–176.

Lee, L., Halpern, C. T., Hertz-Picciotto, I., Martin, S. L., & Suchindran, C. M. (2006). Child care and social support modify the association between maternal depressive symptoms and early childhood behaviour problems: A US national study. *Journal of Epidemiology and Community Health, 60,* 305–310.

Lehmann, U. (2009). Strengthening Human Resources for Primary Health Care. In P. Barron (Ed.), *South African Health Review 2008* (pp. 163–178). Durban: Health Systems Trust.

Lehmann, U., Van Damme, W., Barten, F., & Sanders, D. (2009). Task shifting: the answer to the human resources crisis in Africa? *Human Resources for Health, 7,* 49.

Lopez, A. D., Mathers, C. D., Ezzati, M., Jamison, D. T., & Murray, C. J. (2006). Global and regional burden of disease and risk factors, 2001: systematic analysis of population health data. *Lancet, 367,* 1747–1757.

Manandhar, D. S., Osrin, D., Shrestha, B. P., Mesko, N., Morrison, J., Tumbahangphe, K. M., et al. (2004). Effect of a participatory intervention with women's groups on birth outcomes in Nepal: Cluster-randomised controlled trial. *Lancet, 364,* 970–979.

Max-Neef, M. (1989). *Human scale development: Conception, application and further reflections.* New York: Apex Press.

Milberger, S., Biederman, J., Faraone, S. V., Chen, L., & Jones, J. (1996). Is maternal smoking during pregnancy a risk factor for attention deficit hyperactivity disorder in children? *American Journal of Psychiatry, 153,* 1138–1142.

Miranda, J. J., & Patel, V. (2005). Achieving the Millennium Development Goals: Does Mental Health Play a Role? *PLoS Medicine, 2,* 0962–0965.

Murray, L., Halligan, S. L., & Cooper, P. J. (2010). Effects of postnatal depression on mother-infant interactions, and child development. In T. Wachs and G. Bremner (Eds.), *Handbook of Infant Development.* Hoboken, NJ: Wiley-Blackwell.

Ofosu-Amaah, V. (1983). National experience in the use of community health workers. A review of current issues and problems. *WHO Offset Publications, 71*, 1–49.

Patel, V. (2009). The future of psychiatry in low- and middle-income countries. *Psychological Medicine, 39*, 1759–1762.

Patel, V., & Sumathipala, A. (2001). International Representation in Psychiatric Journals: a survey of 6 leading journals. *British Journal of Psychiatry, 178*, 406–9.

Patel, V., & Thornicroft, G. (2009). Packages of care for mental, neurological, and substance use disorders in low- and middle-income countries. *PLoS Medicine, 6*, 1–2.

Patel, V., Weiss, H.A., Chowdhary, N., Naik, S., Pednekar, S., Chatterjee, S., et al. (2010). Effectiveness of an intervention led by lay health counsellors for depressive and anxiety disorders in primary care in Goa, India (MANAS): a cluster randomised controlled trial. *Lancet, 376*, 2086–2095.

Pelaez-Nogueras, M., Field, T., Cigales, M., Gonzalez, L., & Clasky, S. (1994). Infants of depressed mothers show less "depressed" behavior with their nursery teachers. *Infant Mental Health Journal, 15*, 358–367.

Phillips, M. R., Li, X., & Zhang, Y. (2002). Suicide rates in China, 1995–99. *Lancet, 359*, 835–840.

Philips, M., Zachariah, R., & Venis, S. (2008). Task shifting for antiretroviral treatment delivery in sub-Saharan Africa: Not a panacea. *Lancet, 371*, 682–684.

Prince, M., Patel, V., Saxena, S., Mai, M., Maselko, J., Phillips, M. R., & Rahman, A. (2007). No health without mental health. *Lancet, 370*, 859–877.

Rahman, A. (2005). Maternal depression and child health: The need for holistic health policies in developing countries. *Harvard Health Policy Review, 6*, 70–80.

Rahman, A., Iqbal, Z., Bunn, J., Lovel, H., & Harrington, R. (2004). Impact of maternal depression on infant nutritional status and illness. *Archives of General Psychiatry, 61*, 946–952.

Rahman, A., Malik, A., Sikander, S., Roberts, C., & Creed, F. (2008). Cognitive behaviour therapy-based intervention by community health workers for mothers with depression and their infants in rural Pakistan: A cluster-randomized controlled trial. *Lancet, 372*, 902–909.

Razzouk, D., Sharan, P., Gallo, C., Gureje, O., Lamberte, E., Mari, J. J., et al. (2010). Scarcity and inequity of mental health research resources in low- and middle-income countries: A global survey. *Health Policy, 94*, 211–220.

Rotheram-Borus, M. J., Swendeman, D., & Chovnick, G. (2009). The past, present, and future of HIV prevention: Integrating behavioral, biomedical, and structural intervention strategies for the next generation of HIV prevention. *Annual Review of Clinical Psychology, 5*, 143–167.

Saraceno, B., Van Ommeren, M., Batniji, R., Cohen, A., Gureje, O., Mahoney, J., et al. (2007). Barriers to improvement of mental health services in low-income and middle-income countries. *Lancet, 370*, 1164–1174.

Saxena, S., Paraje, G., Sharan, P., Karam, G., & Sadana, R. (2006). The 10/90 divide in mental health research: Trends over a 10-year period. *British Journal of Psychiatry, 188*, 81–82.

Shah, A. A., & Beinecke, R. H. (2009). Global mental health needs, services, barriers, and challenges. *International Journal of Mental Health, 38*, 14–29.

Sharan, P., Gallo, C., Gureje, O., Lamberte, E., Mari, J. J., Mazzotti, G., et al. (2009). Mental health research priorities in low- and middle-income countries of

Africa, Asia, and Latin America and the Caribbean. *British Journal of Psychiatry, 195*, 354–363. doi: 10.1192/bjp.bp. 108.050187.

Statistics South Africa. (2007). *Mortality and Causes of Death Statistics.* Retrieved from www.statssa.gov.za/.

Stein, D., & Seedat, S. (2007). From research methods to clinical practice in psychiatry: Challenges and opportunities in the developing world. *International Review of Psychiatry, 19*, 573–581.

Tomlinson, M., & Swartz, L. (2003). Imbalances in the knowledge about infancy: the divide between rich and poor countries. *Infant Mental Health Journal, 24*, 547–556.

Tremblay, R. E. (2006). Prevention of youth violence: Why not start at the beginning? *Journal of Abnormal Psychology, 34*, 481–487.

United Nations. (1995). *World Summit of Social Development, Copenhagen.* New York: United Nations.

United Nations. (2009). *The Millennium Development Goals Report.* New York: United Nations.

United Nations Development Programme. (2010). *The Millennium Development Goals.* Retrieved from www.undp.org/mdg/.

United Nations Population Fund. (2008). *State of the world population: Reaching common ground: Culture, gender and human rights.* New York: United Nations.

Wiley-Exley, E. (2007). Evaluations of community mental health care in low- and middle-income countries: A 10-year review of the literature. *Social Science and Medicine, 64*, 1231–1241.

Wilkinson, R.G. (1997). Socioeconomic determinants of health: Health inequalities: relative or absolute material standards? *British Medical Journal, 314*, 591.

World Health Organization. (1995). *Improving the Psychosocial Development of Children.* Geneva: World Health Organization.

World Health Organization. (2006). *The World Health Report 2006: Working together for health.* Geneva: World Health Organzation.

Zachariah, R., Ford, N., Philips, M., Lynch, S., Massaquoi, M., Janssens, V., & Harries, A. D. (2009). Task shifting in HIV/AIDS: Opportunities, challenges and proposed actions for sub-Saharan Africa. *Transactions of the Royal Society for Tropical Medicine and Hygiene, 103*, 549–558.

Zolneirek, C. D. (2008). Mental health policy and integrated care: global perspectives. *Journal of Psychiatric and Mental Health Nursing, 15*, 562–568.

Part III
Public health practice

11 Mental health service utilization in the United States

Past, present, and future

Benjamin G. Druss, Philip S. Wang, and Ronald C. Kessler

Mental health service past and present

Unlike most other countries, the US does not have a national mental health system or any one federal entity that is responsible for overseeing the delivery of mental health services. Rather, the patchwork of services for mental disorders in the US is a de facto system of care made up of a range of financing mechanisms, patient populations, and sectors (Regier, Goldberg, & Taube, 1978; Regier, Narrow, Rae, Manderscheid, Locke, & Goodwin, 1993).

Mental health care is delivered in different service sectors, and this chapter focuses primarily on the two service sectors that are part of the formal health system. The specialty medical sector comprises care by mental health professionals (e.g., psychologists, psychiatrists) in settings dedicated to behavioral health services. The general medical/primary care sector consists of primary care physicians and allied medical professionals (e.g., nurse practitioners) who may provide mental health treatments as part of a broader array of health services. Three additional service sectors, the human services, voluntary support, and complementary and alternative medicine sectors, are not part of the formal health system, but are nonetheless important in the delivery of mental health care. While these will not be a focus of this chapter, we describe them briefly below.

The human services sector consists of religious services as well as social welfare, criminal justice, and educational services. For the general adult population in the US, members of the clergy may be the only point of contact for persons with mental distress and more serious conditions (Wang, Berglund, & Kessler, 2003). The voluntary support network refers to self-help groups and organizations. This sector, which grew out of the Alcoholics Anonymous program developed in the late 1930s, has had growing importance for persons with more serious and persistent mental illness. A total of 13.3% of the US population report having attended a 12-step meeting for alcohol or other conditions (Room & Greenfield, 1993). Mental health consumers who have received certification as peer specialists help train other peers to work towards goals of mental health and recovery. Medicaid programs in 25 states now reimburse services for these peer specialists, who are increasingly moving from the voluntary sector to the formal mental health workforce (Davidson, Chinman, Sells, & Rowe, 2006). The complementary and alternative medicine (CAM) sector is comprised of healers, such as chiropractors, who provide a range of treatments not formally taught in medical schools or reimbursed by health providers. A substantial proportion of persons in mental health treatment also are engaged in CAM treatment (Druss & Rosenheck, 2000).

The mental health specialty sector

The private sector

The history of the private mental health sector in the US tracks the development of health insurance and care in the broader health system. During World War II, a ruling by the Labor Control Board that employer contributions to health insurance were not taxable, coupled with wage controls, led to a widespread expansion of employer-based health insurance in the United States (Starr, 1982). The vast majority of these plans also offered some coverage for mental health services, although these were typically subject to greater restrictions than other types of medical care, including copayments on inpatient and outpatient services and annual caps on total reimbursement (Frank & Glied, 2006). Medicare, which was established in 1965 to provide care for older Americans, adopted these higher copayments and coinsurance rates for mental disorders.

Beginning in the mid-1980s, rising health costs led to the widespread growth of managed care, which used a variety of administrative mechanisms and financial incentives to reduce the use of unnecessary services and improve quality of care. For mental health care, this took the form of managed behavioral care organizations (MBHOs), or "carve outs," which fund or administer mental health benefits separately from general medical insurance. For inpatient mental health care, cost control mechanisms included prior authorization of hospital stays and approval for ongoing treatment. For outpatient services, they involved implementing greater price competition, by driving care to less costly types of services and contracting with groups of providers for discounted fees. Between 1994 and 2006 the number of Americans in managed behavioral health care more than tripled, from 53 million to 170 million (Frank & Garfield, 2007).

Managed care played a major role in changing the nature of service delivery in the mental health private sector. The 1990s saw substantial declines in the number of private hospital beds and in length of stay on general hospital psychiatry units (Sharfstein & Dickerson, 2009; Watanabe-Galloway & Zhang, 2007). In outpatient settings, psychiatrists increasingly provided medications rather than psychotherapy; between

1996 and 2005, the proportion of psychiatrists providing psychotherapy to all of their patients declined by nearly half, from 19.1 to 10.8% (Mojtabai & Olfson, 2008). The nature of psychotherapy also changed, moving from long-term therapy, focused on understanding unconscious processes, to more pragmatic, shorter-term approaches, more focused on interpersonal relationships and challenging and reversing irrational cognitive beliefs (Lambert, Bergin, & Garfield, 2004).

The public sector

The public mental health sector is the safety net provider for individuals without mental health insurance and historically has provided care for persons with the most serious and disabling conditions. The rise of the public sector system for persons with serious mental illness began with the industrial revolution and urbanization of the US, with state governments building large institutions to care for indigent individuals with serious mental disorders (Grob, 1994). By the 1950s, nearly all care for persons with serious mental illness was provided in these state hospitals, and states financed the bulk of care for this population. In 1956, states accounted for 59% of overall mental health spending in the US (Fein, 1958).

In the 1960s, several factors converged to shift the primary locus of public sector mental health treatment from state hospitals into community settings. The development and marketing of antipsychotic medications, beginning with chlorpromazine in 1952, made it possible to stabilize symptoms among long-term residents of hospitals. At the same time, the community mental health movement represented a philosophical shift towards a public health approach, which argued that mental health services could be located in communities rather than in inpatient settings (Morrissey & Goldman, 1984). The Community Mental Health Centers Construction Act of 1963 provided funding to build a national network of community mental health centers that eventually became the backbone of the mental health safety net (Cutler, Bevilacqua, & McFarland, 2003).

Additionally, the enactment of Medicaid in 1965 played an enormous role in changing both the funding and locus of care for serious mental disorders in the US (Frank, Goldman, & Hogan, 2003). This program, under which states and the federal government share payments for indigent and disabled patients, provided states with a strong incentive to shift care out of state hospitals to settings that could be reimbursed by Medicaid, such as general hospital psychiatric units and nursing homes (Gronfein, 1985). The program also provided coverage to individuals who had previously had no insurance, increasing access to mental health services for poor and disabled persons with serious mental illness (Frank et al., 2003). By 2003, Medicaid accounted for 45% of all public mental health spending (Mark, Levit, Buck, Coffey, & Vandivort-Warren, 2007).

The specialty mental health workforce

For the first half of the 20th century, nearly all mental health care in the US was provided by physicians trained as psychiatrists (Menninger & Nemiah, 2000). However, beginning after World War II, there was a rapid growth of other mental health provider groups and with it an expansion and diversification of the mental health workforce. After the war, facing a shortage of psychiatrists, the Veteran's Administration and National Institute of Mental Health supported the funding of programs to train doctoral-level clinical psychologists to help treat returning veterans needing care. By 1950, more than half of PhDs in psychology were being awarded for clinical psychology (Compas & Gotlib, 2002). Social work, which had emerged as a public health-oriented profession at the turn of the 20th century, began to play a role in direct patient counseling (Silverman, 1985). Today, there are more than 122,000 social workers and more than 200,000 licensed counselors providing mental health, substance, or marriage and family services (Bureau of Labor Statistics, 2009). Now psychiatrists, who used to provide nearly all the care in the specialty mental health sector, represent less than 10% of the specialty mental health workforce.

The general medical sector

About three-quarters of the US population make one or more primary care visits in any given year (Ezzati-Rice & Rohde, 2008; Kirby, Machlin, & Thorpe, 2001). Thus, primary care physicians have always had the potential to play an important role in detecting and managing common mental disorders. In contrast with the specialty sector, the general medical sector has historically provided care to persons with common but less disabling conditions, such as anxiety and depression. The vast majority of treatment in general medical settings has been psychotropic medications rather than psychotherapy (Olfson & Klerman, 1993).

During the 1990s, there was a major expansion in the rate of delivery of mental health services in the US, largely driven by an expansion of care in the general medical sector. Between 1990 and 2003, the proportion of individuals receiving mental health services rose from 12.2 to 20.1% of the population, (Kessler, Demler, Frank, Olfson, Pincus, & Walters, 2005), with a nearly threefold increase in the rate of treatment in the general medical sector (Wang, Lane, Olfson, Pincus, Wells, & Kessler, 2006).

The most important factor driving this explosion of growth of mental health delivery in the general health sector was the development of the newer classes of antidepressant medications, beginning with the release of the first selective serotonin reuptake inhibitor (SSRI), Prozac (Fluoxetine), in December 1987. Primary care physicians often had been reluctant to prescribe older classes of antidepressants such as tricyclic medications, due to concerns about side effects and potential suicide risk. When they did recommend these medications, they commonly prescribed them at inadequate dosages. Use of SSRIs was far simpler, with a uniform dosage, relatively few side effects, and minimal risk of overdose. By 2005, antidepressants surpassed antihypertensive agents to become the most commonly prescribed class of medications in office-based medical practice in the US (Cherry, Woodwell, & Rechtsteiner, 2007). Between 1996 and 2005 the number of individuals in the US treated with antidepressants increased from 13.3 to 27 million (Olfson & Marcus, 2009).

Despite the rising rates of treatment for mental disorders, substantial barriers to treatment still exist. In 1990, only 24.3% of individuals with mental disorders in a national survey of the general US population received any treatment. While this proportion increased over time, another national survey carried out in 2003 found that only a minority (40.5%) of individuals with serious mental illness were receiving mental health services.

Among the most common barriers to seeking mental health services reported in the 1990 National Comorbidity Survey were the fact that health insurance would not cover treatment (36.2%), and high out-of-pocket expense (44.3%) (Kessler, Berglund, Bruce, Koch, Laska, & Leaf, 2001). These barriers would be reduced, respectively, by current reform efforts around new parity regulations and insurance expansion. Other barriers to treatment, however, reflect more deep-seated attitudes towards mental disorders and the efficacy of treatments. Two of the most common reasons for not seeking treatment in the 1990 survey among persons with serious mental illness were the belief that the individual did not have a problem requiring treatment (54.6%) and the belief that treatment would not help (38.1%). There is some indication that these attitudes are beginning to change, at least for more common conditions such as major depression. Public opinion surveys found that between 1996 and 2006 the number of Americans who ascribed a biological cause to depression increased from 77 to 88%, and the proportion who regarded biological treatments as a first option for care increased from 48 to 60% (Blumner & Marcus, 2009). These changes are likely to be, in part, both a cause and a consequence of rising rates of antidepressant use.

Once individuals begin mental health treatment, many still do not receive high-quality care. Among individuals already in treatment, Wang, Lane, Olfson, Pincus, Wells, & Kessler (2005) examined the proportion of individuals receiving minimally adequate treatment, defined as two or more treatment visits or being in ongoing treatment at the time of the interview. The study found that only 12.7% of individuals receiving treatment in the general medical sector received minimally adequate care, considerably lower than rate in the specialty mental health sector (48.3%). These quality problems largely reflect broader challenges in effectively treating chronic illnesses in primary care. Managing these problems requires mechanisms for coordinating care across multiple providers and over time (Wagner, Austin, & Von Korff, 1996). Most medical practices in the US are still not equipped to deliver many of these services (Casalino, Gillies, Shortell, Schmittdiel, Bodenheimer, & Robinson, 2003).

The future: New policy initiatives and emerging trends in mental health services

Recent years have seen a number of policy developments and trends that have the potential to reshape the landscape of the current mental health system. At the federal level, the passage of mental health parity legislation in 2008 and comprehensive health reform in 2010 could affect both use and distribution of mental health services. At the state level, fiscal constraints and a reduced role of state authorities in providing mental health services may result in a reduction of responsibility for this population. At a community level, a number of innovative programs are being developed.

Mental health parity

As noted above, ever since the development of the modern health insurance system, coverage for mental health insurance has been more limited than insurance for general medical care (Frank, Koyanagi, & McGuire, 1997). Under fee-for-service plans, consumers typically faced higher copayments and coinsurance for care of mental disorders than physical disorders; for instance, under Medicare, consumers paid 50% coinsurance for outpatient mental health services compared to 20% for other medical care. Several economic considerations led insurance companies to provide less generous mental health services, including concerns about moral hazard (a belief that lower costs would stimulate higher use) and adverse selection (the fear that companies that offered more generous coverage would attract high-cost beneficiaries) (Sharfstein & Taube, 1982). However, the result was a system with higher financial burdens for individuals needing to use mental health services, as well as a payment system that perpetuated inequalities between mental health and general medical services.

Beginning in the early 1990s, mental health advocates made mental health parity – equality of insurance benefits across mental health and medical services – a major focus. In 1999, President Clinton directed the US Office of Personnel Management to enact parity for mental health and substance abuse coverage in the Federal Employees Health Benefits Program by 2001. An evaluation of this program found that parity did not result in an overall increase in plan premiums but did reduce out-of-pocket expenditures for individuals using mental health services (Goldman, Frank, Burnam, Huskamp, Ridgely, & Normand, 2006). This evaluation demonstrated that under current managed care systems parity could be implemented with minimal cost to purchasers, which had been the main concern raised by employers in implementing parity laws.

This data helped set the stage for the passage for the passage of two landmark parity laws in 2008. First, in July of that year the Medicare Improvements for Patients and Providers Act ended Medicare's discriminatory 50% coinsurance for outpatient psychotherapy and services. The bill will phase in the reduction of the copayments through 2014, when it will become 20%, the same as for other medical services. This has the potential to reduce the financial burden and improve follow-through with care for senior and disabled Medicare recipients. Second, on October 3, 2008, the Paul Wellstone and Pete Domenici Mental Health Parity and Addiction Equity Act of 2008 was signed into law, significantly expanding regulations from the Mental Health Parity Act of 1996. These new laws, which go into effect in 2010, require that health benefits be provided at parity with medical/surgical benefits across a range of service types. Importantly, the law also covers Medicaid services.

How will parity affect mental health service delivery in the United States? As noted above, an analysis of the Federal Healthcare Employee Benefit Plan suggests that parity laws have not led to increases in the number of individuals who use mental health services, but these laws do provide important financial protection for individuals already using services (Goldman, 2007). Whether the same result will hold in the larger population remains to be seen.

Health care reform

On March 23, 2010, President Obama signed the Patient Protection and Affordable Care Act (Public Law 111–148), the largest change to the US health system since Medicare and Medicaid were established in 1965. The two pillars of the current reform effort – expansion of insurance coverage and pilot projects to drive delivery system redesign – will likely each have substantial implications for how mental health and substance use services are organized and delivered in the US.

Health reform legislation will require most US citizens to have health insurance and provide subsidies to those who do not. Given high rates of uninsurance and underinsurance among persons with mental disorders (Druss & Rosenheck, 1998), expansion of insurance, particularly in the face of parity, is likely to increase access to mental health services as well as to medical services. For persons with serious mental disorders, this insurance will come in the form of an expansion of Medicaid coverage to 133% of the federal poverty level, translating to a one-third increase in the Medicaid population. As noted previously, mental health parity will ensure a basic Medicaid benefit that includes mental health and substance use services. While this is likely to be a positive development for persons with serious mental disorders, there is already a shortage of community mental health providers who accept Medicaid, and this new entitlement may further stretch this limited capacity.

In addition to an expansion of health insurance, health reform legislation includes a series of demonstration projects and initiatives for reorienting health services to increase provider accountability and strengthen the role of primary care. Perhaps most relevant among these demonstration projects is a series of projects to promote the use of the Patient-Centered Medical Homes (PCMH), "an approach to providing comprehensive primary care ... that facilitates partnerships between individual patients, and their personal physicians, and when appropriate, the patient's family" (American Academy of Family Physicians, American Academy of Pediatrics, American College of Physicians, & American Osteopathic Association, 2007). The new legislation includes provisions for both Medicaid demonstration programs for PCMHs and, within the proposed Center for Medicare and Medicaid Innovation, the opportunity to test new models, including the medical home model within Medicare.

The Patient Protection and Affordable Care Act proposes a new state plan option to permit Medicaid enrollees with at least two chronic conditions, or one serious and persistent mental health condition, to designate a provider as a health home. States are expected to design and implement care models, track costs and avoidable hospitalizations, implement information technology, and monitor and report on quality and outcomes of care, highlighting the need to develop standardized metrics for assessing these indicators. Community Mental Health Centers are explicitly designated as potential health homes, suggesting the importance of supporting organizational strategies – particularly partnerships with community medical providers – that might allow these entities to serve in this capacity for their patients.

New financial mechanisms will be put into place to support these new organized systems of care. The Senate bill has provisions for organizing hospitals, specialists, and primary care providers as Accountable Care Organizations (ACOs), collectives of providers that would take responsibility for a group of patients. Under most ACO proposals, providers would be paid bonuses to the extent that programs meet quality goals or save costs. This may help overcome problems of economies of scale faced by solo primary care and mental health/substance use practitioners, as well as community-based mental health/substance use providers, allowing them to work as part of "virtual" patient centered medical homes. ACOs would not in and of themselves guarantee integration, but they may provide a structure in which integrated models could be supported and incentivized. "Bundling" strategies may be used to pay for episodes of care for individuals across mental and medical conditions.

The role of the states

State mental health authorities, who once held primary responsibility for the care of persons with serious mental illnesses, saw their role diminish after the establishment of Medicaid and the community mental health movement. Several factors may further accelerate these trends in coming years. Of special note, the recent economic recession in the US has left states in financial straits, and mental health expenditures have been subject to major cuts. The expansion of the pool of individuals with Medicaid under health reform will provide opportunities for states to save block grant funds but may also further decentralize responsibility for populations with serious mental illnesses.

Community innovations

At the community level, a number of innovative programs are currently being developed to improve the quality of mental health care. The mental health consumer movement has become more influential in mainstream mental health delivery, and "recovery" has become an organizing principle for improving care. Information technology, such as electronic medical records and registries, is gradually being adopted, although this process has been slower for mental health than for medical care. Community mental health providers are increasingly partnering with general medical organizations to improve care for mental disorders in primary care and to provide primary care for persons with serious mental illnesses.

Conclusions

Recent years have seen an enormous expansion and diversification of mental health service delivery in the US. In the past, most of this change has occurred as a bottom-up process at the provider and patient level. With the passage of federal parity and health insurance reform, these grass-roots efforts will be accompanied by a series of top-down changes, including expansion of insurance and a series of new demonstration projects that are likely to further transform the nature of mental health care delivery.

References

American Academy of Family Physicians, American Academy of Pediatrics, American College of Physicians, & American Osteopathic Association. (2007). *Joint Principles of a Patient-Centered Medical Home*. Retrieved from http://www.pcpcc.net/content/joint-principles-patient-centered-medical-home

Blumner, K. H., & Marcus, S. C. (2009). Changing perceptions of depression: Ten-year trends from the general social survey. *Psychiatry Services, 60*(3), 306–312.

Bureau of Labor Statistics. (2009). *Occupational Outlook Handbook, 2008–09 Edition 2009*. Retrieved from www.bls.gov/oco/.

Casalino, L., Gillies, R. R., Shortell, S. M., Schmittdiel, J. A., Bodenheimer, T., & Robinson, J. C. (2003). External incentives, information technology, and organized processes to improve health care quality for patients with chronic diseases. *JAMA, 289*(4), 434–441.

Cherry, D., Woodwell, D., & Rechtsteiner, E. (2007). *National Ambulatory Medical Care Survey: 2005 Summary*. Hyattsville, MD: National Center for Health Statistics.

Compas, B. E., & Gotlib, I. H. (2002). *Introduction to clinical psychology: Science and practice.* Boston: McGraw-Hill.

Cutler, D. L., Bevilacqua, J., & McFarland, B. H. (2003). Four decades of community mental health: A symphony in four movements. *Community Mental Health Journal, 39*(5), 381–398.

Davidson, L., Chinman, M., Sells, D., & Rowe, M. (2006). Peer support among adults with serious mental illness: A report from the field. *Schizophrenia Bulletin, 32*(3), 443–450.

Druss, B. G., & Rosenheck, R. A. (1998). Mental disorders and access to medical care in the United States. *American Journal of Psychiatry, 155*(12), 1775–1777.

Druss, B. G., & Rosenheck, R. A. (2000). Use of practitioner-based complementary therapies by persons reporting mental conditions in the United States. *Archives of General Psychiatry, 57*(7), 708–714.

Ezzati-Rice, T., & Rohde, F. (2008). *Variation in ambulatory health care visits and visits for general checkup by demographic characteristics and insurance status, US civilian noninstutional population ages 18–64, 2005.* Rockville, MD: Agency for Healthcare Research and Quality.

Fein, R. (1958). *Economics of mental illness: A report to the staff director, Jack R. Ewalt, 1958.* New York: Basic Books.

Frank, R., & Glied, S. (2006). *Better but not well: Mental health policy in the United States since 1950.* Baltimore: Johns Hopkins University Press.

Frank, R., Goldman, H. H., & Hogan, M. (2003). Medicaid and mental health: Be careful what you ask for. *Health Affairs (Millwood), 22*(1), 101–113.

Frank, R. G., & Garfield, R. L. (2007). Managed behavioral health care carve-outs: Past performance and future prospects. *Annual Review of Public Health, 28*, 303–320.

Frank, R. G., Koyanagi, C., & McGuire, T. G. (1997). The politics and economics of mental health 'parity' laws. *Health Affairs (Millwood), 16*(4), 108–119.

Goldman, H. H. (2007). Considering health insurance parity for mental health and substance abuse treatment: The federal employees health benefits experience. *American Journal of Psychiatry, 164*(10), 1473–1474.

Goldman, H. H., Frank, R. G., Burnam, M. A., Huskamp, H. A., Ridgely, M. S., & Normand, S. L. (2006). Behavioral health insurance parity for federal employees. *New England Journal of Medicine, 354*(13), 1378–1386.

Grob, G. N. (1994). *The Mad Among Us: A History of the Care of America's Mentally Ill.* New York Toronto: Free Press; Maxwell Macmillan Canada; Maxwell Macmillan International.

Gronfein, W. (1985). Incentives and intentions in mental health policy: A comparison of the Medicaid and community mental health programs. *Journal of Health and Social Behaviour, 26*(3), 192–206.

Kessler, R. C., Berglund, P. A., Bruce, M. L., Koch, J. R., Laska, E. M., & Leaf, P. J. (2001). The prevalence and correlates of untreated serious mental illness. *Health Services Research Journal, 36*(6 Pt 1), 987–1007.

Kessler, R. C., Demler, O., Frank, R. G., Olfson, M., Pincus, H. A., & Walters, E. E. (2005). Prevalence and treatment of mental disorders, 1990 to 2003. *New England Journal of Medicine, 352*(24), 2515–2523.

Kirby, J., Machlin, S., & Thorpe, J. M. (2001). *Patterns of ambulatory care use: Changes from 1987 to 1996* (No. 01–0026). Rockville, MD: Agency for Healthcare Research and Quality.

Lambert, M. J., Bergin, A. E., & Garfield, S. L. (2004). *Bergin and Garfield's handbook of psychotherapy and behavior change* (5th ed). New York: Wiley.

Mark, T. L., Levit, K. R., Buck, J. A., Coffey, R. M., & Vandivort-Warren, R. (2007). Mental health treatment expenditure trends, 1986–2003. *Psychiatric Services, 58*(8), 1041–1048.

Menninger, R. W., & Nemiah, J. C. (2000). *American psychiatry after World War II: (1944–1994)* (1st ed.). Washington, DC: American Psychiatric Press.

Mojtabai, R., & Olfson, M. (2008). National trends in psychotherapy by office-based psychiatrists. *Archives of General Psychiatry, 65*(8), 962–970.

Morrissey, J. P., & Goldman, H. H. (1984). Cycles of reform in the care of the chronically mentally ill. *Hospital and Community Psychiatry, 35*(8), 785–793.

Olfson, M., & Klerman, G. L. (1993). Trends in the prescription of psychotropic medications. The role of physician specialty. *Medical Care Research and Review, 31*(6), 559–564.

Olfson, M., & Marcus, S. C. (2009). National patterns in antidepressant medication treatment. *Archives of General Psychiatry, 66*(8), 848–856.

Regier, D. A., Goldberg, I. D., & Taube, C. A. (1978). The de facto US mental health services system: a public health perspective. *Archives of General Psychiatry, 35*(6), 685–693.

Regier, D. A., Narrow, W. E., Rae, D. S., Manderscheid, R. W., Locke, B. Z., & Goodwin, F. K. (1993). The de facto US mental and addictive disorders service system. Epidemiologic catchment area prospective 1-year prevalence rates of disorderss and services. *Archives of General Psychiatry, 50*(2), 85–94.

Room, R., & Greenfield, T. (1993). Alcoholics anonymous, other 12-step movements and psychotherapy in the US population, 1990. *Addiction, 88*(4), 555–562.

Sharfstein, S. S., & Dickerson, F. B. (2009). Hospital psychiatry for the twenty-first century. *Health Affairs (Millwood), 28*(3), 685–688.

Sharfstein, S. S., & Taube, C. A. (1982). Reductions in insurance for mental disorders: adverse selection, moral hazard, and consumer demand. *American Journal of Psychiatry, 139*(11), 1425–1430.

Silverman, W. H. (1985). The evolving mental health professions: Psychiatric social work, clinical psychology, psychiatry, and psychiatric nursing. *Journal of Mental Health Administration, 12*(2), 28–31.

Starr, P. (1982). *The social transformation of American medicine.* New York: Basic Books.

Wagner, E. H., Austin, B. T., & Von Korff, M. (1996). Organizing care for patients with chronic illness. *Milbank Quarterly, 74*(4), 511–544.

Wang, P. S., Berglund, P. A., & Kessler, R. C. (2003). Patterns and correlates of contacting clergy for mental disorders in the United States. *Health Services Research, 38*(2), 647–673.

Wang, P. S., Demler, O., Olfson, M., Pincus, H. A., Wells, K. B., & Kessler, R. C. (2006). Changing profiles of service sectors used for mental health care in the United States. *American Journal of Psychiatry, 163*(7), 1187–1198.

Wang, P. S., Lane, M., Olfson, M., Pincus, H. A., Wells, K. B., & Kessler, R. C. (2005). Twelve-month use of mental health services in the United States: Results from the National Comorbidity Survey Replication. *Archives of General Psychiatry, 62*(6), 629–640.

Watanabe-Galloway, S., & Zhang, W. (2007). Analysis of US trends in discharges from general hospitals for episodes of serious mental illness, 1995–2002. *Psychiatric Services, 58*(4), 496–502.

12 Public health approaches to improving population mental health

A local government perspective on integrating mental health promotion into general public health practice

Adam Karpati

Introduction

Formal integration of governmental oversight of physical and behavioral health is uncommon in the U.S. The federal public health agency, the Centers for Disease Control and Prevention (CDC), does not maintain a distinct mental health activity; instead, federal public mental health activities are under the purview of the Substance Abuse and Mental Health Services Administration (SAMHSA). This bifurcation is generally evident at the state and local levels as well. However, in 2002, as the result of a successful popular-ballot measure to amend the New York City Charter, the New York City Department of Health and the Department of Mental Health, Mental Retardation, and Alcoholism Services merged into a single Department of Health and Mental Hygiene (NYC DOHMH). The Commissioner of the newly joined agency, Dr. Thomas Frieden, said at the time,

> At its core, the Department represents a new way of addressing health and behavioral health issues that are so often inextricably linked. No longer will "health" concerns be separate from those of "mental hygiene," a term that encompasses the areas of mental health, developmental disabilities, and chemical dependencies.
> (New York City Department of Health and Mental Hygiene (NYC DOHMH), 2002)

The decade of experience of this unified local public health agency provides an opportunity to reflect on ways in which a public health approach can be brought to bear on issues of mental health and illness. This chapter first describes functional and conceptual frameworks for public health practice and examines their applicability to mental health issues. Then, several specific examples of ways in which public health practice can be applied to mental health promotion are presented, drawing from experience at the NYC DOHMH and from national activities. The chapter then offers two examples of new potential strategic directions, informed by theory and experience.

Overall, applying public health principles to promoting mental health and reducing the burden of mental illness is challenging, given the centrality of services to individuals – clinical and rehabilitative – that characterize the public mental health system and approach, and the paucity of proven prevention strategies. However, insights into the effects of poverty, social disconnection, and trauma, as well as provocative research into larger social and environmental influences, offer a basis for developing a broader public health perspective to address mental health issues.

A framework for integrating mental health into general public health practice

A useful definition of public health is:

> the combination of science, practical skills, and values (or beliefs) directed to the maintenance and improvement of the health of all the people. It is a set of efforts organized by society to protect, promote, and restore the people's health through collective or social action.
>
> (Last, 1998)

The translation of public health's mission and goals into practical and organized activities – ten "essential public health services" (Figure 12.1) – was articulated in the 1990s by governmental and nongovernmental public health leaders convened by the federal Department of Health and Human Services (Public Health Functions Steering Committee, 1995).

- Monitor health status to identify and solve community health problems.
- Diagnose and investigate health problems and health hazards in the community.
- Inform, educate, and empower people about health issues.
- Mobilize community partnerships and action to identify and solve health problems.
- Develop policies and plans that support individual and community health efforts.
- Enforce laws and regulations that protect health and ensure safety.
- Link people to needed personal health services and assure the provision of health care when otherwise unavailable.
- Assure a competent public and personal health care workforce.
- Evaluate effectiveness, accessibility, and quality of personal and population-based health services.
- Research for new insights and innovative solutions to health problems.

Figure 12.1 Ten essential public health services.

Note
Public Health Function Steering Group.

This functional framework provides a useful first step in considering how to better integrate mental health promotion into general public health practice. However, considering some of the more fundamental, conceptual principles that underlie contemporary public health practice is essential to creatively developing new approaches. Three broad (and related) conceptual domains within the public health perspective provide a useful framework within which to develop new interventions to address mental health issues:

1   A focus on prevention of illness.
2   A "population" perspective.
3   An aim to address environmental/contextual influences on health.

Preventing illness is the cornerstone of public health and the guiding principle for the essential services enumerated above. Compelling "secondary prevention" strategies – those that seek to disrupt the onset or course of illness among individuals identified to be at risk or in the early stages – for illnesses such as schizophrenia are emerging, and the potential for applying them widely is exciting (Lieberman & Corcoran, 2007). However, contemporary public mental health practice remains concerned largely with creating and optimizing a system of services and supports for people with serious mental illness and, for those who are more moderately ill, in promoting identification and treatment. The dominant paradigm of "recovery" is oriented toward the period after the development of illness: "Mental health recovery is a journey of healing and transformation enabling a person with a mental health problem to live a meaningful life in a community of his or her choice while striving to achieve his or her full potential" (Substance Abuse and Mental Health Services Administration (SAMHSA), undated). While this goal provides a compelling mission and prompts a clearly actionable agenda, it is not explicitly oriented around an early prevention perspective.

The "population" approach to public health and prevention was articulated by the influential British physician and epidemiologist, Geoffrey Rose, based on his theoretical and empiric epidemiologic work (Rose, 1992). Rose's population approach derives from a number of observations regarding the distribution of disease risks in population groups and the relative rates of disease between groups. One of the many important and actionable aspects of this approach derives from the observation that for certain behaviors or illnesses, rates of extreme manifestations correlate with average population rates. Rose showed, using cross-national studies, that blood pressure, alcohol consumption, and other issues display this phenomenon (Rose & Day, 1990). The implication for practice is that controlling the rate of "extremes" can be achieved by altering population-wide, average levels of risk, even if those levels of risk do not confer a high probability of illness on most individuals within the population. Though this phenomenon has not been clearly established for population means and distributions of mood or anxiety measures and the rates of depression and anxiety disorders (much less the rates of more extreme manifestations of mental illness, such as the non-affective psychoses), a long thread of literature and new insights suggest that prevailing population-level conditions do influence psychiatric disease processes (Mair, Diez-Roux, & Galea, 2008).

At a more fundamental level, and regardless of the association between lower and higher rates of risk within a population, Rose observed that disease risk often does not display a "threshold" effect, but is rather continuous, and the (cumulative) majority of risk actually falls on the moderately exposed. The implication of this observation is, again, that addressing risk across and at the population level, rather than targeting only individuals at highest risk, can potentially produce the greatest public health benefit. Since much of current mental health policymaking involves planning for clinical and rehabilitative services, cost is a central factor, and cost considerations typically lead to a targeted focus on those who use services the most and strategies to manage or prevent that utilization. While often effective at reducing unnecessary use of high-cost services, such as inpatient hospitalization, targeting strategies can avoid addressing the underlying factors that contribute not only to the number of "high-users" of services but to cases of poor outcomes and inappropriate care across the entire population.

In a classic paper, Rose (1985) extended the population perspective by illustrating the importance of focusing beyond individual-level characteristics to identify (and intervene on) the causes of illness. He noted that determinants of differences in the probability of disease between individuals *within* a particular population are distinct from the determinants of the *rate* of disease in that population. He described the phenomenon as distinguishing between the "causes of cases and the causes of incidence." This implies that epidemiologic inquiry into determinants of illness requires inter-group comparisons, since examining differences between groups provides different insights into determinants of illness than does examining differences between individuals. From a practice standpoint, it highlights the need to address influences on health beyond those that are modifiable at the individual level. "Individual-level" approaches to health are based on modifying risk factors that are intrinsic to each person: weight, blood pressure and cholesterol levels, behavior choices, etc. Alternatively, "population-level" approaches focus on risks that are characteristic of the group (and may not even be definable at the individual level). Such risks are often referred to as "contextual" (Diez-Roux, 1998). For example, insurance status is an individual-level characteristic that may influence the likelihood that someone seeks and receives good care for mental illness. In contrast, the level of social stigma in the society in which a person lives may also be an important determinant of access to care, and one that is modifiable (and measurable) only at the group level.

The concept of "upstream" interventions refers to chains in disease causation in which factors can be more proximal ("downstream") or distal ("upstream") to the actual manifestation of disease. In such a heuristic approach, for example, a person's hospitalization for uncontrolled symptoms of schizophrenia can result from downstream (individual-level) causes, such as medication non-adherence and absent outpatient care; midstream (individual-level) causes, such as homelessness and unemployment; and upstream (contextual) causes, such as affordable housing and job availability. Strategies to address upstream, contextual influences on health are attractive to public policymakers, insofar as they are likely to be more effective – and cost-effective – than interventions targeting individuals. However, by their nature – being conceptually "distant" from the problem in need of solution (as the effect of poverty on health), affecting the entire population rather than select individuals, and being frequently entwined with other, non-health issues and agendas – such strategies are often controversial and challenging to implement. That said, contemporary public mental health practice is well-placed and fully engaged with upstream conditions that create a recovery-oriented environment: legal protections against housing and employment discrimination established by the Americans with Disabilities Act and reinforced by the Supreme Court's Olmstead decision, urban affordable housing policies, and supplementary income policies are all examples of powerful contextual influences on the well-being of people with serious mental illness.

The following sections provide examples of how some of these conceptual and functional principles can and have been applied to mental health issues, with a focus on the activities of the NYC DOHMH.

Monitoring health status

Public health practitioners use the term "surveillance" to refer to the response-oriented monitoring of the health of populations. A commonly cited definition of surveillance is: "the ongoing, systematic collection, analysis, interpretation, and dissemination of data regarding a health-related event for use in public health action to reduce morbidity and mortality and to improve health" (Thacker & Berkelman, 1988). A number of surveillance systems, mostly administered by federal agencies, exist to provide national and state-level data regarding a variety of health conditions and health-related behaviors. Most of these systems rely on recurring surveys of non-institutionalized populations and include some items that measure mental illness. Those surveillance systems include annual or otherwise regular telephone or in-person surveys administered by the CDC, such as the Behavioral Risk Factor Surveillance System (www.cdc.gov/brfss/), the National Health Interview Survey (www.cdc.gov/nchs/nhis.htm), the National Health and Nutrition Examination Survey (www.cdc.gov/nchs/nhanes.htm), and the Youth Risk Behavior Survey (www.cdc.gov/HealthyYouth/yrbs/index.htm), and by SAMHSA, such as the National

Survey on Drug Use and Health (https://nsduhweb.rti.org/). In addition, occasional national surveys have been conducted that focused exclusively on mental illness, such as the National Comorbidity Surveys (NCS) (www. hcp.med.harvard.edu/ncs/), although they have not been designed as ongoing monitoring systems.

National surveys are of limited use to local public health agencies that need local data to set priorities, guide the targeting of high-need populations, and evaluate local public health initiatives. Synthetic estimation – the application of measured stratified rates from one population to another, unmeasured population in order to calculate expected rates and case numbers in the second population – can be useful for local jurisdictions to the extent that the derived rates will reflect local demographic distributions. This technique does not capture the impact of other local determinants of prevalence; however, in the absence of locally collected data, this method can produce broad estimates of disease burden. Such estimates can be extremely useful in identifying the scale of intervention needed and in matching resources to needs. An example of such an analysis was conducted by NYC DOHMH, in which data from national surveys and other studies was applied to New York City population estimates in order to estimate the City's prevalence of mental illnesses, substance use disorders, and developmental disabilities (www.nyc.gov/html/doh/downloads/pdf/mh/mh-2003prevalence.pdf).

Ideally, however, local public health agencies should collect local data to not only serve important epidemiologic and planning purposes, but also enhance communication and advocacy with local stakeholders. NYC DOHMH has, since 2002, conducted telephone and in-person examination surveys in order to gather citywide and neighborhood-level data to guide policymaking and the evaluation of public health initiatives. These surveys have allowed for local descriptive epidemiology of mood and anxiety disorders and of nonspecific measures of mental illness, such as psychological distress (Gwynn, McQuiston, McVeigh, Garg, Frieden, & Thorpe, 2008; McVeigh, Mostashari, Wunsch-Hitzig, Kuppin, & King, 2003). These data have, for example, been used to identify target populations and benchmark evaluation of interventions to improve identification and care for depression among, for example, different racial/ethnic groups in New York City (Summers, Cohen, Havusha, Sliger, & Farley, 2009).

The surveys of mental illness mentioned above focus on descriptive epidemiology and also typically include some information on access to and use of clinical care. Their usefulness for planning and policymaking to address the needs of those with the most debilitating mental illnesses is limited by the fact that they typically exclude institutionalized settings, such as jails, hospitals, and long-term care facilities, where a substantial proportion of such individuals reside (Frank & Glied, 2006). More important than these methodologic issues, however, national surveys typically do not include detailed questions on social factors and service needs, since these are so particular to local environments. Moreover, general population-level health surveys are typically multidisciplinary and have limited "space" for detailed queries that can provide essential information – housing status, employment status, incarceration experience, detailed health care access information, community supports and integration, family supports – for planning at the population level. In the face of this gap, such information is often collected from more readily available, though not fully representative sources like service (clinics and other providers) or institutional settings (jails, homeless shelters, hospitals, etc.). While useful, data from these sources cannot provide population-level information and may very well exclude high-need, highly disengaged groups.

Robust population-level data on children's mental health issues are increasingly available (Carter, Wagmiller, Gray, McCarthy, Horwitz, & Briggs-Gowan, 2010; Merikangas, He, Brody, Fisher, Bourdon, & Koretz, 2010). However, most surveys of children's mental health focus on measuring prevalent conditions. Nearly absent from U.S. public health surveillance is population-level measurement of the various domains of early child development. Social-emotional development in early childhood is associated with child and adult mental illness as well as with a variety of physical health and social (educational, criminal justice) outcomes. Tools and methods are available for measuring the domains of early child development; one validated system that has been implemented at the population level in Canada and Australia, for example, is the Early Development Index, a set of scales to assess students administered by kindergarten teachers (Janus, 2007). The assessments provide information on five broad domains of child development and school readiness: physical, social, emotional, cognitive/language, and communication. Importantly, the survey is designed to generate not an individualized assessment of each student but rather an aggregated, normed, result for the community from which the students were sampled. Results can then be aggregated and reported at a group level – school, district, neighborhood, etc. – to identify high-need populations and track the effectiveness of interventions.

Priority-setting

A self-evident intended consequence of the goal of integrating mental health programs and policies into general public health practice is that mental health topics become prioritized and highlighted within the larger public health agenda and not "exceptionalized" as a distinct set of issues independent of larger health promotion activities. In New York, the City's public health agenda was developed in 2004 and updated in 2009 as a succinct and accessible list of priorities accompanied by epidemiologic data and program and policy recommendations (Summers et al., 2009). The principles guiding the choice of topics in this "Take Care New York"

(TCNY) framework were burden of disease and amenability to intervention ("actionability"). Addressing mental illness clearly meets these criteria and was included among the top public health issues for the City in both versions. The value of setting out the TCNY framework extended beyond simply listing important public health issues; it signaled the re-emergence of an activist, agenda-setting, outcome-oriented public health agency. Figure 12.2 shows the 2009 list, highlighting depression and substance misuse as priorities in the agenda.

A long-standing challenge in advocating for increased public health attention to mental illness is difficulty in quantifying the burden of illness; conditions with fatal consequences are easier to measure and their impact is simpler to communicate. The development and adoption of the disability-adjusted life year (DALY) and similar measures that combine morbidity and mortality into a single metric served to highlight mental illness as a leading cause of disability and among the leading contributors to the burden of poor health worldwide (Murray, 1996). In the U.S., updated national estimates of DALYs have not been produced since 1996, when depression ranked fourth among all contributors to DALYs (Michaud, McKenna, Begg, Tomijima, Majmudar, Bulzacchelli, et al., 2006). Also, given limitations of locally available data on prevalence of nonfatal illnesses, local jurisdictions have not typically calculated DALYs for their populations (an exception is Los Angeles (Los Angeles Department of Health Services and the UCLA Center for Health Policy Research, 2000)). Inclusion of mental health issues into local public health priority-setting would be aided by more widespread use of such methods, ideally using as much local data as possible.

Investigating health hazards

Epidemiologic and case investigations of infectious disease and environmental health hazards are critical functions of public health agencies,

Take Care New York framework

New York City aims to:
1. Promote Quality Health Care for All
2. Be Tobacco Free
3. Promote Physical Activity and Healthy Eating
4. Be Heart Healthy
5. Stop the Spread of HIV and Other Sexually Transmitted Infections
6. Recognize and Treat Depression
7. Reduce Risky Alcohol Use and Drug Dependence
8. Prevent and Detect Cancer
9. Raise Healthy Children
10. Make All Neighborhoods Healthy Places to Live

Figure 12.2 Take Care New York framework.

whether for emerging diseases, such as H1N1 influenza, severe acute respiratory syndrome (SARS), West Nile Virus, or long-standing threats, such as tuberculosis, HIV, and lead poisoning. These sorts of investigations entail identifying and interrupting sources of infectious disease transmission or detecting and removing sources of toxic exposure. One approach that adapts these principles to mental illness is to conceptualize poor functioning or adverse outcomes among individuals with mental illness as a product not only of individual-level determinants (such as disease characteristics or the components of a treatment plan) but as the product of the social, physical, and "service" environments with which such individuals interact. As such, epidemiologic and case investigation techniques can be applied to identify opportunities for system improvement.

In 2006 and 2007, following instances of violence involving individuals with mental illness that had generated substantial media coverage, the New York City Mayor's office, New York State Governor's office, and officials from State and City mental health, law enforcement, and other agencies convened to review cases and develop recommendations to improve service and care systems (New York State/New York City Mental Health–Criminal Justice Panel, 2008). Case reviews used techniques similar to those involved in infant and child mortality reviews, with multiple agencies contributing data and a shared appraisal of missed opportunities preceding the critical events. A product of the work was the development of an activity to identify individuals who demonstrate clinical needs yet who are disengaged from the public mental health system. The pilot project, the "Care Monitoring Initiative," was launched in 2008 and entails several notable conceptual and functional components. First, clinical needs and disengagement from care are initially determined via reviews of Medicaid claims data. Individuals with mental illness are identified in the Medicaid claims file by the presence of a mental illness diagnosis or service recorded within the past year and either participation in a high-intensity service (e.g., case management, assertive community treatment, or court-ordered outpatient treatment) or evidence of multiple hospitalizations or emergency department visits within a 12-month period, or a history of receiving treatment while incarcerated in the State prison system. Disengagement is, in turn, defined – via the data – by persistent usage of emergency care or recurring hospitalization, by the absence of visits for outpatient care, or by evidence of unfilled prescriptions. Lists of individuals meeting these criteria are passed to a team of "care monitors" who are responsible for investigating each case via contact with whomever had had previous contact with the patient – emergency department (ED), inpatient, or clinic staff, case manager, etc. Through such investigations, issues, opportunities, and challenges become evident at multiple levels – the individuals themselves, the providers with whom they interact and in whose care they may have been, and the larger system within which the providers operate. Over time, the project will focus on refining the data screening criteria to more efficiently identify patients at highest need and on using the data and investigation information to improve provider accountability and performance.

Addressing mental illness in primary care

Over the past decade, NYC DOHMH has taken an increasingly active role in promoting clinical preventive services – immunization, screening, and early treatment for conditions of significant public health burden – in primary care settings. Several of the priorities highlighted in the TCNY framework refer to such services: HIV testing, influenza vaccination, colonoscopy screening, blood pressure and cholesterol management, screening and brief intervention for alcohol misuse, etc. Included in this list is screening for depression, which is a "B" recommendation of the U.S. Preventive Services Task Force (U.S. Preventive Services Task Force (USPSTF), 2009). TCNY has been the NYC DOHMH's main priority-setting framework, which in a practical sense has meant that NYC DOHMH health promotion activities have been directed toward the TCNY topics. For example, NYC DOHMH has developed a regular, short publication targeting primary care practitioners, providing education and clinical guidance on TCNY and other topics of public health importance. Several of these *City Health Information* documents have focused on depression and other mental health topics (Petit, Cohen, & Lednyak, 2007; Reil, Chisholm, Lednyak, & Cohen, 2010). Another such activity is "public health detailing," which is based upon the pharmaceutical industry's practice of sending representatives directly to practitioners' offices to provide education and practice tools (patient information materials, chart reminders, professional education materials, etc.). This program, in which DOHMH staff develop the materials and conduct the visits, is specifically targeted toward solo or small-practice practitioners in neighborhoods with disproportionately high illness and mortality rates. In a variation on the main goal of bringing information and tools to primary care practitioners, DOHMH also developed a detailing campaign for professionals working in mental health programs around strategies for tobacco cessation among individuals with serious mental illness.

The most ambitious and far-reaching initiative NYC DOHMH has undertaken around clinical practice improvement is the "Primary Care Information Project" (PCIP). PCIP is centered around the principle that in outpatient medical settings, broad implementation of best practices, including preventive services, can only be achieved via electronic systems that provide decision support, practice-level data analysis and reporting, communication with laboratory and other clinical systems, public health reporting, and other such functions. Further, implementation of such electronic health record (EHR) systems necessarily must be accompanied by redesign of policies and procedures within practices and by alignment of financial reimbursement to support these services. The specific activities of

PCIP have included identifying and developing improved functionality of a particular electronic health record product; disseminating the product (subsidizing purchase, providing technical assistance on implementation) to primary care practices across the City; assisting practices with process and policy redesign, and developing practice-level indicators based on data in the record for clinicians to use to monitor and improve performance. The initiative has grown to be the country's largest community-based EHR system, with over 1,500 physicians involved. The decision support and performance indicators have been developed with a focus on the TCNY priorities and, as such, include tools for depression screening and metrics of screening rates, treatment and referral follow-up results, etc. Moreover, NYC DOHMH is interested in leveraging the PCIP model and experience in primary care settings to apply to the specialty mental health sector. In all, there are at least five areas for this future work.

1   Continuing to refine the depression screening and care functionality in the primary care EHR.
2   Recruiting mental health professionals working in practice settings with primary care practitioners to use the EHR and modifying or customizing the primary care-based functionality to facilitate this integration.
3   Developing and disseminating "specialty" EHRs to mental health practitioners.
4   Maximizing information exchange between outpatient primary care, outpatient mental health care, inpatient services, and ancillary services (case management, rehabilitation, etc.).
5   Incorporating mental health topics into patient-oriented interfaces (e.g., patient portals).

New directions

The next sections suggest future directions for a more fully realized public health approach to mental health promotion and disease prevention, building on the work described above and based on the conceptual principles articulated at the beginning of this chapter including a focus on upstream, contextual determinants.

Depression

As described above, NYC DOHMH has prioritized and highlighted depression as a critical public health issue that is both highly prevalent and amenable to intervention. The attendant strategies have been informed by a traditional treatment/service approach and focused almost exclusively on increasing identification (via screening) and access to treatment (in primary care or, if needed, specialty care). While these are appropriate and – if successfully implemented – potentially impactful interventions, a broader "public health" approach to depression based on the principles of population reach, upstream determinants, and environmental influences would entail developing strategies far removed from detection of cases and linkage to care. For example, there is increasing evidence that social connectedness and social supports provide salutary effects on health and mental health (and conversely, that social isolation can have deleterious effects) (Cerdá, Sagdeo, Johnson, & Galea, 2010; Morgan, Burns, Fitzpatrick, Pinfold, & Priebe, 2007). Further, theory-based health promotion strategies for youth and elderly populations often emphasize the positive impact of interpersonal engagement and "purpose"-driven activities (Carlson, Saczynski, Rebok, Seeman, Glass, & McGill, 2008; Kirby, 2002). Efforts to promote civic engagement, reduce isolation, and provide meaningful work for, say, aging populations might be expected to offer comparably cost-effective results on depression rates as individual-level outreach, screening, and referral programs.

Moving further upstream and into the domain of contextual influences, there are also more and increasingly sophisticated insights into neighborhood-level determinants of mental health and illness (Beard, Cerdá, Blaney, Ahern, Vlahov, & Galea, 2009; Mair et al., 2008). As for most health outcomes, neighborhood poverty, economic and racial segregation, and an eroded "built environment" are associated with depression and anxiety. Importantly, these associations are independent of the various individual-level risks neighborhood residents may have for depression. Knowing that the characteristics of the neighborhoods in which people live can affect their mental health provides attractive, though daunting, options for reducing mental illness at the community level. Contemporary public health practitioners are wrestling with the practical implications of similar insights into the negative effects of neighborhood-level conditions on a variety of health domains: cardiovascular disease, diabetes, injuries, HIV/AIDS, sexually transmitted diseases (STDs), etc. And, of course, economic development, residential desegregation, and safe, attractive neighborhoods are worthy goals independent of their public health impact. However, public health (including mental health) researchers and practitioners can play an important role in highlighting the health case for such interventions and bringing unique expertise to the multidisciplinary collaborations that are essential to affecting change.

In New York City, NYC DOHMH has been a key participant in a variety of urban planning and economic development initiatives, and nationally, several public health agencies are playing critical roles in urban development and social change, returning in many ways to the roots of public health as concerned with reducing social disadvantage and promoting social justice. Public mental health agencies and mental health practitioners are well-placed to contribute to these efforts, not only because these issues impact the outcomes they care most about, but because social factors such as housing and employment are already core components of public mental health practice and because public mental health embodies a fundamental social justice perspective rooted in the historical and ongoing human rights issues intrinsic to working with a historically disenfranchised and frequently stigmatized population.

Early child development

There is substantial and growing evidence that influences in early childhood are associated with mental illness later in childhood, adolescence, and adulthood. These insights come both from epidemiologic evidence as well as theory-based models of psychology and behavior. First, a variety of studies have found that adverse experiences in childhood affect such outcomes as mood and behavioral disorders. These include general health studies, such as the Adverse Childhood Experience study conducted by CDC, and new evidence from the National Comorbidity Survey-Replication (NCS-R) (Edwards, Holden, Anda, & Felitti, 2003; Green, McLaughlin, Berglund, Gruber, Sampson, Zaslavsky, & Kessler, 2010). A provocative attributable-fraction estimation from the NCS-R analysis suggested that more than 30% of adolescent and adult mental illness can be explained by adverse experiences in childhood. Second, inquiry into the determinants of maladaptive behaviors, such as drug and alcohol abuse, sexual risk-taking, and eating disorders, are increasingly identifying affect dysregulation as a key mediating characteristic (Bell & McBride, 2010). In turn, evidence is emerging that affect dysregulation is associated with poor attachment in infancy and early childhood (Maunder & Hunter, 2001). Stressful environments (family or community violence, poverty, unemployment, etc.) interacting with this individual-level characteristic can be expected to heighten the likelihood of such behavioral risks.

As with the urban development issues mentioned above, there is substantial evidence and broad consensus that promoting healthy child development has wide-ranging salutary effects on health and social achievement in adolescence and adulthood, well beyond their benefits on mental health and mental illness (Shonkoff, Boyce, & McEwan, 2009). Moreover, successful interventions exist to promote healthy development and mitigate the effects of deprivation and traumatic experiences, ranging from direct family/child programs to developmentally-oriented education programs (The Marmot Review, 2010). In addition, public mental health planning is increasingly focused on addressing impaired social-emotional development (National Center for Mental Health Promotion and Youth Violence Prevention, 2010). Though challenges remain in further refining the range of evidence-based best practices to achieve population-level reach of what are often expensive and intensive services and activities (Lynch, Law, Brinkman, Chittleborough, & Sawyer, 2010), this is an area in which the goals of general public health and public mental health are highly aligned.

Challenges and limitations to the public health approach for mental illness

Public health practice has developed sophisticated and effective methods for addressing health threats from communicable diseases (broadly speaking, by controlling vectors for transmission – e.g., by sanitary strategies in hospitals, herd immunization, water purification, insect control), toxins (broadly speaking, by reducing exposures – e.g., removing lead from gasoline and paint, improving air quality), and other environmental threats (e.g., occupational safety, road and auto safety, gun violence). In recent decades, great advances have also occurred in controlling those conditions influenced by human behavior (by changing the physical and social environments in which behavioral choices, such as smoking, drinking, sex, eating, and physical activity, are made) (Centers for Disease Control and Prevention (CDC), 1999). But mental illness, particularly severe mental illness, does not fit neatly into any of these categories. It is not infectious in origin, and its incidence is not particularly influenced by behavioral patterns. The examples provided in the "New Directions" section above are somewhat, though not directly, analogous to "toxic exposures," in which early childhood experiences and community conditions serve to increase risk, but they are much more causally distal and nonspecific than typical environmental threats. Obviously, then, the "downstream" treatment and service approach to mental illness – complemented by progressive social policy to support that approach – is and will remain central to reducing suffering and promoting recovery.

Also, while there exist provocative epidemiologic insights into the influence of social and physical environments on the incidence of mental illness, the theoretical models of causation are incomplete. Moreover, from a practice standpoint, there are few practical models of applying public health principles to mental health problems and a dearth of evidence on the population-level mental health impact of general public health-informed interventions. As such, to make an integrated public health practice model successful at addressing the substantial and immediate challenges facing individuals with mental illness, not only does public mental health need to seek insights from general public health practice, but the reverse is also true: general public health practitioners need to seek ways to adapt their skills, resources, and perspective – especially around epidemiology and program evaluation – to creatively and collaboratively address mental health issues. This would include developing expertise in medical and rehabilitative service planning and performance improvement and in housing and employment policy.

The 19th century French sociologist, Emile Durkheim, in an early social epidemiologic insight, wrote of patterns of suicide rates across populations,

The victim's act, which at first seems to express only his personal temperament, is really the supplement and prolongation of a social condition which he expresses externally ... his sadness comes ... not from one or another incident of his career but rather from the group to which he belongs.

(Durkheim, 1897)

The interactions between individuals and the groups to which they belong and the environments in which they live are the focus of public health. The compelling challenge to public health and public mental health practitioners is to seek those social levers that can alter the trajectory of even mental illness, the most profoundly personal of afflictions.

Acknowledgments

The author thanks Thomas Farley, Trish Marsik, and Lloyd Sederer for their thoughtful and insightful reviews of earlier drafts of this chapter.

References

Beard, J. R., Cerdá, M., Blaney, S., Ahern, J., Vlahov, D., & Galea, S. (2009). Neighborhood characteristics and change in depressive symptoms among older residents of New York City. *American Journal of Public Health, 99*, 1308–1314. doi:10.2105/AJPH.2007.125104.

Bell, C. C., & McBride, D. F. (2010). Affect regulation and prevention of risky behaviors. *Journal of the American Medical Association, 304*, 565–566. doi:10.1001/jama.2010.1058.

Carlson, M. C., Saczynski, J. S., Rebok, G. W., Seeman, T., Glass, T. A., McGill, S., et al. (2008). Exploring the effects of an "everyday" activity program on executive function and memory in older adults: Experience Corps. *Gerontologist, 48*, 793–801.

Carter, A. S., Wagmiller, R. J., Gray, S. A., McCarthy, K. J., Horwitz, S. M., & Briggs-Gowan, M. J. (2010). Prevalence of DSM-IV disorder in a representative, healthy birth cohort at school entry: Sociodemographic risks and social adaptation. *Journal of the American Academy of Child and Adolescent Psychiatry, 49*, 686–698. doi:10.1016/jaac.2010.03.018.

Centers for Disease Control and Prevention (CDC). (1999). Ten great public health achievements – United States, 1900–1999. *Morbidity and Mortality Weekly Report, 48*, 241–243. Retrieved from www.cdc.gov/mmwr/PDF/wk/mm4812.pdf.

Cerdá, M., Sagdeo, A., Johnson, J., & Galea, S. (2010). Genetic and environmental influences on psychiatric comorbidity: A systematic review. *Journal of Affective Disorders, 126*, 14–38. doi:10.1016.j.jad.2009.22.006.

Diez-Roux, A. V. (1998). Bringing context back into epidemiology: Variables and fallacies in multilevel analysis. *American Journal of Public Health, 88*, 216–222. Retrieved from http://ajph.aphapublications.org/cgi/reprint/88/2/216.

Durkheim, E. (1897). *Suicide*. New York: Free Press.

Edwards, V. J., Holden, G. W., Anda, R. F., & Felitti, V. J. (2003). Experiencing multiple forms of childhood maltreatment and adult mental health: Results from the Adverse Childhood Experiences (ACE) study. *American Journal of Psychiatry, 160*, 1453–1460. Retrieved from http://ajp.psychiatryonline.org/cgi/reprint/160/8/1453.

Frank, R. G., & Glied, S. A. (2006). *Better but not well: Mental health policy in the United States since 1950*. Baltimore, MD: The Johns Hopkins University Press.

Green, J. G., McLaughlin, K. A., Berglund, P. A., Gruber, M. J., Sampson, N. A., Zaslavsky, A. M., & Kessler, R. C. (2010). Childhood adversities and adult psychiatric disorders in the national comorbidity survey replication I: Associations with first onset of DSM-IV disorders. *Archives of General Psychiatry, 67*, 113–123. Retrieved from http://archpsych.ama-assn.org/cgi/reprint/67/2/113.

Gwynn, R. C., McQuistion, H. L., McVeigh, K. H., Garg, R. K., Frieden, T. R., & Thorpe, L. E. (2008). Prevalence, diagnosis, and treatment of depression and generalized anxiety disorder in a diverse urban community. *Psychiatric services, 59*, 641–647. doi:10.1176/appi.ps.59.6.641.

Janus, M. (2007). The Early Development Instrument: A tool for monitoring children's development and readiness for school. In M. E. Young & L. M. Richardson (Eds.), *Early child development – from measurement to action. A priority for growth and equity* (pp. 141–155). Washington, D.C.: World Bank.

Kirby, D. (2002). Effective approaches to reducing adolescent unprotected sex, pregnancy, and childbearing. *Journal of Sex Research, 39*, 51–57.

Last, J. M. (1998). *Public health and human ecology*. Stamford, CT: Appleton and Lange.

Lieberman, J., & Corcoran, C. (2007). The impossible dream: Can psychiatry prevent psychosis? *Early Intervention in Psychiatry, 1*, 219–221. doi:10.1111/j.1751–7893.2007.00031.x.

Los Angeles County Department of Health Services and the UCLA Center for Health Policy Research. (2000). *The burden of disease in Los Angeles County*. Retrieved from www.lapublichealth.org/epi/reports/dburden.pdf.

Lynch, J. W., Law, C., Brinkman, S., Chittleborough, C., & Sawyer, M. (2010). Inequalities in child healthy development: Some challenges for effective implementation. *Social Science & Medicine, 71*, 1244–1248. doi:10.1016/j.socscimed.2010.07.008.

Mair, C., Diez-Roux, A. V., & Galea, S. (2008). Are neighborhood characteristics associated with depressive symptoms? A review of evidence. *Journal of Epidemiology and Community Health, 62*, 940–946.

Maunder, R. G., & Hunter, J. J. (2001). Attachment and psychosomatic medicine: Developmental contributions to stress and disease. *Psychosomatic Medicine, 63*, 556–567. Retrieved from www.psychosomaticmedicine.org/cgi/reprint/63/4/556.

McVeigh, K. H., Mostashari, F., Wunsch-Hitzig, R. A., Kuppin, S. A., King, C. G., Plapinger, J. D., & Sederer, L. I. (2003). There is no health without mental health. *NYC Vital Signs, 2*(3), 1–4. Retrieved from www.nyc.gov/html/doh/downloads/pdf/survey/survey-2003mentalhealth.pdf.

Merikangas, K. R., He, J. P., Brody, D., Fisher, P. W., Bourdon, K., & Koretz, D. S. (2010). Prevalence and treatment of mental disorders among US children in the 2001–2004 NHANES. *Pediatrics, 125*, 75–81. doi:10.1542/peds.2008.2598.

Michaud, C. M., McKenna, M. T., Begg, S., Tomijima, N., Majmudar, M., Bulzac-chelli M. T. et al. (2006). The burden of disease and injury in the United States 1996. *Population Health Metrics, 4*(11). Retrieved from www.pophealthmetrics.com/content/4/1/11 doi: 10.1186/1478–7954–4–11.

Morgan, C., Burns, T., Fitzpatrick, R., Pinfold, V., & Priebe, S. (2007). Social exclusion and mental health: Conceptual and methodological review. *British Journal of Psychiatry, 191*, 477–483. doi:10.1192/bjp.bp. 106.034942.

Murray, C. J. L., & Lopez, A. D. (Eds.). (1996). *The global burden of disease: a comprehensive assessment of mortality and disability from diseases, injuries and risk factors in 1990 and projected to 2020.* Cambridge, MA: Harvard School of Public Health on behalf of the World Health Organization and the World Bank.

Murray, C. J. L. (1996). Rethinking DALYs. In C. J. L. Murray & A. D. Lopez (Eds.), *The global burden of disease: A comprehensive assessment of mortality and disability from diseases, injuries and risk factors in 1990 and projected to 2020.* Cambridge, MA: Harvard School of Public Health on behalf of the World Health Organization and the World Bank.

National Center for Mental Health Promotion and Youth Violence Prevention. (2010). Project *LAUNCH briefing sheet.* Retrieved from http:///projectlaunch.promoteprevent.org/webfm_send/1468.

New York City Department of Health and Mental Hygiene (NYC DOHMH). (2002). Department of Health and Department of Mental Health, Mental Retardation and Alcoholism Services are merged. Retrieved from www.nyc.gov/html/doh/html/press_archive02/pr45–710.shtml.

New York State/New York City Mental Health–Criminal Justice Panel. (2008). *Report and recommendations.* Retrieved from www.omh.state.ny.us/omhweb/justice_panel_report/report.pdf.

Petit, J., Cohen, G., & Lednyak, L. (2007). Detecting and treating depression in adults. *City Health Information, 26*, 59–66. Retrieved from www.nyc.gov/html/doh/downloads/pdf/chi/chi26–9.pdf.

Public Health Functions Steering Committee. (1995). *Public health in America.* Retrieved from: www.health.gov/phfunctions/public.htm.

Reil, M., Chisholm, J., Lednyak, L., & Cohen, G. (2010). Improving the health of adults with serious mental illness. *City Health Information, 29*, 9–16. Retrieved from www.nyc.gov/html/doh/downloads/pdf/chi/chi29–2.pdf.

Rose, G. (1985). Sick individuals and sick populations. *International Journal of Epidemiology, 14*, 32–38. doi:10.1093/ije/14.1.32.

Rose, G. A. (1992). *The strategy of preventive medicine.* London: Oxford University Press.

Rose, G., & Day, S. (1990). The population mean predicts the number of deviant individuals. *British Medical Journal, 301*, 1031–1034. doi:10.1136/bmj.301.6759.1031.

Shonkoff, J. P., Boyce, W. T., & McEwan, B. S. (2009). Neuroscience, molecular biology, and the childhood roots of health disparities: Building a new framework for health promotion and disease prevention. *Journal of the American Medical Association, 301*, 2252–2259. Retrieved from http://jama.ama-assn.org/cgi/reprint/301/21/2252.

Substance Abuse and Mental Health Services Administration (SAMHSA). *National Consensus Statement on Mental Health Recovery.* Retrieved from https://store.samhsa.gov/shin/content/SMA05–4129/SMA05–4129.pdf.

Summers, C., Cohen, L., Havusha, A., Sliger, F., & Farley, T. (2009). *Take Care New York 2012: A policy for a healthier New York City*. New York: New York City Department of Health and Mental Hygiene. Retrieved from www.nyc.gov/html/doh/downloads/pdf/tcny/tcny-2012.pdf.

Thacker, S. B., & Berkelman, R. L. (1988). Public health surveillance in the United States. *Epidemiologic Reviews, 10*, 164–190.

The Marmot Review. (2010). *Fair society, healthy lives*. London: Author. Retrieved from www.marmotreview.org/AssetLibrary/pdfs/Reports/FairSocietyHealthyLives.pdf.

U.S. Preventive Services Task Force (USPSTF). (2009). Screening for depression in adults: U.S. Preventive Services Task Force Recommendation Statement. *Annals of Internal Medicine, 151*, 784–792. Retrieved from www.uspreventiveservices-taskforce.org/uspstf/uspsaddepr.htm.

13 Realizing the possibilities of school mental health across the public health continuum

Carrie Mills, Maura Mulloy, and Mark Weist

Introduction

Investments in our children, particularly those related to their health, mental health, well-being, and education, are investments in our nation's future. Although the primary mission of the US educational system is to promote academic achievement among all students, this system has also been identified as a key setting for the recognition of mental health disorderss and often is the de facto mental health provider for children and adolescents (Burns, Costello, Angold, Tweed, Stangl, Farmer, & Erkanli, 1995; Farmer, Burns, Phillips, Angold, & Costello, 2003; Rones & Hoagwood, 2000; US Department of Health and Human Services, 1999). Considering the role that schools could play in supporting the mental health of children, many unrealized opportunities exist. Currently, a significant number of children with mental health issues are undiagnosed and untreated (Kataoka, Zhang, & Wells, 2002). This unmet need results in schoolchildren with untreated depression, anxiety, eating disorders, and disruptive behavior disorders, which can have a significant and detrimental impact on student's well-being, academic performance, and school outcomes (Kessler, 2009; Roeser, Eccles, & Strobel, 1998; World Health Organization [WHO], 2003).

Consequently, schools have an interest in promoting the health and mental health of students. Beyond individual interventions and treatment, schools have also emerged as a natural setting for prevention efforts. School-wide prevention activities that focus on students' social-emotional development can contribute directly to improvements in academic achievement (e.g., Collaborative for Academic, Social, and Emotional Learning [CASEL], 2008; Payton, Weissberg, Durlak, Dymnicki, Taylor, Schellinger, & Pachan, 2008; Zins, Bloodworth, Weissberg, & Walhberg, 2004).

At the same time, a major paradigm shift is occurring across the social science fields – away from a disorder-focused, deficit-oriented framework and towards a more wellness-focused, strengths-based model that embraces universal and system-wide change. Because students spend so much time in schools, there is a growing realization of the power of school mental health programs not just to effect individual change, but also to lead efforts to bring about positive school-level change that affects all individuals within the school community. This paradigm shift aligns with the tiered public health model, especially when considering the increasing emphasis on health promotion.

Despite the growing evidence of the integral connection between mental health and academic outcomes, schools continue to miss opportunities to promote mental health and prevent or intervene to address children's mental health difficulties. Competing interests, a lack of understanding, and other barriers impede schools from fully embracing mental health as a critical support for school performance. Ironically, school mental health programs can be deprived of resources and access to students due to growing pressure on schools related to accountability and economic challenges. These factors limit the success of efforts to institute school-wide social-emotional supports that can provide the very foundation for academic success – especially for vulnerable, high-risk populations.

In this chapter, we first briefly review the mental health needs of our nation's children and identify opportunities associated with school mental health, with a focus on increasing access to care. Second, we examine the relationship between learning and mental health and emphasize the need for greater integration of public health approaches with mental health in schools. Third, we touch upon the elements that constitute the public health continuum – from mental health promotion, screening and early detection, prevention, and early intervention to intervention and maintenance. To illustrate, we present several examples of how school mental health can connect with larger, coordinated models of care delivered in the school environment, including efforts to improve school culture and connectedness, school-based health care, and early care and education. We assert that these areas exemplify existing school mental health activities, yet they also constitute opportunities for greater involvement from the field.

Following these examples, we address current challenges and opportunities related to mental health intervention in the schools. These include

1   movement toward a common language and vision to facilitate true partnerships with educators;
2   the identification and use of core elements of evidence-based practice and modular approaches to intervention;
3   the importance of building a research base and infrastructure to support quality in school mental health; and
4   consideration of community science approaches and implementation studies to support research and practice in the field.

Next, we reference an emerging opportunity to partner with education and medical providers in the development and implementation of effective prevention interventions to address the epidemic rates of childhood obesity and associated sequelae. The article concludes with a brief discussion of next steps related to advancing research and practice in school mental health using a public health perspective.

The state of children's mental health and disparities in access to care

According to the US Surgeon General, approximately one in five children and adolescents have a mental health disorder that interferes with functioning, yet fewer than 20% of them receive needed services (US Department of Health and Human Services, 1999). Another estimate suggests that the extent of unmet needs ranges from approximately 17 to 33% (Leaf, Alegria, Cohen, Goodman, Horwitz, Hoven, et al., 1996). The consequences of untreated mental health issues can be grave and include suicide (the third leading cause of death among youth from ages 10 to 19), school dropout, substance abuse, teen pregnancy, and recurring adult disorders (Brown & Grumet, 2009; Kessler, 2009). Given the increasing prevalence of mental health conditions among youth and the negative developmental and academic outcomes associated with untreated conditions (Barry & Busch, 2008; Kataoka et al., 2002; Manning, 2009), this is a public health issue that is critical to our nation's welfare.

There appear to be even more barriers to obtaining care for specific subgroups. Compared to white Americans, ethnic and racial minorities are even less likely to have access to or receive mental health services (US Department of Health and Human Services, 2001). In a study of over 5,000 fifth-graders in three metropolitan areas, fewer black (6%) and Hispanic (8%) children accessed mental health services compared to white children (14%) (Coker, Elliott, Kataoka, Schwebel, Mrug, et al., 2009). Explanations for this disparity include being uninsured or underinsured, having issues related to transportation, and feeling stigma associated with seeking mental health care (Dey, Schiller, & Tai, 2004). Rani Elwy, Ranganathan, and Eisen (2008) examined possible reasons for disparities by comparing those who successfully accessed mental health services (i.e., by completing an intake for outpatient treatment) and found no racial or ethnic differences in rates of subsequent treatment. They concluded that racial and ethnic differences occur in regards to seeking treatment and recommended that treatment should be made as available and accessible as possible in order to have the best chance of reaching those in need.

Movement toward school mental health

In response to this growing awareness of unmet needs, there has been a national movement towards providing a full continuum of health and mental health services in schools (New Freedom Commission on Mental

Health, 2003). The advantages of providing mental health services within schools are numerous. The provision of services within a school enables outreach to a greater number of children, with schools providing unparalleled access to youth. School-based services are also delivered in a natural, familiar environment (Adelman & Taylor, 2000), which may reduce the sense of stigma associated with seeking mental health care (Mufson, Dorta, Olfson, Weissman, & Hoagwood, 2004). Indeed, most children who access mental health care do so in schools (US Department of Health & Human Services, 1999), as school mental health services are commonly available and accessible (Slade, 2002). Furthermore, the location provides greater opportunities for observations in the natural environment, *in vivo* practice of learned strategies, consultation with teachers and school staff, efficient use of limited resources, and enhanced capacity to institute school-wide interventions that can promote the well-being and academic success for all students.

While a number of models exist, the expanded school mental health model promotes collaborative partnerships among schools, community organizations, and universities to provide a full continuum of mental health promotion and intervention services for youth in regular and special education (Weist, 2003). Research on expanded school mental health programs has provided evidence of a positive impact on a number of outcomes, including decreased incidence of special education referrals, absences, discipline referrals, suspension, grade retention, increased test scores, and a reduction in symptoms (Bruns, Walrath, Glass-Siegel, & Weist, 2004; Hussey & Guo, 2003; Jennings, Pearson, & Harris, 2000; National Research Council and Institute of Medicine, 2000; Substance Abuse and Mental Health Services Administration, 2005). The success of this model is due, in part, to the growing recognition of the inseparable links between mental health and learning.

The relationship between mental health and learning

Researchers, policymakers, administrators, educators, clinicians, and families have come to realize the interdependent relationships between mental health and achievement (CASEL, 2008; Greenberg et al., 2003; Zins et al., 2004). Children experiencing high levels of distress, experienced internally or demonstrated externally, have poorer academic functioning and achievement (Roeser et al., 1998). However, students who receive social-emotional support and services demonstrate higher levels of achievement and more positive school outcomes (Greenberg, Weissberg, O'Brien, Zins, Fredericks, Resnik, & Elias, 2003; Jennings et al., 2000; Zins et al., 2004). The focus on students' overall developmental needs, particularly among at-risk populations, builds an important foundation for academic success in school (Comer, 2005). Students' internalization of social-emotional skills makes them less likely to engage in high-risk behavior and more likely to persevere through academic challenges (Osher & Fleischman, 2005; Solomon, Battistich, Watson, Schaps, & Lewis, 2000; Zins & Elias, 2006). As Masten, Roisman, Long, Burt, Obradovic, and Riley (2005) noted, "developmental competence" is integrally linked to "academic competence," and this relationship should be a primary focus of efforts to support healthy childhood development.

Integrating public health approaches with mental health in the context of schools

In the schools, public health approaches to mental health prevention and intervention are becoming increasingly influential and are undergoing rapid development, coalescing into organized, well-articulated, and integrated models; however, much work remains in this area. Adelman and Taylor (2006) described the public health approach to intervention as the provision of a coordinated continuum of services that adapts to changing needs and facilitates transitions among levels of care. School-based prevention and intervention efforts are increasingly developed, implemented, and evaluated using rigorous methodology, as evidenced by the prevention science framework (Domitrovich, Bradshaw, Greenberg, Embry, Poduska, & Ialongo, 2010; Kellam & Langevin, 2003) and advances in the area of positive behavior supports (Lewis & Sugai, 1999; McIntosh, Filter, Bennett, Ryan, & Sugai, 2010; Sugai & Horner, 2006).

Despite these advances, there remain a number of challenges to the implementation of these models, including a lack of infrastructure for providing interventions in the schools, particularly proactive behavior supports for all students. Many schools continue to struggle to implement a comprehensive system of mental health promotion, prevention, and intervention. This presents a significant opportunity for school mental health to support the design, selection, implementation, and evaluation of these efforts. In the section below, examples of programs that facilitate mental health promotion, screening and early detection of problems, prevention and early intervention, and intervention are presented. We recognize that these examples may address multiple areas of the public health continuum, such as conducting screening and then providing further assessment or treatment when indicated. However, these programs were selected to illustrate existing relations to school mental health and, in many schools, opportunities for greater involvement across the full continuum.

Mental health promotion

Schools continue to miss opportunities to promote mental health and to prevent or intervene to address children's mental health difficulties. The importance of each of these areas was illuminated in a recent report by the National Research Council and Institute of Medicine (2009), Preventing

Mental, Emotional, and Behavioral Disorders among Young People. This report expanded the traditional three-tier approach to prevention by adding mental health promotion as an important element of the continuum. The authors conceptualized mental health promotion as the pursuit of well-being or positive states, such as competence, and not merely the absence of disease or disorder. While mental health promotion frequently occurs in school settings and has been explored elsewhere (e.g., Durlak, Taylor, Kawashima, Pachan, DuPre, Celio, et al., 2007; Weist, Paternite, Wheatley-Rowe, & Gall, 2009; Wells, Barlow, & Stewart-Brown, 2003), it represents a significant agenda that can often be overlooked by schools that are under growing pressure related to accountability and economic challenges. One way to promote mental health is through the development of positive school environments.

An example: Enhancing school climate and supporting connectedness

One of the ways to bring about positive school-level change that affects all individuals within is improving the school's climate. There is growing evidence that improvements in school climate – defined in large part by how students, staff, and parents "feel" about being in the school and the quality of relationships between students and staff – enhances student achievement (Cohen, McCabe, Michelli, & Pickeral, 2009; Gonder & Hymes, 1994; Scales & Leffert, 1999). In a review of studies on the impact of school climate upon academic performance, Scales and Leffert (1999) found that a caring school climate is linked with higher grades, increased attendance, decreased drop-out rates, higher self-esteem, and less anxiety, depression, and substance use.

Studies show that positive school environments foster students' sense of school connectedness and function as a protective factor that increases the likelihood of positive outcomes (Battistich, Schaps, & Wilson, 2004; Centers for Disease Control and Prevention, 2009; Reinke & Herman, 2002). School connectedness refers to a "belief by students that adults and peers in the school care about their learning as well as about them as individuals" (Centers for Disease Control and Prevention, 2009, p. 3) and derives from a positive school climate characterized by positive relationships among school staff and students (Weiss, Cunningham, Lewis, & Clark, 2005). Students who report feeling connected perform better academically, earn higher grades and test scores, have better attendance, and are less likely to drop out (Battin-Pearson, Newcomb, Abbot, Hill, Catalano, & Hawkins, 2000; Klem & Connell, 2004; Wang, Haertel, & Walberg, 1997). Among adolescents, school connectedness also is associated with reduced high-risk behaviors for both males and females, including substance use, absenteeism, early sexual behavior, violence, emotional distress, suicidal ideation, and number of attempted suicides (Blum,

McNeeley, & Rinehart, 2002; Catalano, Haggerty, Oesterle, Fleming, & Hawkins, 2004; Resnick, Bearman, Blum, Bauman, Harris, & Jones, 1997; Resnick, Harris, & Blum, 1993).

Significant advances in the development of school-wide positive behavior supports focus on improving school climate, building supportive classroom environments through consultation and coaching, and supporting the needs of individual students. Following a public health model, this tiered framework for prevention and intervention has witnessed significant increases in rates of adoption and implementation in recent years and has demonstrated positive effects on the school climate (Bradshaw, Koth, Thornton, & Leaf, 2009). The presence of school mental health programs has also been found to be directly associated with improvements in school climate (Bruns et al., 2004).

Screening and early detection

Although somewhat controversial, valid screening efforts to detect persistent mental health difficulties in school-aged children allows for early intervention and treatment, increasing the likelihood of positive outcomes. Evidence suggests that mental health difficulties can be detected early in the school career and that these difficulties tend to persist into later years (Essex, Kraemer, Slattery, Burk, Boyce, & Woodward, 2009). However, screening in schools is not without barriers and challenges, and requires thoughtful consideration and careful implementation (Weist, Rubin, Moore, Adelsheim, & Wrobel, 2007). Weist et al. (2007) have identified two primary areas for consideration, including

1   whether knowledgeable staff trained in screening, assessment, and treatment are available; and
2   whether appropriate methods exist for selecting screening instruments, obtaining consent/assent, ensuring confidentiality, and managing liability.

Important work has recently begun to provide cost estimates of effective screening, a necessary consideration in challenging economic times (Kuo, VanderStoep, McCauley, & Kernic, 2009). In addition, the use of technology to facilitate screening and early identification efforts is also an area for continued exploration (e.g., Nemeroff, Levitt, Faul, Wonpat-Borja, Bufferd, Setterberg, & Jensen, 2008).

An example: Supporting holistic development through school-based health care

While a number of different models of school mental health exist, the growth of school-based health centers (SBHC) presents an opportunity to build a continuum of coordinated health and mental health services. A recent survey by the National Association of School Based Health Care (NASBHC, 2007) indicates that there are over 1,700 SBHCs across the nation, a rapid increase from approximately 100 in the late 1980s (Lear, 2007). SBHCs are primarily located in urban environments (59%) or rural settings (29%), and the racial/ethnic profiles for students served include 34% Hispanic, 30% black, and 30% white students (NASBHC, 2007).

Preliminary evidence suggests that providing health care in schools not only offers greater access to care for somatic and physical needs, but also provides greater opportunity for screening, early detection, and intervention related to mental health needs. A study by Guo, Wade, and Keller (2008) found that SBHCs provide access to mental health services for a higher proportion of students across both rural and urban environments. This may be particularly true for children and youth residing in disadvantaged environments and seems that it may, with time, be an acceptable way for children and youth to access mental health services. One study found that mental health related visits to new SBHCs in rural and urban areas increased from 1 to 22% over a three-year period (Wade, Mansour, Guo, Huentlemen, Line, & Keller, 2008).

Of the SBHCs surveyed by NASBHC from 2004 to 2005, 67% reported having a mental health provider on staff (NASBHC, 2007). Although the survey also indicated that the majority of SBHCs without mental health providers on staff still provide mental health referrals, screening, and diagnostic services, a number of advantages arise from the integration of school-based health care and expanded school mental health services. These include greater opportunities for successful referrals and a team-based approach, increased screening, enhanced confidentiality and privacy, decreased need for more intensive care, and, likely, cost savings through integration of care (Weist, Goldstein, Morris, & Bryant, 2003).

In addition to the improvements in health and mental health access and outcomes, there is also evidence suggesting that increased use of SBHCs and greater access to care result in improvements in academic indicators (Gall, Pagano, Desmond, Perrin, & Murphy; McCord, Klein, Foy, & Fothergill, 1993). While rigorous implementation and evaluation of these models have yet to be completed, there is promising evidence of the potential for positive impact of coordinated school health programs on student achievement (Murray, Low, Hollis, Cross, & Davis, 2007).

Prevention and early intervention

Similar to the positive changes evident in meta-analyses of mental health prevention programs (Durlak & Wells, 1997; Durlak & Wells, 1998), school-based preventive interventions can also promote positive outcomes among children and adolescents (Greenberg, 2004; Greenberg, Domitrovich, & Bumbarger, 2001; Hoagwood, Olin, Kerker, Kratochwill, Crowe,

& Saka, 2007). Comprehensive reviews of school-based prevention programs found that interventions linking social, emotional, and academic learning were significantly associated with improved social and academic outcomes (Elias, Zins, Graczyk, & Weissberg, 2003; Wilson, Gottfredson, & Najaka, 2001). An extensive review of over 200 school-based research studies found that intervention efforts aimed at bolstering social and emotional skills in children and adolescents resulted in an approximately 11% increase in achievement test scores (CASEL, 2008). Given these findings, it is clear that this area warrants further development and investigation, ideally through collaborations between educators and mental health researchers and practitioners.

An example: Prevention and early intervention in early childhood

Research over the past several decades has shown that early intervention programs can have a significant impact on the later academic achievement, mental health, and functioning of participants (National Research Council and Institute of Medicine, 2000). Early childhood is a significant and influential period for life trajectories of health and development (e.g., Guyer, Ma, Grason, Frick, Perry, Sharkey, & McIntosh, 2009; National Scientific Council on the Developing Child, 2008). Long-term positive effects have been found for mental health indicators for participants of several early childhood programs, including the Brookline Early Education Project (Palfrey, Hauser-Cram, Bronson, Warfield, Sirin, & Chan, 2005), the Abecedarian Project (McLaughlin, Campbell, Pungello, & Skinner, 2007), the Chicago Child-Parent Centers (Reynolds, Temple, Ou, Robertson, Mersky, Topitzes, & Niles, 2007), and the Seattle Social Development Project (Hawkins, Kosterman, Catalano, Hill, & Abbott, 2008). These programs demonstrate the importance of positive experiences in early childhood, particularly those focused on social and emotional development, for outcomes in adulthood. Recent conceptualizations, including the "School of the 21st Century," build upon this evidence to support the continued development of models and programs that address specific early care and educational needs during this sensitive period (Zigler & Finn-Stevenson, 2007). Studies estimate significant potential cost savings from these programs (e.g., Barnett, 1998; Reynolds & Temple, 2008), indicating that investments in our disadvantaged children at a young age will lead not only to improved outcomes, but also to economic benefits for society over time.

Early childhood and family support programs offer opportunities for the extension of mental health services beyond traditional K-12 programs. The advantages of building stronger connections between these programs and school mental health include opportunities to

1   enhance protective factors, such as school readiness and parent involvement;

2   provide education and consultation related to the emotional and behavioral needs of young children; and
3   develop integrated, seamless systems to support children and their families.

Despite documented need, early childhood mental health continues to be an area in need of significant interdisciplinary attention and action (Knitzer, 2000). School mental health providers already familiar with the interrelations among areas of development possess many of the requisite skills needed to advance this agenda, and they are already involved with multiple child-serving systems providing coordinated support to children, families, and early child care and education providers.

Mental health interventions in a school-based setting

Addressing the "research-to-practice gap" in children's mental health will require an increased focus on the adaptation, implementation, and evaluation of evidence-based interventions delivered in school settings (Ringeisen, Henderson, & Hoagwood, 2003; Rones & Hoagwood, 2000). Similar to those faced in the field of children's mental health more generally, multiple challenges limit the provision of high-quality, evidence-based school mental health interventions. While numerous reviews of these challenges exist (e.g., Schaeffer, Bruns, Weist, Stephan, Goldstein, & Simpson, 2005), three specific opportunities to address these challenges are presented below.

First, manualized, evidence-based interventions are difficult, if not impossible, to implement with high fidelity in the school setting. For example, the 90-minute sessions found in many manuals are often not practical for implementation in school settings. Other challenges include the chaotic nature of the school environment, limitations in personnel preparation and supervision practices, and a lack of awareness among consumers and the general public as to the value of empirically supported interventions (Evans & Weist, 2004; Schaeffer et al., 2005). Thus, the use of modular interventions, developed through the use of distillation and matching protocols, presents an alternate method to identify effective components of evidence-based interventions (Chorpita & Daleiden, 2009; Chorpita, Daleiden, & Weisz, 2005a; Chorpita, Daleiden, & Weisz, 2005b). Next, the discrepancy between research-supported programs and services and the everyday practice of school mental health is significant (Weist, 2005). The issue of quality assessment and improvement, including more rigorous and consistent implementation and evaluation, must be a primary focus to advance the field. This area requires substantial research and development. Finally, continued exploration of different models to support development, implementation, and evaluation is important. Top-down versus bottom-up models have been proposed to close the gap between research and practice. While both approaches have value, the need exists to address the enduring inquiry of "what works" and "for whom" in the school setting. Other questions that are just as critical include issues of acceptability, feasibility, and sustainability.

Challenges and opportunities in implementing school mental health

The following sections address current challenges and opportunities in the field of school mental health, including the need to further develop partnerships across disciplines; increase the effectiveness of school mental health through implementation of high-quality, evidence-based interventions; and apply innovative models to bridge the research-to-practice divide.

Partnering with educators: establishing a common vision and language

Although there is a long history between the fields of education and mental health, this link is often tenuous (Sedlak, 1997). However, educators have been referred to as the "linchpins" of school mental health due to their proximity to students, which gives them opportunities to promote mental health through their day-to-day interactions (Paternite, 2004). Despite the central role that teachers play in supporting students, several barriers to true collaboration remain, including competing demands for limited resources, varying definitions as to the "scope" of practice or professional roles, and communication barriers, often related to the establishment of hierarchal consultative relationships (Burke & Paternite, 2007; Paternite & Johnston, 2005). To engage teachers as full partners in promoting the mental health of students, a number of organizational factors, along with teacher characteristics, must be considered (Han & Weiss, 2005; Ransford, Greenberg, Domitrovich, Small, & Jacobson, 2009). Recommendations to enhance school mental health consistently reference the critical importance of building positive, working relationships with educators (Paternite & Johnston, 2005; Rones & Hoagwood, 2000).

For consultation to effectively address the needs of students with challenging behavior, there is evidence that "buy in" from educators, particularly those that are influential or highly regarded by their peers, is critical (Atkins, Frazier, Leathers, Graczyk, Talbott, & Adil, 2008; Lynn, McKay, & Atkins, 2003). Building a mutual understanding between educational staff and administration and mental health providers is important not as a means to an end, but with respect to the process itself. Not only is this alignment valuable for a particular student, but also for the development of innovative approaches to larger programmatic, systemic, and institutional issues. Educators and mental health providers in the schools are uniquely positioned to identify common challenges, identify areas for mental health promotion, and to develop, implement, and evaluate preventive interventions. It is only through the development of a shared understanding, facilitated by a shared language, that true partnerships can occur. Eloquently stated, Atkins and colleagues (2010) note that true integration in mental health and education will occur "when the goal of mental health includes effective schooling and the goal of effective schools includes the healthy functioning of students" (Abstract).

Implementation of evidence-based practices: the promise of modular approaches

Recent advances in bridging the research-to-practice gap utilize distillation and matching methods to identify core practice elements of evidence-based mental health interventions (Chorpita & Daleiden, 2009; Chorpita et al., 2005a; 2005b). Many of the challenges identified by clinicians to implementing evidence-based practices, particularly in the schools, cite the lack of flexibility in implementation (Schaeffer et al., 2005). Therefore, identification of core practice elements eliminates many of the concerns about using efficacious, manualized programs by allowing for a modularized approach to intervention for common mental health disorders that increases flexibility in therapeutic practice and considers child characteristics and context. While this is a relatively new area, this approach holds significant promise. As the methodology evolves, there will be a corresponding need for greater clarity and understanding of the supports needed to implement modular approaches, including the development of best practices in areas such as training and coaching for clinicians, the monitoring of fidelity, and the development of clinical decision-making supports. This work will be complemented by advances in the studies on implementation and dissemination (Domitrovich, Bradshaw, Poduska, Hoagwood, Buckley, & Olin, 2008; Durlak & DuPre, 2008).

A continued emphasis on quality in school mental health

The growing need for mental health services, the limited resources that lead to competing demands, and the weak infrastructure for training and implementation support all create a challenging context in which to implement educational and mental health interventions (Elias et al., 2003; Foster, Rollefson, Doksum, Noonan, Robinson, G., & Teich, 2005; Weist, 2005). Therefore, a commitment to quality assessment and improvement that supports effectiveness and efficiency is essential to promote mental health and positive educational outcomes among children and youth in schools. Quality assessment and improvement in school mental health includes the development of a "shared" agenda that involves all stakeholders, with a particular focus on family support and engagement; provision of a full continuum of services and supports for all students to promote school success; appropriate personnel selection and preparation, with ongoing staff development; implementation of empirically-based interventions with consideration of the specific school context; monitoring of key outcomes for use in data-based decision-making; and iterative evaluation focused on continuous program improvement, policy development, and advocacy efforts (Nabors, Weist, Tashman, & Meyers, 1999; Weist, Sander, Lever, Link, Christodulu, & Rosner, 2002; Weist, Stephan, Lever, Moore, Flaspohler, & Maras, 2007).

Continued effort to develop each of these aspects of quality assessment and improvement is needed to move beyond merely aspirations to embed these elements into standard practice in the field.

Drawing upon community science and implementation studies to support systemic change

The community science approach (Wandersman, 2003), along with increased awareness of the role of organizational factors and advances in implementation science (Fixen, Naoom, Blasé, Friedman, & Wallace, 2005; Graczyk, Domitrovich, & Zins, 2003; Huang, Macbeth, Dodge, & Jacobstein, 2004), will guide the development of theory and best practices to support quality in school mental health. The community science approach represents an interdisciplinary paradigm that supports the integration and involvement of community stakeholders in the translation of research-to-practice. A recent framework to support action in school mental health, guided by the community science perspective, involves consideration of policies, infrastructure, resources, and practices (Flaspohler, Anderson-Butcher, Paternite, Weist, & Wandersman, 2006). These authors note that a critical element of working within the research-to-practice gap is to support the diffusion of innovation into the school setting; however, little systematic work has been conducted on the systems required to do this.

Expanding upon an existing model for evaluating public health impact, Merrell and Buchanan (2006) developed an innovative model to guide schools in the selection and evaluation of interventions that encourages the consideration of factors such as reach, efficacy, adoption, implementation, and maintenance. While further examination of existing models that attempt to bridge the research-to-practice gap (e.g., deployment-focused models; see Weisz et al., 2005) will likely reveal many commonalities, this effort requires careful consideration and continued collaboration and discussion among researchers, practitioners, and other key stakeholders.

While these four areas related to school-based interventions present challenges, they also bring opportunity. School mental health is well-positioned to collaborate with other health providers and educators to address issues that impact the health, mental health, and functioning of children and adolescents. One example of an area for growth and development is related to childhood obesity and the associated sequelae.

Childhood obesity: An opportunity to partner with medical providers and educators

National attention has focused on the alarming prevalence rates of overweight and obese children and youth in America. The rates have reached epidemic proportions, with estimates that as much as 35% of children meet criteria for being overweight or obese (Lobstein & Jackson-Leach, 2007). Obesity places children at an increased risk of developing a number of secondary health conditions, including diabetes, hypertension, and heart disease (Daniels, 2006), and tends to persist into adulthood (Whitlock, Williams, Gold, Smith, & Shipman, 2005). This health risk has both short-term and long-term implications for children's physical, mental, and social development (Daniels, 2006; Doak, Visscher, Rendel, & Seidell, 2006). Furthermore, overweight and obesity status is associated with poorer academic outcomes (e.g., Datar, Sturm, & Magnabosco, 2004; Taras & Potts-Datema, 2005). For these reasons, this issue has become an international "public health crisis" (Lobstein, Baur, & Uauy, 2004) and, as such, deserves the attention of all child-serving systems.

Recent calls for an integrated approach to the prevention and treatment of childhood obesity have focused on collaboration among families and communities, with particular emphasis on the role of health care providers and schools (Flohr & Williams, 2007). Although this approach is not without controversy (Katz, 2009), schools have been involved in many of the current intervention studies designed to prevent or reduce obesity (Summerbell, Waters, Edmunds, Kelly, Brown, & Campbell, 2005), and there is growing evidence of the effectiveness of such interventions (Gonzalez-Suarez, Worley, Grimmer-Somers, & Dones, 2009; Yetter, 2009). As described above, school-based health centers may be in a unique position to identify and address obesity among students (Oetzel, Scott, & McGrath, 2009; Peterson & Fox, 2007). One study found that high-school students identified obesity as a significant impetus that led them to seek mental health services through a school-based clinic (Jepson, Juszczak, & Fisher, 1998). While the links between mental health, overweight and obesity status, and the school environment are clear, the critical mechanisms to effective prevention and intervention are less clear. In past school-based studies of this issue, mental health indicators largely have been neglected (van Wijnen, Wendel-Vos, Wammes, & Bemelmans, 2009) and are thus an important element of future research.

Next steps

The promotion of well-being and the prevention and treatment of mental health disorders remains a significant public health need that warrants continued development, research, and innovation. Cooper (2008) proposed that a critical factor is for schools and mental health sevices to establish an egalitarian relationship in recognition of shared goals to advance the school mental health agenda. Cooper asserts that such a partnership would provide a basis for collaborative efforts to

1   provide support for teachers when working with students with challenging behavior;
2   build a shared framework between schools and mental health; and
3   establish joint accountability for improving child mental health outcomes.

Partnerships guided by these principles will begin to break down the "silos" that continue to exist between and within systems and optimize the likelihood of positive impact on the health, mental health, and well-being of children.

To facilitate improvements in child health and mental health outcomes using a public health framework, Kazak and colleagues (2010) assert that the most basic critical elements must include

> rapid translation of research findings into practice, continued advocacy for effective services, ongoing monitoring of outcomes, accountability standards to ensure that quality services are delivered, and collaborative partnerships among families, providers, researchers, and policymakers in the shared pursuit of optimal care for children.
>
> (p. 95)

While school environments are facing notable challenges related to increased expectations for demonstrating student outcomes and limited fiscal resources, it is paramount that the robust findings supporting the integral relations between mental health and learning are communicated along with the potential for school mental health services to support both of these areas.

References

Adelman, H. S., & Taylor, L. (2000). Shaping the future of mental health in schools. *Psychology in the Schools, 37*, 49–60.

Adelman, H. S., & Taylor, L. (2006). *The current status of mental health in schools: A policy and practice brief*. Los Angeles, CA: University of Los Angeles, California School Mental Health Project.

Atkins, M., Frazier, S., Leathers, S., Graczyk, P., Talbott, E., Adil, J., et al. (2008). Teacher key opinion leaders and mental health consultation in urban low-income schools. *Journal of Consulting and Clinical Psychology, 76*, 905–908.

Atkins, M. S., Hoagwood, K. E., Kutash, K., & Seidman, E. (2010). Toward the integration of education and mental health in schools. *Administration and Policy in Mental Health and Mental Health Services Research*. doi: 10.1007/s10488-010-0299-7.

Barnett, W. S. (1998). Long-term cognitive and academic effects of early childhood education on children in poverty. *Prevention Science, 27*, 204–207.

Barry, C. L., & Busch, S. H. (2008). Caring for children with mental disorders: Do state parity laws increase access to treatment? *Journal of Mental Health Policy and Economics, 11*(2), 57–66.

Battin-Pearson, S., Newcomb, M. D., Abbot, R. D., Hill, K. G., Catalano, R. F., & Hawkins, J. D. (2000). Predictors of early high school dropout: A test of five theories. *Journal of Educational Psychology, 92*(3), 568–582.

Battistich, V., Schaps, E., & Wilson, N. (2004). Effects of an elementary school intervention on students' "connectedness" to school and social adjustment during middle school. *Journal of Primary Prevention, 24*, 243–262.

Blum, R. W., McNeely, C., & Rinehart, P. M. (2002). *Improving the odds: The untapped power of schools to improve the health of teens.* Minneapolis: Center for Adolescent Health and Development, University of Minnesota.

Bradshaw, C. P., Koth, C. W., Thornton, L. A., & Leaf, P. J. (2009). Altering school climate through school-wide positive behavioral interventions and supports: Findings from a group-randomized effectiveness trial. *Prevention Science, 10*, 100–115.

Brown, M. M., & Grumet, J. G. (2009). School-based suicide prevention with African American youth in an urban setting. *Professional Psychology: Research and Practice, 40*(2), 111–117.

Bruns, E. J., Walrath, C., Glass-Siegel, M., & Weist, M. D. (2004). School-based mental health services in Baltimore: Association with school climate and special education referrals. *Behavior Modification, 28*, 491–512.

Burke, R. W., & Paternite, C. E. (2007). Teacher engagement in expanded school mental health. In S. W. Evans, M. D. Weist, & Z. N. Serpell (Eds.), *Advances in school-based mental health interventions: Best practices and program models, vol. II*, (pp. 21:1–21:15). Kingston, NJ: Civic Research Institute.

Burns, B. J., Costello, E. J., Angold, A., Tweed, D., Stangl, D., Farmer, E. M., & Erkanli, A. (1995). Children's mental health service use across service sectors. *Health Affairs, 14*, 147–159.

Capella, E., Frazier, S. L., Atkins, M. S., Schoenwald, S. K., & Glisson, C. (2008). Enhancing schools' capacity to support children in poverty: An ecological model of school-based mental health services. *Administration and Policy in Mental Health and Mental Health Services Research, 35*, 395–409.

Catalano, R. F., Haggerty, K. P., Oesterle, S., Fleming, C. B., & Hawkins, J. D. (2004). The importance of bonding to school for healthy development: Findings from the Social Development Research Group. *Journal of School Health, 74*, 252–261.

Centers for Disease Control and Prevention. (2009). *School connectedness: Strategies for increasing protective factors among youth.* Atlanta, GA: US Department of Health and Human Services.

Chorpita, B. F., Daleiden, E. L., & Weisz, J. R. (2005a). Identifying and selecting the common elements of evidence-based interventions: A distillation and matching model. *Mental Health Services Research, 7*, 5–20.

Chorpita, B. F., Daleiden, E. L., & Weisz, J. R. (2005b). Modularity in the design and application of therapeutic interventions. *Applied and Preventive Psychology, 11*, 141–156.

Chorpita, B. F., & Daheden, E. L. (2009). Mapping evidence-based treatments for children and adolescents: Application of the distillation and matching model to 615 treatments from 322 randomized trials. *Journal of Consulting and Clinical Psychology, 77,* 566–578.

Cohen, J., McCabe, E. M., Michelli, N. M., & Pickeral, T. (2009). School climate: Research, policy, teacher education and practice. *Teachers College Record, 111,* 180–213.

Coker, T. R., Elliott, M. N., Kataoka, S., Schwebel, D. C., Mrug, S., Grunbaum, J. A. et al. (2009). Racial/Ethnic disparities in the mental health care utilization of fifth grade children. *Academic Pediatrics, 9*(2), 89–96.

Collaborative for Academic, Social, and Emotional Learning (2008). *Social and emotional learning (SEL) and student benefits: Implications for the Safe Schools/Healthy Students core elements.* Chicago, IL: Author. Retrieved from www.casel.org/downloads/EDC_CASELSELResearchBrief.pdf.

Comer, J. (2005). *Leave no child behind: Preparing today's youth for tomorrow's world.* New Haven, CT: Yale University Press.

Cooper, J. L. (2008). The federal case for school-based mental health services and supports. *Journal of the American Academy of Child and Adolescent Psychiatry, 47,* 4–8.

Daniels, S. R. (2006). The consequences of childhood overweight and obesity. *The Future of Children, 16,* 47–67.

Datar, A., Sturm, R., & Magnabosco, J. (2004). Childhood overweight and academic performance: National study of kindergartners and first graders. *Obesity Research, 12,* 58–68.

Dey, A. N., Schiller, J. S., & Tai, D. A. (2004). Summary Health Statistics for US Children: National Health Interview Survey, 2002. *National Center for Health Statistics. Vital Health Statistics, 10,* 221.

Doak, C. M., Visscher, T. L. S., Renders, C. M., & Seidell, J. C. (2006). The prevention of overweight and obesity in children and adolescents: A review of interventions and programmes. *Obesity Review, 7,* 111–136.

Domitrovich, C. E., Bradshaw, C. P., Greenberg, M. T., Embry, D., Poduska, J. M., & Ialongo, N. S. (2010). Integrated models of school-based prevention: Logic and theory. *Psychology in the Schools, 47,* 71–88.

Domitrovich, C. E., Bradshaw, C. P., Poduska, J., Hoagwood, K., Buckley, J., Olin, S., et al. (2008). Maximizing the implementation quality of evidence-based preventive interventions in schools: A conceptual framework. *Advances in School Mental Health Promotion, 1,* 6–18.

Durlak, J. A., Taylor, R. D., Kawashima, K., Pachan, M. K., DuPre, E. P., Celio, C. I., et al. (2007). Effects of positive youth development programs on school, family, and community systems. *American Journal of Community Psychology, 39,* 269–286.

Durlak, J. A., & DuPre, E. P. (2008). Implementation matters: A review of research on the influence of implementation on program outcomes and the factors affecting implementation. *American Journal of Community Psychology, 41,* 327–350.

Durlak, J. A., & Wells, A. M. (1997). Primary prevention mental health programs for children and adolescents: A meta-analytic review. *American Journal of Community Psychology, 25,* 115–152.

Durlak, J. A., & Wells, A. M. (1998). Evaluation of indicated preventive intervention (secondary prevention) mental health programs for children and adolescents. *American Journal of Community Psychology, 26,* 775–802.

Elias, M. J., Zins, J. E., Graczyk, P. A., & Weissberg, R. P. (2003). Implementation, sustainability, and scaling up of social-emotional and academic innovations in public schools. *School Psychology Review, 32*, 303–319.

Essex, M. J., Kraemer, H. C., Slattery, M. J., Burk, L. R., Boyce, W. T., & Woodward, H. R. (2009). Screening for childhood mental health problems: Outcomes and early identification. *Journal of Child Psychology & Psychiatry, 50*, 562–570.

Evans, S. W., & Weist, M. D. (2004). Implementing empirically supported treatments in the schools: What are we asking? *Clinical Child and Family Psychology Review, 7*, 263–267.

Farmer, E., Burns, B., Phillips, S., Angold, A., & Costello, E. (2003). Pathways into and through mental health services for children and adolescents. *Psychiatric Services, 54*, 60–66.

Fixen, D. L., Naoom, S. F., Blasé, K. A., Friedman, R. M., & Wallace, F. (2005). *Implementation research: A synthesis of the literature.* Tampa: University of South Florida, Louis de la Parte Florida Mental Health Institute.

Flaspohler, P. D., Anderson-Butcher, D., Paternite, C. E., Weist, M., & Wandersman, A. (2006). Community science and expanded school mental health: Bridging the research-to-practice gap to promote child well-being and academic success. *Educational and Child Psychology, 23*, 27–41.

Flohr, J. A., & Williams, J. A. (2007). Childhood obesity: The consequences and the role of schools. In S. W. Evans, M. D. Weist, & Z. N. Serpell (Eds.), *Advances in school-based mental health interventions: Best practices and program models, vol. II* (pp. 14:1–14:16). Kingston, NJ: Civic Research Institute.

Foster, S., Rollefson, M., Doksum, T., Noonan, D., Robinson, G., & Teich, J. (2005). *School mental health services in the United States, 2002–2003* (DHHS Publication No. (SMA) 05–4068). Rockville, MD: Center for Mental Health Services, Substance Abuse and Mental Health Services Administration.

Gall, G., Pagano, M. E., Desmond, S., Perrin, J. M., & Murphy, J. M. (2000). Utility of psychosocial screening at a school-based health center. *Journal of School Health, 70*, 292–298.

Gonder, P. O., & Hymes, D. (1994). *Improving school climate and culture: Critical issues report.* Arlington, VA: American Association of School Administrators.

Gonzalez-Suarez, C., Worley, A., Grimmer-Somers, K., & Dones, V. (2009). School-based interventions on childhood obesity: A meta-analysis. *American Journal of Preventive Medicine, 37*(5), 418–27.

Graczyk, P. A., Domitrovich, C. E., & Zins, J. E. (2003). Facilitating the implementation of evidence-based prevention and mental health promotion efforts in schools. In M. D. Weist, S. W. Evans, & N. A. Lever (Eds.), *Handbook of school mental health: Advancing practice and research* (pp. 301–318). New York: Kluwer Academic/Plenum Press.

Greenberg, M. T. (2004). Current and future challenges in school-based prevention: The researcher perspective. *Prevention Science, 5*, 5–13.

Greenberg, M. T., Domitrovich, C., & Bumbarger, B. (2001). The prevention of mental disorders in school-aged children: Current state of the field. *Prevention & Treatment, 4*, no pagination specified.

Greenberg, M. T., Weissberg, R. P., O'Brien, M. U., Zins, J. E., Fredericks, L., Resnik, H., & Elias, M. J. (2003). Enhancing school-based prevention and youth development through coordinated, social, emotional, and academic learning. *American Psychologist, 58*, 466–474.

Guo, J. J., Wade, T. J., & Keller, K. N. (2008). Impact of school-based health centers on students with mental health problems. *Public Health Reports, 123,* 768–780.

Guyer, B., Ma, S., Grason, H., Frick, K. D., Perry, D. F., Sharkey, A., & McIntosh, J. (2009). Early childhood health promotion and its life course health consequences. *Academic Pediatrics, 9,* 133–135.

Han, S. S., & Weiss, B. (2005). Sustainability of teacher implementation of school-based mental health programs. *Journal of Abnormal Child Psychology, 33,* 665–679.

Hawkins, D. J., Kosterman, R., Catalano, R. F., Hill, K. G., & Abbott, R. D. (2008). Effects of social development intervention in childhood 15 years later. *Archives of Pediatric and Adolescent Medicine, 162,* 1133–1141.

Hoagwood, K. E., Olin, S. S., Kerker, B. D., Kratochwill, T. R., Crowe, M., & Saka, N. (2007). Empirically based school interventions target academic and mental health functioning. *Journal of Emotional and Behavioral Disorders, 15,* 66–94.

Hussey, D. L., & Guo, S. (2003). Measuring behavior change in young children receiving intensive school-based mental health services. *Journal of Community Psychology, 31,* 629–639.

Huang, L., Macbeth, G., Dodge, J., & Jacobstein, D. (2004). Transforming the workforce in children's mental health. *Administration and Policy in Mental Health and Mental Health Services Research, 32*(2), 167–187.

Jennings, J., Pearson, G., & Harris, M. (2000). Implementing and maintaining a school-based mental health services in a large, urban school district. *Journal of School Health, 70,* 201–205.

Jepson, L., Juszczak, L., & Fisher, M. (1998). Mental health care in a high school-based health service. *Adolescence, 33,* 1–15.

Kaplan, D., Brindis, C., Naylor, K., Phibbs, S., Ahlstrand, K., & Melinkovich, P. (1998). Elementary school-based health center use. *Pediatrics, 101*(6), 12.

Kataoka, S. H., Zhang, L., & Wells, K. B. (2002). Unmet need for mental health care among US children: Variation by ethnicity and insurance status. *American Journal of Psychiatry, 159,* 1548–1555.

Katz, D. L. (2009). School-based interventions for health promotion and weight control: Not just waiting on the world to change. *Annual Review of Public Health, 30,* 353–372.

Kazak, A. E., Hoagwood, K., Weisz, J. R., Hood, K., Kratochwill, T. R., Vargas, L. A., & Banez, G. A. (2010). A meta-systems approach to evidence-based practice for children and adolescents. *American Psychologist, 65,* 85–97.

Kellam, S., & Langevin, D. (2003). A framework for understanding "evidence" in prevention research and programs. *Prevention Science, 4,* 137–153.

Kessler, R. (2009). Identifying and screening for psychological and comorbid medical and psychological disorders in medical settings. *Journal of Clinical Psychology, 65*(3), 253–267.

Klem, A., & Connell, J. (2004). Relationships matter: Linking teacher support to student engagement and achievement. *Journal of School Health, 74*(7), 262–273.

Knitzer, J. (2000). Early childhood mental health services: A policy and systems development perspective. In J. P. Shonkoff, & S. J. Meisels, *Handbook of Early Childhood Intervention (2nd ed.)* (pp. 416–438). New York: Cambridge University Press.

Kuo, E., VanderStoep, A., McCauley, E., & Kernic, M. A. (2009). Cost-effectiveness of a school-based emotional health screening program. *Journal of School Health, 79,* 277–285.

Leaf, P. J., Alegria, M., Cohen, P., Goodman, S. H., Horwitz, S. M., Hoven, C. W., et al. (1996). Mental health service use in the community and schools. *Journal of the American Academy of Child and Adolescent Psychiatry, 35,* 889–897.

Lear, J. G. (2007). Health at school: A hidden health care system emerges from the shadows. *Health Affairs, 26,* 409–419.

Lewis, T. J., & Sugai, W. (1999). Effective behavior support: A systems approach to proactive school-wide management. *Focus on Exceptional Children, 31,* 1–24.

Lobstein, T., & Jackson-Leach, R. (2007). Child overweight and obesity in the USA: Prevalence rates according to IOTF definitions. *International Journal of Pediatric Obesity, 2,* 62–64.

Lobstein, T., Baur, L., & Uauy, R. (2004). Obesity in children and young people: A crisis in public health. *Obesity Review, 5*(Suppl 1), 4–85.

Lynn, C. J., McKay, M. M., & Atkins, M. S. (2003). School social work: Meeting the mental health needs of students through collaboration with teachers. *Children and Schools, 25,* 197–204.

Manning, A. R. (2009). Bridging the gap from availability to accessibility: Providing health and mental health services in schools. *Journal of Evidence Based Social Work, 6*(1), 40–57.

Marx, E., Wooley, S. F., & Northrup, D. (1998). *Health is academic: A guide to coordinated school health programs.* New York: Teachers College Press.

Masten, A. S., Best, K. J., & Garmezy, N. (1990). Resilience and development: Contributions from the study of children who overcome adversity. *Development and Psychopathology, 2,* 425–444.

Masten, A. S., Roisman, G. I., Long, J. D., Burt, K. B., Obradovic, J., Riley, J. R., et al. (2005). Developmental cascades: Linking academic achievement and externalizing and internalizing symptoms over 20 years. *Developmental Psychology, 41,* 733–746.

McCord, M. T., Klein, J. D., Foy, J. M., & Fothergill, K. (1993). School-based clinic use and school performance. *Journal of Adolescent Health, 14,* 91–98.

McIntosh, K., Filter, K. J., Bennett, J. L., Ryan, C., & Sugai, G. (2010). Principles of sustainable prevention: Designing scale-up of school-wide positive behavior support to promote durable systems. *Psychology in the Schools, 47,* 5–21.

McLaughlin, A. E., Campbell, F. A., Pungello, E. P., & Skinner, M. (2007). Depressive symptoms in young adults: The influences of the early home environment and early educational child care. *Child Development, 78,* 746–756.

Merrell, K. W., & Buchanan, R. (2006). Intervention selection in school-based practice: Using public health models to enhance systems capacity of schools. *School Psychology Review, 35,* 167–180.

Mufson, L. H., Dorta, K. P., Olfson, M., Weissman, M. M., & Hoagwood, K. (2004). Effectiveness research: Transporting Interpersonal Psychotherapy for Depressed Adolescents (IPT-A) from the lab to school-based health clinics. *Clinical Child and Family Psychology Review, 7*(4), 251–261.

Murray, N. G., Low, B. J., Hollis, C., Cross, A. W., & Davis, S. M. (2007). Coordinated school health programs and academic achievement: A systematic review of the literature. *Journal of School Health, 77,* 589–600.

Nabors, L. A., Weist, M. D., Tashman, N. A., & Meyer, C. P. (1999). Quality assurance and school-based mental health services. *Psychology in the Schools, 36*, 485–493.

National Assembly on School-Based Health Care. (2007). *School-based health center census: National census school year 2004–05.* Retrieved from http://ww2.nasbhc.org/RoadMap/Public/EQ_2005census.pdf.

National Research Council and Institute of Medicine. (2000). From Neurons to Neighborhoods: The Science of Early Childhood Development. In J. P. Shonkoff & D. A. Phillips (Eds.), *Board on Children, Youth, and Families, Commission on Behavioral and Social Sciences and Education.* Washington, DC: National Academy Press.

National Research Council and Institute of Medicine. (2009). Preventing mental, emotional, and behavioral disorders among young people: Progress and possibilities. In M. E. O'Connell, T. Boat, & K. E. Warner (Eds.), *Committee on the prevention of mental disorders and substance abuse among children, youth, and young adults: Research advances and promising interventions.* Washington DC: National Academies Press.

National Scientific Council on the Developing Child. (2008). *Mental health problems in early childhood can impair learning and behavior for life: Working paper no. 6.* Retrieved from www.developingchild.harvard.edu.

Nemeroff, R., Levitt, J. M., Faul, L., Wonpat-Borja, A., Bufferd, S., Setterberg, S., & Jensen, P. S. (2008). Establishing ongoing, early identification programs for mental health problems in our schools: A feasibility study. *Journal of the American Academy of Child & Adolescent Psychiatry, 47*, 328–338.

New Freedom Commission on Mental Health. (2003). *Achieving the promise: Transforming mental health care in America: Final report* (DHHS Pub. No. SMA-03–3832). Rockville, MD.

Oetzel, K. B., Scott, A. A., & McGrath, J. (2009). School-based health centers and obesity prevention: Changing practice through quality improvement. *Pediatrics, 123*(Suppl 5), S267–S271.

Osher, D., & Fleischman, S. (2005). Research matters: Positive culture in urban schools. *Learning from Urban Schools, 62*(6), 84–85.

Palfrey, J. S., Hauser-Cram, P., Bronson, M. B., Warfield, M. E., Sirin, S., & Chan, E. (2005). The Brookline Early Education Project: A 25-year follow-up study of a family-centered early health and development intervention. *Pediatrics, 116*, 144–152.

Paternite, C. E. (2004). Involving educators in school-based mental health programs. In K. E. Robinson (Ed.), *Advances in school-based mental health interventions: Best practices and program models*, (pp. 6:1–6:21). Kingston, NJ: Civic Research Institute.

Paternite, C. E., & Johnston, T. C. (2005). Rationale and strategies for central involvement of educators in effective school-based mental health programs. *Journal of Youth and Adolescence, 34*, 41–49.

Payton, J., Weissberg, R. P., Durlak, J. A., Dymnicki, A. B., Taylor, R. D., Schellinger, K. B., & Pachan, M. (2008). *The positive impact of social and emotional learning for kindergarten to eighth-grade students: Findings from three scientific reviews.* Chicago, IL: Collaborative for Academic, Social, and Emotional Learning.

Peterson, K. E., & Fox, M. (2007). Addressing the epidemic of childhood obesity through school-based interventions: What has been done and where do we go from here? *The Journal of Law, Medicine & Ethics, 35*, 113–130.

Rani Elwy, A., Ranganathan, G., & Eisen, S. (2008). Race-Ethnicity and diagnosis as predictors of outpatient service use among treatment initiators. *Psychiatric Services, 59*, 1285–1291.

Ransford, C. R., Greenberg, M. T., Domitrovich, C. E., Small, M., & Jacobson, L. (2009). The role of teachers' psychological experiences and perceptions of curriculum supports on the implementation of a social and emotional learning curriculum. *School Psychology Review, 38*, 510–532.

Reinke, W. M., & Herman, K. C. (2002). Creating school environments that deter antisocial behaviors in youth. *Psychology in the Schools, 39*, 549–559.

Resnick, M. D., Bearman, P. S., Blum, R. W., Bauman, K. E., Harris, K. M., Jones, J., et al. (1997). Protecting adolescents from harm: Findings from the National Longitudinal Study on Adolescent Health. *Journal of the American Medical Association, 278*, 823–832.

Resnick, M. D., Harris, L. J., & Blum, R. W. (1993). The impact of caring and connectedness on adolescent health and well-being. *Journal of Paediatrics & Child Health, 29*, S3–9.

Reynolds, A. J., & Temple, J. A. (2008). Cost-effective early childhood development programs from preschool to third grade. *Annual Review of Clinical Psychology, 4*, 109–139.

Reynolds, A. J., Temple, J. A., Ou, S., Robertson, D. L., Mersky, J. P., Topitzes, J. W., & Niles, M. D. (2007). Effects of a school-based, early childhood intervention on adult health and well-being: A 19-year follow-up of low-income families. *Archives of Pediatric and Adolescent Medicine, 161*, 730–739.

Ringeisen, H., Henderson, K., & Hoagwood, K. (2003). Context matters: Schools and the "research-to-practice gap" in children's mental health. *School Psychology Review, 32*, 153–168.

Roeser, R. W., Eccles, J. S., & Strobel, K. R. (1998). Linking the study of schooling and mental health: Selected issues and empirical illustrations at the level of the individual. *Educational Psychologist, 33*, 153–176.

Rones, M., & Hoagwood, K. (2000). School-based mental health services: A research review. *Clinical Child and Family Psychology Review, 3*, 223–241.

Scales, P., & Leffert, N. (1999). *Developmental assets: A synthesis of scientific research on adolescent development.* Minneapolis, MN: Search Institute.

Schaeffer, C. M., Bruns, E., Weist, M., Stephan, S. H., Goldstein, J., & Simpson, Y. (2005). Overcoming challenges to using evidence-based interventions in schools. *Journal of Youth and Adolescence, 34*, 15–22.

Sedlak, M. W. (1997). The uneasy alliance of mental health services and the schools: An historical perspective. *American Journal of Orthopsychiatry, 67*, 349–362.

Slade, E. P. (2002). Effects of school-based mental health programs on mental health service use by adolescents at school and in the community. *Mental Health Services Research, 4*, 151–166.

Smith, B. H., Molina, B. S. G., Massetti, G. M., Waschbusch, D. A., & Pelham, W. E. (2007). School-wide interventions: The foundation of a public health approach to school-based mental health. In S. Evans, M. Weist, & Serpell, Z. (Eds.), *Advances in school-based mental health interventions: Best practices and program models, vol. II* (pp. 7:1–7:21). Kingston, NJ: Civic Research Institute.

Solomon, D., Battistich, V., Watson, M., Schaps, E., & Lewis, C. (2000). A six-district study of educational change. *Social Psychology of Education, 4*, 3–51.

Strein, W., Hoagwood, K., & Cohn, A. (2003). School psychology: A public health perspective I. Prevention, population, and systems change. *Journal of School Psychology, 41*, 23–38.

Substance Abuse and Mental Health Services Administration. (2005). *Depression among Adolescents: The NSDUH Report.* Rockville, MD: Author.

Sugai, G., & Horner, R. H. (2006). A promising approach for expanding and sustaining the implementation of school-wide positive behavior support. *School Psychology Review, 35*, 245–259.

Summerbell, C. D., Waters, E., Edmunds, L. D., Kelly, S., Brown, T., & Campbell, K. J. (2005). Interventions for preventing obesity in children. *The Cochrane Database of Systematic Reviews, 3*, 1–70.

Taras, H., & Potts-Datema, W. (2005). Obesity and student performance at school. *Journal of School Health, 75*, 291–295.

US Department of Health and Human Services. (1999). *Mental health: A report of the Surgeon General.* Rockville, MD: US Department of Health and Human Services, Substance Abuse and Mental Health Services Administration, Center for Mental Health Services, National Institutes of Health, National Institute of Mental Health.

US Department of Health and Human Services. (2001). *Mental health: Culture, race, and ethnicity – a supplement to mental health: A report of the Surgeon General.* Rockville, MD: US Department of Health and Human Services, Substance Abuse and Mental Health Services Administration, Center for Mental Health Services.

Van Wijen, L. G., Wendel-Vos, G. C., Wammes, B. M., & Bemelmans, W. J. (2009). The impact of school-based prevention of overweight on psychosocial well-being of children. *Obesity Review, 10*(3), 298–312.

Wade, T. J., Mansour, M. E., Guo, J. J., Huentelman, T., Line, K., & Keller, K. N. (2008). Access and utilization patterns of school-based health centers at urban and rural elementary and middle schools. *Public Health Reports, 123*, 739–750.

Wandersman, A. (2003). Community science: Bridging the gap between science and practice with community-centered models. *American Journal of Community Psychology, 31*, 227–242.

Wang, M. C., Haertel, G. D., & Walberg, H. J. (1997). Learning influences. In H. J. Walberg and G. D. Haertel (Eds.), *Psychology and educational practice* (pp. 199–211). Berkley, CA: McCuthan.

Weiss, C. L. A., Cunningham, D. L., Lewis, C. P., & Clark, M. G. (2005). *Enhancing Student Connectedness to Schools.* Baltimore, MD: Center for School Mental Health Analysis and Action, Department of Psychiatry, University of Maryland School of Medicine.

Weist, M. (2001). Toward a public mental health promotion and intervention system for youth. Journal of School Health, 71(3), 101–104.

Weist, M. (2003). Challenges and opportunities in moving toward a public health approach in school mental health. *Journal of School Psychology, 41*, 77–82.

Weist, M. D. (2005). Fulfilling the promise of school-based mental health: Moving toward a public mental health promotion approach. *Journal of Abnormal Psychology, 33*, 735–741.

Weist, M. D., Paternite, C. E., Wheatley-Rowe, D., & Gall, G. (2009). From thought to action in school mental health promotion. *The International Journal of Mental Health Promotion, 11*, 32–41.

Weist, M. D., Goldstein, A., Morris, L., & Bryant, T. (2003). Integrating expanded school mental health programs and school-based health centers. *Psychology in the Schools, 40*, 297–308.

Weist, M. D., Rubin, M., Moore, E., Adelsheim, S., & Wrobel, G. (2007). Mental health screening in schools. *Journal of School Health, 77*, 53–58.

Weist, M. D., Sander, M. A., Lever, N. A., Link, B., Christodulu, K. V., & Rosner, L. E. (2002). Advancing the quality agenda in expanded school mental health. *Emotional and Behavioral Disorders in Youth, 2*, 59–70.

Weist, M.D., Stephan, S., Lever, N., Moore, E., Flaspohler, P., Maras, M., … Cosgrove, T. (2007). Quality and school mental health. In S. Evans, M. Weist, & Z. Serpell (Eds.), *Advances in school-based mental health interventions: Best practices and program models, vol. II* (pp. 4:1–4:19). Kingston, NJ: Civic Research Institute.

Weisz, J. R., Sandler, I. N., Durlak, J. A., & Anton, B. S. (2005). Promoting and protecting youth mental health through evidence-based prevention and treatment. *American Psychologist, 60*, 628–648.

Wells, J., Barlow, J., & Stewart-Brown, S. (2003). A systematic review of universal approaches to mental health promotion in schools. *Health Education, 103*, 197–220.

Werner, E. E., & Smith, R. S. (Eds.). (1992). *Overcoming the odds: High risk children from birth to adulthood*. Ithaca, NY: Cornell University Press.

Whitlock, E. P., Williams, S. B., Gold, R., Smith, P. R., & Shipman, S. A. (2005). Screening and interventions for childhood overweight: A summary of evidence for the US Preventive Services Task Force. *Pediatrics, 116*, e125–e144.

Wilson, D. B., Gottfredson, D. C., & Najaka, S. S. (2001). School-based prevention of problem behaviors: A meta-analysis. *Journal of Quantitative Criminology, 17*, 247–272.

World Health Organization. (2003). *Caring for children and adolescents with mental health disorders: Setting WHO directions*. Geneva, Switzerland: Author.

Yetter, G. (2009). Exercise-based school obesity prevention programs: An overview. *Psychology in the Schools, 46*, 739–747.

Zigler, E., & Finn-Stevenson, M. (2007). From research to policy and practice: The school of the 21st century. *American Journal of Orthopsychiatry, 77*, 175–81.

Zins, J. E., Bloodworth, M. R., Weissberg, R. P., & Walhberg, H. J. (2004). The scientific base linking social and emotional learning to school success. In J. Zins, R. Weissberg, M. Wang, & H. L. Walberg (Eds.), *Building academic success on social and emotional learning: What does the research say?* (pp. 3–22). NY: Teachers College Press.

Zins, J. E., & Elias, M. E. (2006). Social and emotional learning. In G. G. Bear & K. M. Minke (Eds.), *Children's needs III: Development, prevention, and intervention* (pp. 1–13). Bethesda, MD: National Association of School Psychologists.

14 Healthy aging and mental health

A public health challenge for the 21st century

Marianne C. Fahs, William Cabin, and William T. Gallo

Introduction

Population aging is a major trend shaping the 21st century. Due in large part to public health effectiveness in infectious disease surveillance and control, an unparalleled increase in life expectancy ranks among the greatest achievements of the 20th century. Between 1900 and 2000 in the United States (US), life expectancy improved by almost 60%, increasing from 49 to 77 years (Arias, 2002). This extraordinary public health achievement now presents unprecedented challenges for public health policy in the 21st century.

During the first half of the 21st century, this increased life expectancy will be accompanied by exponential growth in the population of older adults (see Figure 14.1). In the US, the first "baby boomers" turn 65 years

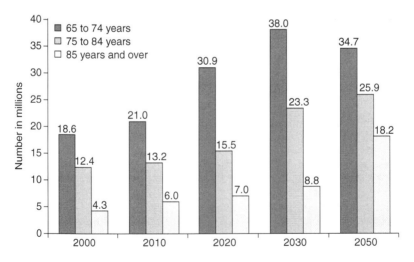

Figure 14.1 Projected growth of older population by age cohort: 2000 to 2050 (source: U.S. Bureau of the Census. (2000). Population projections of the United States by age, sex, race and Hispanic origin: 1995–2050, Current Population Reports, P25–1130).

old in 2011, soon to be followed by 76 million others, doubling the size of the older population by 2030 (US Census Bureau, 2008). Between 2010 and 2050, the US population of older adults, persons aged 65 years and over, will increase from 13 to 20% of the total population (US Census Bureau, 2008). Most significantly, the fastest growing population group will be the "oldest old", adults aged 85 years and older. This population group is projected to double from four million in 2000 to 8.8 million in 2030 and to double again to 18.2 million in 2050 (US Census Bureau, 2008).

These trends will influence nearly every aspect of public health policy development in the 21st century. Healthy aging is vital to economic productivity, yet population aging and mental health remain critically important areas for public health to tackle. The complex interaction of biological, clinical, social, economic, and environmental factors affecting healthy aging and mental health for older adults calls for a new translational public health policy framework. Recently, multilevel ecological models have been introduced in the literature both to outline important linkages across the fields of public health and healthy aging and to help guide researchers, policy makers, and practitioners interested in establishing such linkages (Bodenheimer, Wagner, & Grumbach, 2002; Fahs, Viladrich, & Parikh, 2009; Vlahov, Freudenberg, Proietti, Ompad, Quinn, Nandi, & Galea, 2007; Warner, 2000). However, absent from the literature to date is a comprehensive conceptual model integrating aging, mental health, and public health. While the specification of such a model is beyond the scope of this chapter, a public health framework for developing one is presented. We hope that by using this framework as a roadmap, researchers and policy makers interested in bridging the disciplinary divides among aging, mental health, and public health can contribute to further advances in the development of a comprehensive public health approach to healthy aging.

In the first section of the chapter, we review the prevalence and burden of mental illness and chronic mental health conditions among older adults. We focus in particular on Alzheimer's disease and late-life depression, as these age-related disorders are of enormous and increasing public health significance. We also discuss related mental health issues for caregivers of older adults with Alzheimer's disease and address the exceptional impact of chronic disease co-morbidity on depression for older adults, underscoring an urgent need for a new comprehensive public health approach that bridges mental and physical health. Finally, we present a preliminary framework for a public health/mental health model, summarizing the complex set of factors that influence healthy aging. Building on prior conceptual models, the framework illustrates important population-based components of a comprehensive public health approach to addressing the simultaneous physical and mental health challenges and opportunities for older adults in the 21st century.

The burden of mental illness and cognitive decline among older adults

The estimated prevalence of mental illness among older adults is 20% (US Department of Health and Human Services (DHHS), 1999; 2000). Yet despite the disproportionate prevalence compared with younger populations, older Americans' mental illnesses are less commonly recognized, diagnosed, and treated than those of younger patients (United States Department of Health and Human Services [US DHHS], 1999). Mental illness conditions among older adults reflect the same range of mental disorders found among younger populations, including early-onset conditions (i.e., schizophrenia and recurrent major affective disorders), which continue into old age (Brenes, Guralnik, Williamson, Fried, Simpson, Simonsick, & Penninx, 2005; Kessler, Berglund, Demler, Jin, Merikangas, & Walters, 2005). Affective disorders may have special relevance for older adults. The National Comorbidity Survey Replication (NCS-R) found 7% of adults aged 65 and older meet criteria for experiencing an anxiety disorder within a 12-month span (Kessler et al., 2005), and Depp, Woodruff-Borden, Meeks, Gretarsdottir, and DeKryger (2005) found 26.2% of adults aged 60 to 95 report experiencing at least one panic attack in the past year, with the average number of attacks in the previous year being 3.23. Grenier, Preville, Boyer, and O'Connor (2009) found a 12-month prevalence rate of 1.5% among adults aged 65 years and older for obsessive-compulsive disorder.

Chronic mental illness among the older adult population is substantially augmented by later-onset conditions – cognitive impairment and depression. Thus, the next sections focus on these two conditions in more detail. Nonetheless, it is important to emphasize that age-related depression and dementia, the two conditions that most significantly affect the mental health of older adults, are not a normal part of aging (Centers for Disease Control and Prevention [CDC], 2007).

Cognitive impairment and Alzheimer's disease

Cognitive impairment can be mild, moderate, or severe. Mild cognitive impairment – cognitive impairment without dementia – may affect 16 to 25% of older adults (Graham, Rockwood, Beattie, Eastwood, Gauthier, Tuokko, & McDowell, 1997; Lopez, Jagust, DeKosky, Becker, Fitzpatrick, & Dulberg, 2003; Unverzagt, Gao, Baiyewu, Ogunniyi, Gureje, & Perkins, 2001). More severe cognitive impairment is associated with various dementias, such as vascular dementia and Alzheimer's disease. According to a recent survey reported by the CDC, adults are more than twice as likely to fear losing their mental capacity (62%) as their physical ability (29%) (Research!America, 2006). In 2000, between three and seven million persons experienced various types of dementia (Sloane, Zimmerman, Suchindran,

Reed, Wang, Boustani, & Sudha, 2002), and Alzheimer's disease is now ranked the 8th leading cause of death (Heron & Smith, 2007).

Without scientific advances to alter the incidence and progression of cognitive disorders such as Alzheimer's disease, the aging of the US population will be accompanied by a dramatic rise in the prevalence of dementia, reaching epidemic proportions. Prevalence rates for Alzheimer's disease increase sharply with age, approximately doubling with each decade of later life. Population-based estimates range from three to 11% for persons over age 65 years and 10 to 20% for persons over 75 years (Boustani, Baker, Campbell, Munger, Hui, & Castelluccio, 2003), reaching an astonishing 42% among those aged 85 years or older (Hebert, Scherr, Bienias, Bennett, & Evans, 2003). With the oldest old expected to increase from 29.5% of all older people in the US in 2010 to 35.5% in 2050, 16 million people are predicted to have Alzheimer's disease by the year 2050 (Hebert et al., 2003; Kinsella & He, 2009).

Alzheimer's disease and other dementias cause an extremely high burden of suffering. According to the Global Burden of Disease estimates for the 2003 World Health Report, Alzheimer's disease contributed to 11% of total years lived with disability in people aged 60 years and older – more than cancer, stroke, and cardiovascular disease (Ferri, Prince, Brayne, Brodaty, Fratiglioni, & Ganguli, 2005). Cognitive problems include memory impairment, aphasia (limitation in ability to speak or comprehend language), apraxia (a voluntary movement disorder), disorientation, visual-spatial dysfunction, and impaired judgment. Behavioral problems include personality changes, irritability, anxiety, depression, delusions, hallucinations, aggression, and wandering (Small, Rabins, Barry, Buckholtz, DeKosky, & Ferris, 1997). Functional problems include difficulty performing or an inability to perform activities of daily living, such as eating, dressing, bathing, toileting, walking, grooming, and getting in/out of bed, or instrumental activities of daily living, such as meal preparation, shopping, moving within and outside the house, money management, using the telephone or computer, and taking medication (Dunkle, Roberts, & Haug, 2001). In addition to cognitive and functional deterioration, Alzheimer's disease is associated with a host of related problems, including behavioral and psychological complications, increased risks for falls, higher rates of motor vehicle accidents, complicated clinical management of comorbid conditions, and infections (Boustani et al., 2003; Schubert, Boustani, Callahan, Perkins, Carney, & Fox, 2006; Schubert, Boustani, Callahan, Perkins, Hui, & Hendrie, 2008).

Over the past several decades, numerous studies have identified cognitive impairment in general, and Alzheimer's disease in particular, as independent risk factors for high acute care utilization, including frequent emergency room visits, greater probability of hospitalization, more frequent 30-day rehospitalizations, and longer hospital stays (Boustani, Baker, Campbell, Munger, Hui, et al., 2010; Boustani, Schubert, & Sennour, 2007; Bynum, Rabins, Weller, Niefeld, Anderson, & Wu, 2004;

Hill, Futterman, Mastey, & Fillit, 2002; Phelan, Borson, Grothaus, Balch, & Larson, 2009; Schubert et al., 2008). The majority of dementia patients and their families are cared for in primary care clinics (Borson, Scanlan, Watanabe, Tu, & Lessig, 2006; Boustani, Sachs, & Callahan, 2007; Callahan, Weiner, & Counsell, 2008; Ganguli, Rodriguez, Mulsant, Richards, Pandav, Bilt, et al., 2004; Sachs, Shega, & Cox-Hayley, 2004). In the primary care setting, between 10 and 20% of patients aged 75 and older are estimated to have dementia (Boustani, Callahan, Unverzagt, Austrom, Perkins, Fultz, et al., 2005; Boustani, Peterson, Hanson, Harris, Lohr, & US Preventive Services Task Force, 2003; Holsinger, Deveau, Boustani, & Williams, 2007). Furthermore, on average, these patients have 2.4 chronic conditions and receive 5.1 medications (Bynum et al., 2004; Chodosh, Mittman, Connor, Vassar, Lee, DeMonte, et al., 2007; Schubert et al., 2006; Schubert et al., 2008). Medicare beneficiaries with Alzheimer's disease cost Medicare three times more than other older beneficiaries and account for 34% of Medicare spending, even though they constitute only 13% of the beneficiaries aged 65 and older (Bynum et al., 2004). By 2050, actuarial forecasts predict Medicare will be spending over $1 trillion on beneficiaries with this syndrome (Lewin Group, 2004).

There is at present no effective treatment for Alzheimer's disease. Recent microbiologic research posits an association between certain infectious agents and Alzheimer's (Honjo, van Reekum, & Verhoeff, 2009), and these preliminary findings suggest interventions against chronic infection may delay or even prevent the future development of Alzheimer's, at least in some cases. However, currently available pharmacological interventions for dementia are limited in their clinical impact on the syndrome progression, and there are no approved preventive methods (Boustani et al., 2003; Jedrziewski, Lee, & Trojanowski, 2005; Raina, Santaguida, Ismaila, Patterson, Cowan, Levine, et al., 2008; Saddichha & Pandey, 2008).

Effective community-based supportive programs can reduce the potentially tremendous negative impact of Alzheimer's, presenting some cause for optimism about improvements in the management of the disease. There are numerous psychosocial and non-pharmacological interventions, which target both patients and family caregivers, that are capable of meaningfully reducing the burden and healthcare utilization consequences of dementia-related symptoms (Bates, Boote, & Beverley, 2004; Boustani et al., 2003; Kong, Evans, & Guevara, 2009; Livingston, Johnston, Katona, Paton, & Lyketsos, 2005; Saddichha & Pandey, 2008; Spijker, Vernooij-Dassen, Vasse, Adang, Wollersheim, Grol, & Verhey, 2008). The efficacy of collaborative care management programs has been documented (Callahan, Boustani, Unverzagt, Austrom, Damush, & Perkins, 2006; Vickrey, Mittman, Connor, Pearson, Della Penna, Ganiats, et al., 2006), and is reviewed in the next subsection on caregivers.

Decreasing the impending burden of Alzheimer's disease and other dementia disorders will require substantial efforts and investment at a public health level. First and foremost, effective management requires early recognition of dementia, and recently there has been an increased interest in routine screening for cognitive impairment. However, dementia remains underdiagnosed among primary care patients, and quality of care for dementia remains low, with less than one-third of dementia patients receiving recommended dementia care (Chodosh et al., 2007). Moreover, studies suggest only 20 to 34% of dementia cases are recognized by a routine history and physical examination (Borson et al., 2006; Boustani et al., 2003; Boustani et al., 2005), and unfortunately, the majority of the unrecognized cases have significant levels of cognitive, behavioral, and functional disability (Boustani et al., 2005; Callahan et al., 2006; Schubert et al., 2008). Barriers to quality care include the failure to recognize and respond to symptoms of dementia, time constraints, provider ageism, stigma, and negative attitudes toward the importance of making a diagnosis (Boise, Camicioli, Morgan, Rose, & Congleton, 1999; Boustani et al., 2005; Boustani et al., 2007; Chodosh, Seeman, Keeler, Sewall, Hirsch, Guralnik, & Reuben, 2004; Chodosh, Berry, Lee, Connor, DeMonte, Ganiats, et al., 2006; Harris, Chodosh, Vassar, Vickrey, & Shapiro, 2009; Iliffe & Manthorpe, 2004; Iliffe, Wilcock, & Hayworth, 2006; Ostbye, Yarnall, Krause, Pollak, Gradison, & Michener, 2005).

While diagnosis and specialist referral are necessary and important first steps, they do not necessarily address or represent the scope, process, or goals of dementia management. Primary care currently has no system in place to facilitate successful connections to community resources that can aid in education and complex management required for patients with dementia (Boustani et al., 2005; Boustani et al., 2007; Chodosh et al., 2007; Iliffe & Manthorpe, 2004; Iliffe et al., 2006). A community-based public health approach involving primary and specialty care, as well as patients, families, and social service resources, is required.

Caregivers

The impact of dementia on acute care utilization extends to informal caregivers who support and provide care for patients with dementia (Schubert et al., 2008). For caregivers, the burden of coping with the cognitive, behavioral, and functional symptoms of Alzheimer's disease is enormous. The number of caregivers in the US was estimated to be 44.4 million in 2003 (National Alliance for Caregiving, 2004); this number is expected to rise dramatically with the aging of the population (CDC, 2007). Unpaid, informal care provided by families accounts for a large proportion of the economic costs of treating Alzheimer's disease, increasing sharply as the patient's cognitive impairment worsens (Prigerson, 2003). The magnitude of these economic costs is astounding, totaling over $143 billion (Alzheimer's Association, 2010).

The physical and mental costs associated with caregiving are devastating. Caregivers cope with the burden of adjusting to patient changes in diet and exercise, ability to drive, loss of personal identity, sleep disturbance, inclination to engage in sex or intimacy, urinary incontinence, and restlessness (Small, Rabins, Barry, Buckholtz, DeKosky, Ferris, et al., 1997). Often, the result is increased stress, depression, substance abuse, loss of sleep, increased personal isolation, identity loss, increased physical and mental health problems, and a perceived decline in quality of life (Eisdorfer, Czaja, Loewenstein, Rubert, Argüelles, Mitrani, & Szapocznik, 2003; Levine, 2000; Sadik & Wilcock, 2003; Sands, Ferreira, Stewart, Brod, & Yaffe, 2004; Schulz et al., 2003; Wisniewski et al., 2003). In one study, nearly 43% of the family members providing care to relatives with Alzheimer's disease manifested clinically significant levels of depression during the last few months of the patient's life (Schulz et al., 2003b). There is extensive literature on successful evidence-based interventions that limit the adverse physical and mental health impacts of caregiver and care recipient burden, particularly Alzheimer's disease and dementia more generally. These studies validate the interaction of individual-level characteristics, neighborhood-level characteristics, and community linkages, implying the need for a public health framework to elucidate and understand the context within which interventions can more effectively prevent, diagnose, and treat these age-related mental health conditions and their consequences.

The nearly decade-long, federally-funded, multi-site *Resources for Enhancing Alzheimer's Caregiver Health* (REACH) project, Phase I, tested five interventions, finding "a rich array of effective intervention strategies that can be used to enhance different outcomes for caregivers of persons with dementia" (Schulz et al., 2003b, p. 518). These interventions included individual information and support strategies, group support and family systems therapy, psycho-educational and skill-based training approaches, home-based environmental interventions, and enhanced technology support systems. Results of these interventions included decreased patient and caregiver depression and sense of social isolation, improved relationships and patient self identity, and improved in-home patient mobility (Burgio, Stevens, Guy, Roth, & Haley, 2003; Gallagher-Thompson, Coon, Solano, Ambler, Rabinowitz, & Thompson, 2003; Gitlin, Winter, Corcoran, Dennis, Schinfeld, & Hauck, 2003; Mahoney, Turlow, & Jones, 2003; Schulz et al., 2003; Wisniewski, Belle, Marcus, Burgio, Coon, Ory, et al., 2003).

Gitlin (2003) and Gitlin et al. (2003) conducted multiple REACH I studies, demonstrating that in-home environmental assessments, skills-building training, and home modifications increase patient mobility, decrease caregiver and patient stress, and improve both caregiver and patient quality of life. The results included improved activities of daily living capability and reduced risks of falls and related injuries. Over the course of 17 years at the New York University Medical Center, Mittelman (2002, 2004) and Mittelman, Ferris, Steinberg, Shulman, Mackell, Ambinder, and Cohen, (1993); Mittelman, Ferris, Shulman, Steinberg,

Ambinder, Mackell, and Cohen (1995); Mittelman, Ferris, Shulman, Steinberg, and Levin (1996); Mittelman, Epstein, and Pierzchala (2003); Mittelman, Roth, Coon, and Haley (2004a); and Mittelman, Roth, Haley, and Zarit (2004b) conducted studies of support and counseling intervention programs with Alzheimer's patients residing at home and their caregivers. Most of their studies used randomly-assigned control and treatment groups. Overall, their "results have been consistently positive with reduced [caregiver] depression and burden and increased time to institutionalization of the care recipient" (Zarit & Femia, 2008, p. 51). Furthermore, Mittelman and colleagues' research is considered so effective that SAMHSA has listed the intervention on the National Registry of Evidence-based Programs and Practices (National Registry of Evidence-based Programs and Practice [NREPP], 2010).

Depression

Depression among older adults in the US is a significant problem, though there is wide variation in estimates and types of depression. According to the American Association of Geriatric Psychiatry (American Association of Geriatric Psychiatry [AAGP], 2006), the overall prevalence of late-life depression is between 15 and 30% of community-dwelling older persons, who represent about 90% of the older population (Administration on Aging, 2009). Among this group, 8 to 20% face minor depression, while another 2.1% have dysthymia, a less severe type of depression (Hooyman & Kiyak, 2005). For more severe depression, conservative estimates are that 1 to 5% of all community-dwelling older adults endure clinically-defined major depression, with the rate rising to seven to 36% among older medical outpatients, 11.5 to 40% among hospitalized older adults, up to 50% in long-term care facilities, and 13.5 to 27.5% of older adults receiving home health care (Bruce, McAvay, Raue, Brown, Meyers, Keohane, et al., 2002; Gellis, McGinty, Tierney, Jordan, Burton, Misener, & Bruce, 2005; Gellis & Kim, 2004; Hybels & Blazer, 2003; National Institute of Mental Health [NIMH], 2009; Sirey, Bruce, Carpenter, Booker, Reid, Newell, & Alexopoulos, 2008). Estimates of the prevalence of depression among older adults are considered conservative because late-life depression often goes undetected or is undertreated (Gellis, 2006; Sirey et al., 2008; Wang, Lane, Olfson, Pincus, Wells, & Kessler, 2005).

Factors associated with late-life depression include female gender (Andreescu, Chang, Mulsant, & Ganguli, 2007; Heo et al., 2008), functional disability (Andreescu et al., 2007; Bryant, Jackson, & Ames, 2009; Lenze, Munin, Skidmore, Dew, Rogers, Whyte, et al., 2007), persistent insomnia (Bluestein, Rutledge, & Healey, 2010; Kim, Stewart, Kim, Yang, Shin, & Yoon, 2009; Perlis, Smith, Lyness, Matteson, Pigeon, Jungquist, & Tu, 2006), loneliness (Cacioppo, Hughes, Waite, Hawkley, & Thisted, 2006), and vascular conditions (Mast, Miles, Penninx, Yaffe, Rosano,

Satterfield, et al., 2008). Depression is a major contributor to functional decline, disability, perceptions of poor health, diminished productivity, and mortality (Birrer & Vemuri, 2004; Stuck, Walthert, Nikolaus, Büla, Hohmann, & Beck, 1999). In addition, depression among older persons is associated with increases in nursing home placement, burden on caregivers, inappropriate utilization of medical services, and increased health care costs (Andreescu et al., 2007; Charney, Nemeroff, Lewis, Laden, Gorman, Laska, et al., 2002; Katon, Bush, & Ormal, 1992; Unützer, Patrick, Simon, Grembowski, Walker, Rutter, & Katon, 1997; Wells, Rogers, Burnam, Greenfield, & Ware, 1991). As in younger populations, suicide is associated with depression among older adults (Holland, Schutte, Brennan, & Moos, 2010; Liu & Chiu, 2009; Pfaff & Almeida, 2005; Sirey et al., 2008). From 2001 to 2005 the rate of suicide for all older adults was 14.8 per 100,000, nearly 50% higher than the rate for the general population, with older men being more likely to complete a suicidal attempt than older women (Dombrovski, Szanto, Duberstein, Conner, Houck, & Conwell, 2008).

Depression often co-occurs with medical illness, increasing the complexity of health care treatment and management. Depressive disorders have been associated with multiple chronic conditions, including asthma, arthritis, cardiovascular disease, cancer, diabetes, obesity, and myocardial infarction (Chapman, Perry, & Strine, 2005; Sharp & Lipsky, 2002; Wells et al., 1991). This association is particularly significant in the older adult population. According to the CDC, 80% of older adults have at least one chronic condition, and 50% have at least two (CDC, 2010), which simultaneously complicates chronic disease management and treatment of both major and minor depression. The proportion of geriatric primary care patients who have some type of clinically or symptom-assessed depression may be as high as 37% (Garrard, Rolnick, Nitz, Luepke, Jackson, Fischer, et al., 1998; Glasser & Gravdal, 1997). Among the almost 2.5 million hospitalizations in the US with depression as a secondary diagnosis, older adults are disproportionately represented, accounting for almost 40% (Russo, Hambrick, & Owens, 2007).

The relationship between chronic disease and depression is a reciprocal one; that is, chronic disease increases the risk of depression, and likewise, depression increases the risks associated with chronic disease. Older persons who suffer from depression have worse outcomes for hip fractures, heart attacks, or cancer than those who do not. In unpublished research, frequent chronic conditions endured by older adults, but less commonly recognized in the public health literature than in the geriatric literature, appear to be associated with depression (Cabin & Fahs, 2010). These conditions include visual impairment, falls, lack of physical activity, hearing loss, arthritis/rheumatoid arthritis, and functional disability. Furthermore, ample evidence suggests that mental illness adversely impacts the effectiveness and cost-effectiveness of community-based public health initiatives, such as diabetes self-management initiatives. Depression has a negative impact on glycemic control, increasing the risk of diabetic complications (e.g., peripheral neuropathy, retinopathy, nephropathy, macrovascular complications, and sexual dysfunction), and the complexity of diabetic care (de Groot, Anderson, Freedland, Clouse, & Lustman, 2001). As a result, co-morbid depression with diabetes increases health care use and expenditures (Thomson, Rankin, Ashcroft, Yates, McQueen, & Cummings, 1982). Unless immediate action is taken, the aging of the population will increase the overall prevalence of Americans experiencing mental illness, taxing already scarce health and mental health resources (Compton, Conway, Stinson, & Grant, 2006; Heo, Murphy, Fontaine, Bruce, & Alexopoulos, 2008). Therefore, the comorbidy of mental illness and chronic disease among older persons is an issue of pressing concern for public health.

Primary care providers remain the principal physicians for older Americans. To reduce the risk of depression among older adults, primary care providers must recognize and treat depression. Currently, the ability of such providers to recognize and properly identify mental disorders is low (United States Public Health Service [USPHS], 1999). In one study of primary care physicians, only 55% felt confident diagnosing depression. Still fewer (35%) were at ease prescribing antidepressants to older people (Callahan, Nienaber, Hendrie, & Tierney, 1992).

However, training in depression for primary care providers leads to increased detection of depression in older adults (McCabe, Russo, Mellor, Davison, & George, 2008), and the Patient Health Questionnaire 2 (PHQ-2) has been shown to be a valid initial screening tool for major depression in older people (Li, Friedman, Conwell, & Fiscella, 2007). Long and short forms of the Geriatric Depression Scale (GDS) may also used to screen older adults at risk for depression (Pedraza, Dotson, Willis, Graff-Radford, & Lucas, 2009) and suicide (Heisel, Duberstein, Lyness, & Feldman, 2010).

Given the significant negative consequences of depression for both older adults and for society, accurate measurement of depressive symptoms among older adults is vital (Chapman & Perry, 2008). However, population-based research suggests that only 10% of depressed older adults obtain formal evaluation or treatment (Weisman, Bruce, Leaf, Florio, & Holzer, 1991). It is well known that primary care screening for depression has no significant effect on patient outcomes unless it is linked to effective, coordinated care management protocols (US Preventive Services Task Force, 2009). Several effective treatment options are available for the treatment of late-life depression, including antidepressant medications and psychotherapy (Frazer, Christensen, & Griffiths, 2005; Pinquart, Duberstein, & Lyness, 2006; Snowden, Steinman, & Frederick, 2008). While antidepressants are most commonly used to treat depression in primary care settings, research suggests that depressed older primary care patients may prefer counseling (57%) to medication (43%), with preferences differing by gender. Men are more likely to prefer medication; women are more likely to prefer counseling (Gum et al., 2006). Lin, Campbell, Chaney, Liu, Heagerty, Felker, and Hedrick (2005) concluded that linking individuals to their preferred treatment type has a positive impact on depression treatment outcome.

However, there are several perceived barriers that deter the utilization of mental health care among older adults, including cost, transportation, mobility, and insurance (Ojeda & McGuire, 2006; Weinberger, Mateo, & Sirey, 2009). Moreover, older adults are likely to attribute the development of depression to medical illness, financial trouble, or a recent loss. Perceived stigma toward individuals with mental illness is also a barrier, and may influence early treatment discontinuation among older patients with major depression (Sirey, Bruce, Alexopoulos, Perlick, Raue, Friedman, & Meyers 2001). Nevertheless, public health campaigns can change social norms and reduce health risks (Freudenberg, Brantley, & Serrano, 2009; Shelley, Fahs, Yerneni, Das, Nguyen, Hung, et al., 2008), and a major public health campaign is needed to reduce age-related stigmatization, as was recently recommended by the CDC (2008). Finally, despite the fact that effective models exist for the treatment of depression, such as Psychogeriatric Assessment and Treatment in City Housing (PATCH), and Improving Mood: Promoting Access to Collaborative Treatment for Late Life Depression (IMPACT) (Chapman & Perry, 2008; Katz & Coyne, 2000), the current system of primary care does not provide the reimbursement incentives or the tools to facilitate appropriate diagnosis and evaluation. The lack thereof imposes a significant barrier to appropriate mental health care for both patients and health care providers.

Toward a conceptual framework

A public health model that specifically addresses the mental health of older adults is necessary if we are to systematically address the challenges posed to our society by an aging population (Katz & Coyne, 2000). The purpose of this section is to synthesize the emerging body of theoretical and empirical research into an integrated conceptual framework for a public health model of mental health among older adults. A number of the studies reviewed in the previous sections signal a trend toward the integration of essential co-occurring factors in models of mental health; nevertheless, prior research has not fully assimilated the interaction of older persons' individual, neighborhood-level, and system-level characteristics. Therefore, as the literature increasingly suggests that this interaction defines the risk of and protection from mental health conditions, the proposed framework offers a means to consider links between these various domains. Extending the structure of existing models (Auchincloss & Diez-Roux, 2008; Fahs et al., 2009; Kim, 2008; Mair, Diez-Roux, & Galea, 2008; World Health

Organization [WHO], 2007), we present a multidirectional, multilevel framework that can both guide empirical investigation and motivate program and practice innovation, each of which is critical to supporting the well-being of older adults in the community.

Our model is particularly influenced by a conceptual framework recently advanced by the WHO. The WHO model seeks to encourage active aging by "optimizing opportunities for health, participation and security in order to enhance quality of life as people age" so as to "tap the potential that older people represent for humanity" (WHO, 2007, p. 1). With data gathered from focus groups in 33 cities around the world, the WHO project defined eight community-level characteristics of particular concern to older people: outdoor spaces and buildings, transportation, housing, social participation, respect and social inclusion, civic participation and employment, communication and information, and community support and health services. Although the WHO project specifically focuses on urban communities, it provides a useful checklist of core "age-friendly" features in each of the eight areas and can thus serve as a more general blueprint for the development of specific public health policy goals for older adults' mental health.

In the following sections, we first introduce our model, which elucidates elements of the domains in some detail. Second, we review existing studies of mental health at the contextual/neighborhood, individual, and health-system levels, giving detailed attention to interrelations of key mental health determinants within and across model domains. Neighborhood research is a rather nascent field, and investigations of the association between neighborhood factors and mental health are therefore rare in their application to older individuals. For this reason, we provide a broad base of evidence for neighborhood determinants, while maintaining a focus on studies of mental health and older adults.

The conceptual model

Our conceptual model, presented in Figure 14.2 below, builds on fundamental cause theory, wherein individually-based risk factors are contextualized to examine "what puts people at risk of risks" (Link & Phelan, 1995). The model posits that determinants of mental health among older adults are broad-based and multilevel. The major structural components, or domains, of the model are public and private policies, neighborhoods, individuals, and mental health care delivery models. Public and private policies form the structure for mental health, within which neighborhood and individual characteristics interact with mental health care delivery features to influence mental health outcomes among older adults. For example, national and local public policies, such as Medicare and Medicaid eligibility for mental health care, housing conditions, options for long-term care, and access to transportation, interact with the social and physical

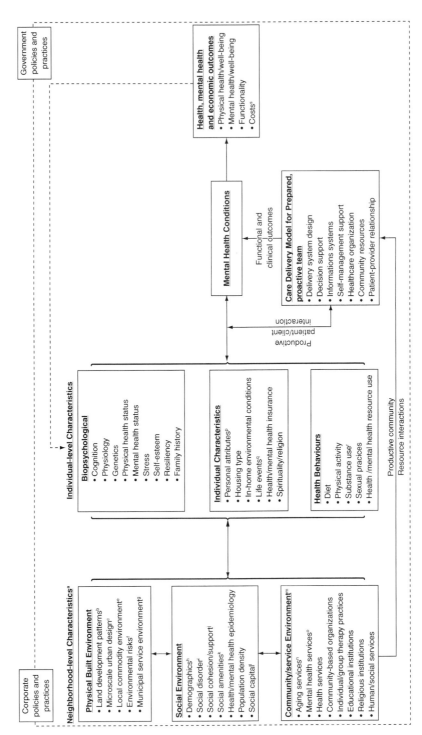

Figure 14.2 Conceptual framework for public health, mental health, and older adults

Notes

a Neighborhood characteristics, definitions and measures will vary.

b Land development patterns include land-use mix, residential density, housing (type and condition), green layer space, and educational facilities.

c Micro-scale urban design includes street connectivity, sidewalks, walking, infrastructure, walkability, bike lanes, pedestrian safety, and street lights.

d Transportation includes motor vehicles, public transportation such as buses and subways, taxis, and private vehicle services.

e Local commodity environment includes distribution of, types of, and access to commercial and retail establishments, including food, alcohol, and tobacco outlets.

f Environmental risks include air, water, and ground pollution, distribution of risk producing facilities/plants, and noise levels.

g Municipal services environment includes police, fire, and sanitation (public and private) facilities.

h Demographics include distribution of age, gender, education level, income level, homelessness, and employment.

i Social disorder includes crime rate, juvenile delinquency, graffiti, violence, and drug use.

j Social cohesion includes social networks and social support.

k Social amenities include libraries, museums, parks and other recreational facilities.

l Social capital includes voting participation and other measures of civic engagement.

m Community/service environment includes private and public entities.

n Aging services include senior centers, adult day care services, and other services by local area agencies on aging and community-based organizations serving older adults.

o Mental health services include inpatient, outpatient, and community-based.

p Personal attributes include age, gender, income level, education level, marital status, sexual orientation, family size, ethnicity/race, employment status, and immigration status.

q Life events include adverse childhood experiences, caregiver burden, care recipient burden, loss/grief/bereavement (i.e., death, major injury), and divorce/ separation.

r Substance abuse includes drugs, alcohol, and tobacco use.

s Costs include both direct and indirect costs, including productivity.

characteristics of neighborhoods, such as food availability, living conditions and public parks, as well as with the availability of quality and accessible mental health care programs and services, to influence mental health outcomes, which are influenced at the individual level by social, psychological and biologic characteristics.

Thus, the conceptual framework posits that within these domains, specific elements, identified in the footnotes to Figure 14.2, are the key factors shaping a multilayered complexity of interactions. These interactions in turn influence individual pathways to mental health, suggesting societal interventions could be more effective than individual interventions in producing substantial mental health benefits. The following sections elucidate interactions among these domains and elements, as presented thus far in the literature.

Neighborhood-level characteristics

A substantial body of literature has recently emerged exploring individual-level and neighborhood-level effects on mental health across all age groups (Henderson, Diez-Roux, Jacobs, Kiefe, West, & Williams, 2005; Truong & Ma, 2006; Kim, 2008; Mair et al., 2008). The literature supports a significant role for neighborhood-level and individual-level interactions on mental health. These findings are further supported by recent studies addressing mental health and depression among older adults in particular (Beard, Tracy, Vlahov, & Galea, 2008; Beard, Cerda, Blaney, Ahern, Vlahov, & Galea, 2009).

Physical/built environment

The importance of the physical/built environment – which includes land development patterns, micro-scale urban design, transportation, municipal service environment, local commodity environment, and environmental risks – to healthy aging has been highlighted in numerous studies, several of which have documented an association between elements of the built environment and mental health. Features such as neighborhood noise levels (environmental risk) and the convenience of shopping establishments (local commodity environment) have been linked both to the likelihood and levels of depressive symptoms (Evans, 2003; Galea, Ahern, & Karpati, 2005). Related studies have demonstrated that elements of the physical environment may adversely affect willingness to leave home, which affects the propensity to socialize; to access food, health, and mental health services; and to be physically active (Dannenburg et al., 2003; Evans, 2003; Frank, Engelke, & Schmid, 2003; Frumkin, Frank, & Jackson, 2004; Jackson, 2003; Northridge, Sclar, & Biswas, 2003). All may have adverse consequences for mental health. One assessment suggested that the effect of neighborhood deterioration on depressive symptoms and emotional stress is mediated through perceptions of crime and reduced social contact and social capital (Kruger, Reischl, & Gee, 2007).

The potential risks and benefits of the neighborhood on the mental health may be more concentrated for older persons because they spend more time in neighborhoods than do younger individuals, whose employment often necessitates leaving their residential communities for a substantial proportion of the week. Several investigations have exclusively studied older persons' mental health in relation to the physical environment. Two studies have assessed micro-scale urban design elements; one found a protective effect of neighborhood walkability on depressive symptoms among men over age 65 (Berke, Gottlieb, Moudon, & Larson, 2007), while the other reported that perceived environmental dissatisfaction and transportation limitations are associated with greater depressive symptoms among Alabamians over age 55, especially the for low-income individuals (LaGory & Fitpatrick, 1992). Research on Hispanic elders in Florida (Brown, Mason, Lombard, Martinez, Plater-Zyberk, Spokane, et al., 2009) has suggested that architectural features that promote visibility are associated with higher perceived social support, which reduces psychological distress. Somewhat similar findings were reported by Galea, Ahern, Rudenstine, Wallace, and Vlahov (2005), who indicated a significant adverse impact of residential deficiencies on the probability of recent and lifetime depression.

Social environment

The social environment, broadly defined, appears to be a major predictor of mental health. A good deal of evidence supports the notion that neighborhood socioeconomic status (SES) is an important correlate of individual well-being and mortality. Studies have suggested a relationship between aggregate neighborhood SES and such diverse measures of health as self-rated health, chronic disease, physical functioning, depression, anxiety and mood disorders, life satisfaction, and substance abuse (Lang, Hubbard, Andrew, Llewellyn, Melzer, & Rockwood, 2009; Lynch & Kaplan, 2000; Marmot & Wilkinson, 2001; Murali & Oyebode, 2004; Pearlin, 1999; Schoeni, House, Kaplan, & Pollack, 2008; Seedat, Nyamai, Njenga, Vythilingum, & Stein, 2004; Sundaram, Helweg-Larsen, Laursen, & Bjerregaard, 2004). Evidence on the SES-mental health association is bolstered by a natural experiment involving the relocation of families from public housing in poor neighborhoods to private housing in less poverty-stricken neighborhoods, which found significant decreases in psychological distress (Leventhal & Brooks-Gunn, 2003).

Evidence of mental health effects of SES among older individuals is substantial. In a contextual analysis in New Haven, Connecticut, Kubzansky, Subramanian, Kawachi, Fay, Soobader, and Berkman (2005) found that poorer neighborhoods were associated with greater individual depressive symptoms among older persons, a finding reinforced in work by Ostir,

Eschbach, Markides, and Goodwin (2003) among older Mexican-Americans in Southwestern US. Using longitudinal data on New York City residents over age 50, Beard and colleagues (2009) found that neighborhood affluence was found to be a protective factor against worsening depression. In addition to depression, Yen and Kaplan (1999) reported an association between neighborhood poverty and unhealthy behaviors (i.e., smoking and alcohol consumption), which have been shown to be indicators of mental illness (Dufour, 2010; Kleinschmidt, Hills, & Elliott, 1995; Hill, Ross, & Angel, 2005; Husten, 2010; Reijneveld, 1998). Somewhat anomalous findings are those of Hybels and Blazer (2003) and Wight, Cummings, Karlamangla, and Aneshensel (2009), whose results suggested that among older individuals, census tract-level socioeconomic disadvantage was not associated with depressive symptoms.

Research on neighborhood social components offers a compelling case for contextual determination of emotional well-being. Social disorder, population density, and social cohesion and support have each been linked to mental health outcomes. A longitudinal examination of a convenience sample of 818 participants in an AIDS outreach intervention reported that perceptions of social disorder (e.g., vandalism, litter, vacant housing, crime) were predictive of depressive symptoms at nine-month follow-up (Latkin & Curry, 2003), a finding supported by the results of another local-area follow-up study, which included individuals 65 and older in the Washington, DC, metropolitan area (Bierman, 2009). The Bierman research further suggested a protective effect of household social support, wherein the effect of neighborhood physical and social disorder on subsequent depression and mastery/perceived control is concentrated among the non-married. Research by Kim and Ross (2009) confirmed the buffering effect of individual social support and further isolated neighborhood social cohesion as a moderator in the neighborhood disorder-depression relationship. LaGory and Fitpatrick (1992) likewise found that limited social support exacerbated the built environment effects among older Alabamians described above. Direct effects of neighborhood social support also have been demonstrated. Beard and colleagues (2009) showed that low social support at the neighborhood-level was associated with risk of late-life depression, while research by emphasizes the relevance of social capital as a protective factor for the mental health of older adults. Residential stability, which often proxies social support, also has been inversely associated with depressive symptoms in a national sample (Aneshensel, Wight, Miller-Martinez, Botticello, Karlamangla, & Seeman, 2007). Finally, the distal outcomes of social isolation are dire. Yen and Kaplan (1999) cite multiple studies showing an increased risk of death associated with social isolation among older adults.

The results of studies assessing compositional effects are also intriguing. Neighborhoods with higher density of older individuals (Kubzansky et al., 2005) and Mexican-Americans (Ostir et al., 2003) are associated with lower depressive symptoms. These results suggest that age-related and ethnic clustering may confer a type of social or cultural advantage to residents.

Community/service environment

The community/service environment comprises the number, distribution, and accessibility of private and public community-based and human/social service organizations, including educational, religious, social service, aging, health, and mental health organizations. These neighborhood-level characteristics have not previously been studied in the public health literature except indirectly as related to social cohesion and social capital. Nevertheless, community-based organizations are likely quite important to the mental health of older adults. An integrated public health model should include these organizations as potential resource partners, and further research should be undertaken to advance evidence of their association with mental health.

Bio-psychological characteristics

As noted in previous sections, biological and physiological factors feature prominently in our current understanding of mental illness. Biological, physiological, and psychological factors of relevance include cognition, physiology, genetics, physical health status, mental health status, family history, resiliency, self-esteem, and stress level. The growth of antipsychotic medications, selective serotonin reuptake inhibitors, and serotonin and norepinephine reuptake inhibitors is based on the chemical imbalance hypothesis of mental illness. Evidence supports the relevance of genetics in major mental illnesses, such as schizophrenia and bipolar disorder, and, to a lesser extent, suicide, severe alcoholism, and sociopathy (Kety, 1986; Murrary, Jones, Susser, van Os, & Cannon, 2003; Smith & Susser, 2002; Susser, Hoek, & Brown, 1998).

Also as noted previously, the increased occurrence of comorbid physical and mental health conditions associated with aging is of critical importance to public health (NIMH, 2009; Satariano, 2006). Depression is frequently comorbid with chronic disease, particularly for older adults; medical and psychiatric comorbidities for cardiovascular disease, diabetes mellitus, and geriatric depression are common among older adults (Eaton, 2006).

Demographic characteristics

A consistent body of research demonstrates significant variation in health and mental health by demographic characteristics (US DHHS, 1999; Fiscella & Williams, 2004; Marmot, 2005; Marmot & Wilkinson, 2001;

Williams, Yu, Jackson, & Anderson, 1997). These characteristics include age, gender, race, ethnicity, culture, income, education level, birth location, family size, marital status, sexual orientation, occupation, and employment status (Eaton, 2001; Lynch & Kaplan, 2000; McLeod & Kessler, 1990; Mirowsky & Ross, 2003). Also included, and particularly applicable to older adults, are housing type, caregiver/care recipient status, in-home living environment, spirituality/religiosity, health and mental health insurance; and life events (i.e., adverse childhood experiences; exposure to trauma, loss, grief or bereavement; caregiver or care recipient burden). Little research has systematically examined the relationship of these characteristics to mental health among older adults, with the exception of caregiver stress, and no research to date has investigated mechanisms and underlying causes for socioeconomic variation in mental health. Link and Phelan (1995) hypothesize that intervening risk and protective factors, highly correlated with SES, are the fundamental causes. These are flexible resources people actively use to gain health advantages, including, know-ledge, money, power, prestige, and beneficial social connections. These associations may be particularly important for older adults.

Gender inequality also has been cited as a factor in propensity for mental health issues, with women reporting more psychological distress than men, regardless of class (Kessler & McRae, 1981; Mirowsky & Ross, 2003). There is debate as to whether such reporting is merely a measure-ment artifact, a reflection of differences in gender-based roles (the sex role hypothesis), or a reflection of social and economic advantage, itself pos-sibly linked to roles (Belle & Doucet, 2003; Miranda & Green, 1999; Mirowsky & Ross, 2003). Similarly, ethnicity has been shown to be related to mental health, with ethnicity being reflected through ethnic/race-based roles, socioeconomic factors, and racial discrimination (Berkman, 2009; US DHHS, 1999; Williams, 1986; 2002).

Health behaviors

The health behaviors component of the model reflects individual behav-iors, such as diet, physical activity, substance use, sexual practices, and health and mental health resource use. Ainsworth and Mcera (2010) present extensive literature supporting the association between physical activity and physical and mental health. Balfour and Kaplan (2002) and Prohaska, Belansky, Belza, Buchner, Marshall, McTigue, et al. (2006) con-firmed the linkage between built environment, physical activity, and health among older Americans. Sherrington, Whitney, Lord, Herbert, Cumming, and Close (2008) conducted a meta-analysis confirming the protective effect of physical activity in falls prevention, which is correlated with depression and other mental health issues of older Americans. Further-more, diet and nutrition are associated with mental health (Malas, Tharp, & Foerster, 2010).

Health, mental health, and economic outcomes

The primary health, mental health, and economic outcomes affected by mental health conditions are physical health and well-being, mental health and well-being, functionality (i.e., activities and instrumental activities of daily life), and costs. Fortunately, evidence is accumulating that mental health care and support is effective for older Americans and can reduce costs and improve daily functioning (Borson, McDonald, Gayle, Deffebach, Lakshminarayan, & VanTuinen, 1992; McEvoy & Barnes, 2007; Oslin, Streim, Katz, Edell, & TenHave, 2000; Rabins, Black, Roca, German, McGuire, Robbins, et al., 2000; Schneider, 1995). However, unmet need for mental health services remains high, with as much as 63% of adults aged 65 years and older with a mental disorder experiencing unmet need (Rabins, 1996). Moreover, mental health care accounts for only five percent of the Medicare budget (Mark, McKusick, King, Harwood, & Genuardi, 1998).

Care delivery model for a prepared proactive team

The final aspect of the model represents the diagnostic, preventive, and treatment interventions for mental health conditions that affect health, mental health, and economic outcomes. An effective intervention model to promote and maintain optimal mental health among older adults is one that follows established principals for effective management of long-term chronic care (Wagner, Austin, & Von Korff, 1996; Wagner, Davis, Schaefer, von Korf, & Austin, 2002). This model stresses the importance of collaboration between relevant public health, general medical, and mental health care professionals; the patient; and the patient's family/caregivers. It also includes linkages to community resources. The model calls for decision support for an effective care delivery system through collaboration and practice guidelines, appropriate information technology, and support for patient self-management. This model has been applied successfully among older adults with long-term physical conditions facing depression (McEvoy & Barnes, 2007).

Conclusion

Supporting and promoting optimal mental health among older adults demands increased public health attention as more people join the population group known as "older adults aging in place" in neighborhoods and communities across the nation. However, currently there is a dearth of gerontological theory underpinning public health approaches, and new theoretical developments are needed to expand the boundaries of the field to address social priorities and provide direction for education, policy, and practice. As Achenbaum and Levin (1989) stated in the 50th Anniversary issue of the Gerontologist, "In the face of globalization, US gerontologists need to reach out to disciplines and professions here and abroad with a stake in investigating labor force and health care issues embedded in the political economies and institutions of aging societies" (Achenbaum & Levin, 1989, p. 3).

Preventive gerontology, a field first introduced in the early 1980s, is an example of a discipline within gerontology that could contribute important lessons for public health, mental health, and aging. Significant insights will emerge as the boundaries of preventive gerontology expand to include the vital determinants for healthy aging and the interactions at the confluence of public health and mental health, including the social and physical environment, health care delivery, and mental health care. The conceptual framework presented in this chapter is one approach to elucidating underlying determinants of these relationships. The systematic expansion of gerontology, taking into account these fundamental determinants of health, is a necessary foundation to advance integrated theoretical and policy approaches.

The unprecedented increase in longevity associated with public health innovation in the 20th century has created exciting opportunities for social advancement in the 21st century. To realize these opportunities, we must address the individual, organizational, and societal challenges that have evolved with an aging society. On the cusp of a major demographic shift in the US, it is a propitious time for public health to engage new theoretical and practical approaches to the challenges of mental health promotion in an aging population. It is only through addressing these challenges that the new longevity will be accompanied by the realization of its full potential – not only the achievement of longer life, but improved quality of life for all.

Acknowledgments

The authors thank Maureen Canavan and Porsha Hall for research assistance, Mathew Caron, MS, for graphic design, and Nuzhat Mirza for administrative assistance and manuscript production.

References

Achenbaum, W. A., & Levin, J. S. (1989). What does gerontology mean. *Gerontologist*, 29(3), 393–400.

Administration on Aging. (2009). A profile of older Americans: 2009. Washington, DC: Administration on Aging, US Department of Health and Human Services.

Ainsworth, A. E., & Mcera, C. A. (2010). Physical activity. In P. L. Remington, R. C. Brownson, and M. V. Wegner (Eds.), *Chronic disease epidemiology and control* (pp. 199–228). Washington, DC: American Public Health Association.

Alzheimer's Association. (2010). Alzheimer's Disease Facts and Figures. In Alzheimer's & Dementia (Vol. 6). Chicago, IL: Alzheimer's Association.

American Association for Geriatric Psychiatry. (2006). *Treatment available and effective for late-life depression, according to AAGP*. Retrieved from www.aagoonline.org/news//pressreleases.asp?viewfull=112.

Andreescu, C., Chang, C. H., Mulsant, B. H., & Ganguli, M. (2007). Twelve-year depression symptom trajectories and their predictors in a community sample of older adults. *International Psychogeriatrics, 20*(2), 221–236.

Aneshensel, C. S., Wight, R. G., Miller-Martinez, D., Botticello, A. L., Karlamangla, A. S., & Seeman, T. E. (2007). Urban neighborhoods and depressive symptoms among older adults. *Journal of Gerontology: Social Science, 62B*(1), S52–S59.

Arias, E. (2002). *United States life tables, 2000. In National vital statistics reports* (Vol. 51, no 3). Hyattsville, Maryland: National Center for Health Statistics.

Auchincloss, A. H., & Diez-Roux, A. V. (2008). A new tool for epidemiology: The usefulness of dynamic-agent models in understanding place effects on health. *American Journal of Epidemiology, 168*(1), 1–8.

Balfour, J. L., & Kaplan, G. A. (2002). Neighborhood environment and loss of physical function in older adults: Evidence from the Alameda County Study. *American Journal of Epidemiology, 155*(6), 507–515.

Bates, J., Boote, J., & Beverley, C. (2004). Psychosocial interventions for people with a milder dementing illness: A systematic review. *Journal of Advanced Nursing, 45*(6), 644–658.

Beard, J. R., Cerda, M., Blaney, S., Ahern, J., Vlahov, D., & Galea, S. (2009). Neighborhood characteristics and change in depressive symptoms among older residents of New York City. *American Journal of Public Health, 99*(7), 1308–1314.

Beard, J. R., Tracy, M., Vlahov, D., & Galea, S. (2008). Trajectory and socio-economic predictors of depression in a prospective study of residents of New York City. *Annals of Epidemiology, 18*(3), 235–243.

Belle, D., & Doucet, J. (2003). Poverty, inequality and discrimination as sources of depression among U. S. women. *Psychology of Women Quarterly, 27*, 101–113.

Berke, E. M., Gottlieb, L. M., Moudon, A. V., & Larson, E. B. (2007). Protective association between neighborhood walkability and depression in older men. *Journal of the American Geriatric Society, 55*(4), 526–533.

Berkman, L. F. (2009). Social epidemiology: Social determinants of health in the United States: Are we losing ground? *Annual Review of Public Health, 30*, 27–41.

Bierman, A. (2009). Marital status as contingency for the effects of neighborhood disorder on older adults' mental health. *Journals of Gerontology, Series B: Psychological Sciences and Social Sciences, 64*(3), 425–434.

Birrer, R. B., & Vemuri, S. P. (2004). Depression in later life: A diagnostic and therapeutic challenge. *American Family Physician, 69*(10), 2375–2382.

Bluestein, D., Rutledge, C. M., & Healey, A. C. (2010). Psychosocial correlates of insomnia severity in primary care. *Journal of the American Board of Family Medicine, 23*(2), 204–211.

Bodenheimer, T., Wagner, E., & Grumbach, K. (2002). Improving primary care for patients with chronic illness: The chronic care model. *JAMA*, 288, 1775–1779.

Boise, L., Camicioli, R., Morgan, D. L., Rose, J. H., & Congleton, L. (1999). Diagnosing dementia: Perspectives of primary care physicians. *Gerontologist, 39*(4), 457–464.

Borson, S., McDonald, G. J., Gayle, T., Deffebach, M., Lakshminarayan, S., & VanTuinen, C. (1992). Improvement in mood, physical symptoms, and function with nortriptyline for depression in patients with chronic obstructive pulmonary disease. *Psychosomatics*, *33*(2), 190–201.

Borson, S., Scanlan, J. M., Watanabe, J., Tu, S. P., & Lessig, M. (2006). Improving identification of cognitive impairment in primary care. *International Journal of Geriatric Psychiatry*, *21*(4), 349–355.

Boustani, M., Baker, M. S., Campbell, N., Munger, S., Hui, S. L., Castelluccio, P., et al. (2010). Impact and recognition of cognitive impairment among hospitalized elders. *Journal of Hospital Medicine*, *5*(2), 69–75.

Boustani, M., Callahan, C. M., Unverzagt, F. W., Austrom, M. G., Perkins, A. J., Fultz, B. A., et al. (2005). Implementing a screening and diagnosis program for dementia in primary care. *Journal of General Internal Medicine*, *20*(7), 572–577.

Boustani, M., Peterson, B., Hanson, L., Harris, R., Lohr, K. N., & US Preventive Services Task Force. (2003). Screening for dementia in primary care: A summary of the evidence for the U.S. Preventive Services Task Force. *Annals of Internal Medicine*, *138*(11), 927–937.

Boustani, M., Sachs, G., & Callahan, C. M. (2007). Can primary care meet the biopsychosocial needs of older adults with dementia? *Journal of General Internal Medicine*, *22*(11), 1625–1627.

Boustani, M., Schubert, C., & Sennour, Y. (2007). The challenge of supporting care for dementia in primary care. *Journal of Clinical Interventions in Aging*, *2*, 631–636.

Brenes, G. A., Guralnik, J. M., Williamson, J. D., Fried, L. P., Simpson, C., Simonsick, E. M., & Penninx, B. W. J. H. (2005). The influence of anxiety on the progression of disability. *Journal of the American Geriatric Society*, *53*(1), 34–39.

Brown, S. C., Mason, C. A., Lombard, J. L., Martinez, F., Plater-Zyberk, E., Spokane, A. R., et al. (2009). The relationship of built environment to perceived social support and psychological distress in hispanic elders: The role of "eyes on the street". *Journals of Gerontology: Social Sciences*, *64B*(2), 234–246.

Bruce, M. L., McAvay, G. J., Raue, P. J., Brown, E. L., Meyers, B. S., Keohane, D. J., et al. (2002). Major depression in elderly home health care patients. *American Journal of Psychiatry*, *159*(8), 1367–1374.

Bryant, C., Jackson, H., & Ames, D. (2009). Depression and anxiety in medically unwell older adults: Prevalence and short-term course. *International Psychogeriatrics*, *21*(4), 754–763.

Burgio, L., Stevens, A., Guy, D., Roth, D. L., & Haley, W. E. (2003). Impact of two psychosocial interventions on white and African American family caregivers of individuals with dementia. *Gerontologist*, *43*(4), 568–579.

Bynum, J. P. W., Rabins, P. V., Weller, W. E., Niefeld, M., Anderson, G. F., & Wu, A. (2004).The impact of dementia and chronic illness on Medicare expenditures and hospital use. *Journal of the American Geriatric Society*, *52*,187–194.

Cabin, W., & Fahs, M. (2010). Developing a predictive model for depression among seniors attending senior centers in NYC neighborhoods. Unpublished Manuscript. Brookdale Center for Healthy Aging and Longevity of Hunter College. New York: City University of New York.

Cacioppo, J. T., Hughes, M. E., Waite, L. J., Hawkley, L. C., & Thisted, R. A. (2006). Loneliness as a specific risk factor for depressive symptoms: Cross-sectional and longitudinal analyses. *Psychology of Aging*, *21*(1), 140–151.

Callahan, C. M., Boustani, M. A., Unverzagt, F. W., Austrom, M. G., Damush, T. M., Perkins, A. J., et al. (2006). Effectiveness of collaborative care for older adults with Alzheimer disease in primary care. A randomized controlled trial. *JAMA, 295*, 2148–2157.

Callahan, C. M., Nienaber, N. A., Hendrie, H. C., & Tierney, W. M. (1992). Depression of elderly outpatients: Primary care physicians' attitudes and practice patterns. *Journal of General Internal Medicine, 7*(1), 26–31.

Callahan, C. M., Weiner, M., & Counsell, S. R. (2008). Defining the domain of geriatric medicine in an urban public health system affiliated with an academic medical center. *Journal of the American Geriatric Society, 56*(10), 1802–1806.

Centers for Disease Control. (2010). *Healthy aging: Improving and extending quality of life among older Americans: At a glance.* Retrieved from www.cdc. gov/chronicdisease/resources/publications/AAG/aging.htm.

Centers for Disease Control and Prevention, & National Association of Chronic Disease Directors. (2008). *The State of Mental Health and Aging in America Issue Brief 1: What Do the Data Tell Us?* Atlanta, GA: National Association of Chronic Disease Directors.

Centers for Disease Control, & the Alzheimer's Association. (2007). *The healthy brain initiative: A national public health road map to maintaining cognitive health.* Chicago, IL: Alzheimer's Association. Retrieved from www.cdc.gov/aging/pdf/TheHealthyBrainInitiative.pdf.

Chapman, D. P., Perry, G. S., & Strine, T. W. (2005). The vital link between chronic disease and depressive disorders. *Preventing Chronic Disease: Public Health Research, Practice Policy, 2*(1), 1–10.

Chapman, D. L. P., & Perry, G. S. (2008). Depression as a major component of public health for older adults. *Preventing Chronic Disease: Public Health Research, Practice Policy, 5*(1), A22.

Charney, D. S., Nemeroff, C. B., Lewis, L., Laden, S. K., Gorman, J. M., Laska, E. M., et al. (2002). National depressive and manic-depressive association consensus statement on the use of placebo in clinical trials of mood disorders. *Archives of General Psychiatry, 59*(3), 262–270.

Chodosh, J., Berry, E., Lee, M., Connor, K., DeMonte, R., Ganiats, T., et al. (2006). Effect of a dementia care management intervention on primary care provider knowledge, attitudes, and perceptions of quality of care. *Journal of the American Geriatric Society, 54*(2), 311–317.

Chodosh, J., Mittman, B. S., Connor, K. I., Vassar, S. D., Lee, M. L., DeMonte, R. W., et al. (2007). Caring for patients with dementia: How good is the quality of care? Results from three health systems. *Journal of the American Geriatric Society, 55*(8), 1260–1268.

Chodosh, J., Seeman, T. E., Keeler, E., Sewall, A., Hirsch, S. H., Guralnik, M., & Reuben, D. B. (2004). Cognitive decline in high-functioning older persons is associated with an increased risk of hospitalization. *Journal of the American Geriatric Society, 52*(9), 1456–1462.

Compton, W. M., Conway, K. P., Stinson, F. S., & Grant, B. F. (2006). Changes in the prevalence of major depression and comorbid substance use disorders in the United States between 1991–1992 and 2001–2002. *American Journal of Psychiatry, 163*(12), 2141–2147.

Dannenberg, A. L., Jackson, R. J., Frumkin, H., Schieber, R. A., Pratt, M., Kochtitzky, C., & Tilson, H. H. (2003). The impact of community design and land-use choices on public health: A scientific research agenda. *American Journal of Public Health*, 93(9), 1500–1508.

De Groot, M., Anderson, R., Freedland, K. E., Clouse, R. E., & Lustman, P. J. (2001). Association of depression and diabetes complications: A meta-analysis. *Psychosomatic Medicine*, 63, 619–630.

Depp, C., Woodruff-Borden, J., Meeks, S., Gretarsdottir, E., & DeKryger, N. (2005). The phenomenology of non-clinical panic in older adults in comparison to adults. *Journal of Anxiety Disorders*, 19(5), 503–519.

Dombrovski, A. Y., Szanto, K., Duberstein, P., Conner, K. R., Houck, P. R., & Conwell, Y. (2008). Sex differences in correlates of suicide attempt lethality in late life. *American Journal of Geriatric Psychiatry*, 6(11), 905–913.

Dufour, M. A. (2010). Alochol use. In P. L. Remington, R. C. Brownson, & M. V. Wegner (Eds.), *Chronic disease epidemiology and control* (pp. 229–268). Washington, DC: American Public Health Association.

Dunkle, R., Roberts, B., & Haug, M. (2001). *The oldest old in everyday life: Self perception, coping with change, and stress*. New York: Springer Publishing Company.

Eaton, W. W. (2001). *The sociology of mental disorders*. Westport, CT: Praeger.

Eaton, W. W. (Ed.) (2006). *Medical and psychiatric comorbidity over the course of life*. Washington, DC: American Psychiatric Publishing.

Eisdorfer, C., Czaja, S. J., Loewenstein, D. A., Rubert, M. P., Argüelles, S., Mitrani, V. B., & Szapocznik, J. (2003). The effect of a family therapy and technology-based intervention on caregiver depression. *Gerontologist*, 43(4), 521–531.

Evans, G. W. (2003). The built environment and mental health. *Journal of Urban Health*, 80(4), 536–555.

Fahs, M., Viladrich, A., & Parikh, N. S. (2009). Immigrants and urban aging: Toward a policy framework. In N. Freudenberg, S. Klitzman, & S. Saegert (Eds.), *Urban health and society: Interdisciplinary approaches to research and practice* (pp. 239–270). San Francisco, CA: Jossey-Bass.

Ferri, C. P., Prince, M., Brayne, C., Brodaty, H., Fratiglioni, L., Ganguli, M., et al. (2005). Global prevalence of dementia: A Delphi consensus study. *Lancet*, 366(9503), 2112–2117.

Fiscella, K., & Williams, D. R. (2004). Health disparities based on socioeconomic inequities: Implications for urban health care. *Academic Medicine*, 79(12), 1139–1147.

Frank, L. D., Engelke, P. O., & Schmid, L. T. (2003). *Health and community design: The impact of the built environment on physical activity*. Washington, DC: Island Press.

Frazer, C. J., Christensen, H., & Griffiths, K. M. (2005). Effectiveness of treatments for depression in older people. *Medical Journal of Australia*, 182(12), 627–632.

Freudenberg, N., Brantley, P., & Serrano, M. (2009). Public health campaigns to change industry practices that damage health: An analysis of 12 case studies. *Health Education and Behaviour*, 36(2), 230–249.

Frumkin, H., Frank, L., & Jackson, R. (2004). Urban sprawl and public health: Designing, planning and building for healthy communities. Washington, DC: Island Press.

Galea, S., Ahern, J., Rudenstine, S., Wallace, Z., & Vlahov, D. (2005). Urban built environment and depression: A multilevel analysis. *Journal of Epidemiology and Community Health*, 59, 822–827.

Gallagher-Thompson, D., Coon, D. W., Solano, N., Ambler, C., Rabinowitz, Y., & Thompson, L. W. (2003). Change in indices of distress among Latino and Anglo female caregivers of elderly relatives with dementia: Site-specific results from the REACH national collaborative study. *Gerontologist, 43*(4), 580–591.

Ganguli, M., Rodriguez, E., Mulsant, B., Richards, S., Pandav, R., Bilt, J. V., et al. (2004). Detection and management of cognitive impairment in primary care: The Steel Valley Seniors Survey. *Journal of the American Geriatric Society, 52*(10), 1668–1675.

Garrard, J., Rolnick, S. J., Nitz, N. M., Luepke, L., Jackson, J., Fischer, L. R., et al. (1998). Clinical detection of depression among community-based elderly people with self-reported symptoms of depression. *Journal of Gerontology, Series A: Biological Sciences and Medical Sciences, 53*(2), M92-M101.

Gellis, Z. D. (2006). Mental and emotional disorders in older adults. In B. Berkman (Ed.), *Handbook of social work in health and aging* (pp. 129–139). New York: Oxford University Press.

Gellis, Z. D., & Kim, J. (2004). Confirmatory factor analysis of the CES-D Short form as a screening measure of depression in an elderly home health care population. Paper presented at the 57th Gerontological Society of America annual conference. Washington, DC.

Gellis, Z. D., McGinty, J., Tierney, L., Jordan, C., Burton, J., Misener, E., & Bruce, M. (2005). *Home care professional's recognition of depression and anxiety in older cardiac patients.* Paper presented at the 58th Gerontoloical Society of America annual conference. Washington, DC.

Gitlin, L. N. (2003). Conducting research on home environments: lessons learned and new directions. *Gerontologist, 43*(5), 628–637.

Gitlin, L. N., Winter, L., Corcoran, M., Dennis, M. P., Schinfeld, S., & Hauck, W. W. (2003). Effects of the home environmental skill-building program on the caregiver-care recipient dyad: 6-month outcomes from the Philadelphia REACH Initiative. *Gerontologist, 43*(4), 532–546.

Glasser, M., & Gravdal, J. A. (1997). Assessment and treatment of geriatric depression in primary care settings. *Archives of Family Medicine, 6*(5), 433–438.

Graham, J. E., Rockwood, K., Beattie, B. L., Eastwood, R., Gauthier, S., Tuokko, H., & McDowell, I. (1997). Prevalence and severity of cognitive impairment with and without dementia in an elderly population. *Lancet, 349*(9068), 1793–1796.

Grenier, S., Preville, M., Boyer, R., & O'Connor, K. (2009). Prevalence and correlates of obsessive-compulsive disorder among older adults living in the community. *Journal of Anxiety Disorders, 23*(7), 858–865.

Gum, A. M., Arean, P. A., Enid Hunkeler, E., Tang, L., Katon, W., Hitchcock, P., et al. (2006). Depression treatment preferences in older primary care patients. *Gerontologist, 46*(1), 14–22.

Harris, D. P., Chodosh, J., Vassar, S. D., Vickrey, B. G., & Shapiro, M. F. (2009). Primary care providers' views of challenges and rewards of dementia care relative to other conditions. *Journal of the American Geriatric Society, 57*(12), 2209–2216. Hebert, L. E., Scherr, P. A., Bienias, J. L., Bennett, D. A., & Evans, D. A. (2003). Alzheimer disease in the U.S. population: Prevalence estimates using the 2000 Census. *Archives of Neurology, 60*, 1119–1122.

Heisel, M. J., Duberstein, P. R., Lyness, J. M., & Feldman, M. D. (2010). Screening for suicide ideation among older primary care patients. *Journal of the American Board of Family Medicine, 23*(2), 260–269.

Heo, M., Murphy, C. F., Fontaine, K. R., Martha, L., Bruce, M. L., & Alexopoulos, G. S. (2008). Population projection of US adults with lifetime experience of depressive disorder by age and sex from year 2005 to 2050. *International Journal of Geriatric Psychiatry*, 23(12), 1266–1270.

Henderson, C., Diez-Roux, A., Jacobs, D. R., Kiefe, C., West, D., & Williams, D. R. (2005) Neighborhood characteristics, individual-level socioeconomic factors, and depressive symptoms in young adults: The CARDIA Study. *Journal of Epidemiology and Community Health*, 59(4), 322–328.

Heron, M. P., & Smith, B. L. (2007). *Deaths: Leading causes for 2003* (National vital statistics reports, vol. 55, no 10). Hyattsville, MD: National Center for Health Statistics.

Hill, J. W., Futterman, R., Mastey, V., & Fillit, H. (2002). The effect of donepezil therapy on health costs in a Medicare managed care plan. *Managed Care Interface*, 15, 63–70.

Hill, T. D., Ross, C. E., & Angel, R. J. (2005). Neighborhood disorder, psychophysiological distress, and health. *Journal of Health and Social Behaviour*, 46(2), 170–186.

Holland, J. M., Schutte, K. K., Brennan, P. L., & Moos, R. H. (2010). The structure of late-life depressive symptoms across a 20-year span: A taxometric investigation. *Psychology of Aging*, 25(1), 142–156.

Holsinger, T., Deveau, J., Boustani, M., & Williams, J. W. (2007). Rational clinical examination: Is this patient demented? *JAMA*, 297, 2391–2404.

Honjo, K., van Reekum, R., & Verhoeff, N. P. (2009). Alzheimer's disease and infection: Do infectious agents contribute to progression of Alzheimer's disease? *Alzheimer's and Dementia*, 5(4), 348–360.

Hooyman, N. R., & Kiyak, H. A. (2005). *Social gerontology: A multidisciplinary perspective* (7th ed.). Boston: Allyn and Bacon.

Husten, C. G. (2010). Tobacco use. In P. L. Remington, R. C. Brownson, & M. V. Wegner (Eds.), *Chronic disease epidemiology and control* (pp. 117–158). Washington, DC: American Public Health Association.

Hybels, C. F., & Blazer, D. G. (2003). Epidemiology of late-life mental disorders. *Clinics inGeriatric Medicine*, 19(4), 663–696.

Iliffe, S., & Manthorpe, J. (2004). The recognition of and response to dementia in primary care: Lessons for professional development. *Learning in Health and Social Care*, 3(1), 5–16.

Iliffe, S., Wilcock, J., & Hayworth, D. (2006). Obstacles to shared care for patients with dementia: A qualitative study. *Family Practice*, 23(3), 353–362.

Jackson, R. J. (2003). The impact of the built environment on health: An emerging field. *American Journal of Public Health*, 93(9), 1382–1384.

Jedrziewski, M. K., Lee, V. M. Y., & Trojanowski, J. Q. (2005). Lowering the risk of Alzheimer's disease: Evidence-based practices emerge from new research. *Alzheimer's and Dementia: Journal of Alzheimer's Association*, 1(2), 152–160.

Katon, V., Bush, L., & Ormel. (1992). Adequacy and duration of antidepressant treatment in primary care. *Medical Care*, 30(1), 67–76.

Katz, I. R., & Coyne, J. C. (2000). The public health model for mental health care for the elderly. *JAMA*, 283(21), 2844–2845.

Kessler, R. C., Berglund, P., Demler, O., Jin, R., Merikangas, K. R., & Walters, E. E. (2005). Lifetime prevalence and age-of-onset distributions of DSM-IV disorders in the national comorbidity survey replication. *Archives of General Psychiatry*, 62(6), 593–602.

Kessler, R. C., & McRae, J. A. (1981). Trends in the relationship between sex and psychological distress: 1957–1976. *American Sociology Review, 46,* 443–452.

Kety, S. S. (1986). The interface between neuroscience and psychiatry. In R. Rosenberg, F. Schulsinger, and E. Stomgren (Eds.), *Psychiatry and its related disciplines* (pp. 21–28). Copenhagen, The Netherlands: World Psychiatric Association.

Kim, D. (2008). Blues from the neighborhood: Neighborhood characteristics and depression. *Epidemiologic Reviews, 30,* 101–117.

Kim, J., & Ross, C. E. (2009). Neighborhood-specific and general social support: Which buffers the effect of neighborhood disorder on depression? *Journal of Community Psychology, 37*(6), 725–736.

Kim, J. M., Stewart, R., Kim, S. W., Yang, S. J., Shin, I. S., & Yoon, J. S. (2009). Insomnia, depression, and physical disorders in late life: A 2-year longitudinal community study in Koreans. *SLEEP, 32*(9), 1221–1228.

Kinsella, K., & He, W. (2009). *An Aging World.* U.S. Census Bureau, International Population Reports. Washington, DC: US Government Printing Office.

Kleinschmidt, I., Hills, M., & Elliott, P. (1995). Smoking behaviour can be predicted by neighbourhood deprivation measures. *Journal of Epidemiology and Community Health, 49*(Suppl 2), S72–S77.

Kong, E. H., Evans, L. K., & Guevara, J. P. (2009). Nonpharmacological intervention for agitation in dementia: A systematic review and meta-analysis. *Aging and Mental Health, 13*(4), 512–20.

Kruger, D. J., Reischl, T. M., & Gee, G. C. (2007). Neighborhood social conditions mediate the association between physical deterioration and mental health. *American Journal of Community Psychology, 40*(3–4), 261–271.

Kubzansky, L. D., Subramanian, S. V., Kawachi, I., Fay, M. E., Soobader, M. J., & Berkman, L. F. (2005). Neighborhood contextual influences on depressive symptoms in the elderly. *American Journal of Epidemiology, 162*(3), 253–260.

LaGory, M., & Fitpatrick, K. (1992). The effects of environmental context on elderly depression. *Journal of Aging and Health, 4*(4), 459–479.

Lang, I. A., Hubbard, R. E., Andrew, M. K., Llewellyn, D. J., Melzer, D., & Rockwood, K. (2009). Neighborhood deprivation, individual socioeconomic status, and frailty in older adults. *Journal of the American Geriatric Society, 57*(10), 1776–1780.

Latkin, C. A., & Curry, A. D. (2003). Stressful neighborhoods and depression: A prospective study of the impact of neighborhood disorder. *Journal of Health and Social Behaviour, 44*(1), 34–44.

Lenze, E. J., Munin, M. C., Skidmore, E. R., Dew, M. A., Rogers, J. C., Whyte, E. M., et al. (2007). Onset of depression in elderly persons after hip fracture: Implications for prevention and early intervention of late-life depression. *Journal of the American Geriatric Society, 55*(10), 81–86.

Leventhal, T., & Brooks-Gunn, J. (2003). Moving to opportunity: An experimental study of neighborhood effects on mental health. *American Journal of Public Health, 93*(9), 1576–1582.

Levine, C. (2000). The many worlds of family caregivers. In C. Levine (Ed.) *Always on call: When illness turns families into caregivers* (pp. 1–17). New York: United Hospital Fund of New York.

Lewin Group. (2004). Saving lives, Saving money: Dividends for Americans investing in Alzheimer's research. Report of the Lewin Group to the Alzheimer's Association. Chigago, IL: Alzheimer's Association.

Li, C., Friedman, B., Conwell, Y., & Fiscella, K. (2007). Validity of the patient health questionnaire 2 (PHQ-2) in identifying major depression in older people. *Journal of the American Geriatric Society, 55*(4), 596–602.

Lin, P., Campbell, D. G., Chaney, E. F., Liu, C., Heagerty, P., Felker, B. L., & Hedrick, S. C. (2005). The influence of patient preference of depression treatment in primary care. *Annals of Behavioural Medicine, 30*(2), 164–173.

Link, B. G., & Phelan, J. (1995). Social conditions as fundamental causes of disease. *Journal of Health and Social Behavior, 35*:80–94.

Liu, L., & Chiu, C. (2009). Case-control study of suicide attempts in the elderly. *International Psychogeriatrics, 21*(5), 896–902.

Livingston, G., Johnston, K., Katona, C., Paton, J., & Lyketsos, C. G. (2005). Systematic review of psychological approaches to the management of neuropsychiatric symptoms of dementia. *American Journal of Psychiatry, 162*(11), 1996–2021.

Lopez, O. L., Jagust, W. J., DeKosky, S. T., Becker, J. T., Fitzpatrick, A., Dulberg, C., et al. (2003). Prevalence and classification of mild cognitive impairment in the Cardiovascular Health Study Cognition Study. *Archives of Neurology, 60*, 1385–1389.

Lynch, J. W., & Kaplan, G. A. (2000). Socioeconomic position. In L. F. Berman and I. Kawachi (Eds.), *Social epidemiology* (pp. 13–35). New York: Oxford University Press.

Mahoney, D. F., Turlow, B. T. & Jones, R. N. (2003). Effects of an automated telephone support system on caregiver burden and anxiety: Findings from the REACH for TLC intervention study. *The Gerontologist, 43*(4), 556–567.

Mair, C., Diez-Roux, A., & Galea, S. (2008). Are neighborhood characteristics associated with depressive symptoms? A review of evidence. *Journal of Epidemiology and Community Health, 62*, 940–946.

Malas, N., Tharp, K. M., & Foerster, S. B. (2010). Diet and nutrition. In P. L. Remington, R. C. Brownson, & M. V. Wegner (Eds.), *Chronic disease epidemiology and control* (pp. 159–198). Washington, DC: American Public Health Association.

Mark, T., McKusick, D., King, E., Harwood, H., & Genuardi, J. (1998). *National expenditures for mental health, alcohol, and other drug abuse treatment, 1996.* Rockville, MD: Substance Abuse and Mental Health Services Administration.

Marmot, M. (2005). Social determinants of health inequalities. *Lancet, 365*(9464), 1099–1104.

Marmot, M., & Wilkinson, R. G. (2001). Psychosocial and material pathways in the relation between income and health: A response to Lynch et al. *BMJ, 322*(7296), 1233–1236.

Mast, B. T., Miles, T., Penninx, B. W., Yaffe, K., Rosano, C., Satterfield, S., et al. (2008). Vascular disease and future risk of depressive symptomatology in older adults: Findings from the health, aging, and body composition study. *Biological Psychiatry, 64*(4), 320–326.

McCabe, M. P., Russo, S., Mellor, D., Davison, T. E., & George, K. (2008). Effectiveness of a training program for caregivers to recognize depression among older people. *International Journal of Geriatric Psychiatry, 23*(12), 1290–1296.

McEvoy, P., & Barnes, P. (2007). Using the chronic care model to tackle depression among older adults who have long-term physical conditions. *Journal of Psychiatric and Mental Health Nursing, 14*(3), 233–238.

McLeod, J.D., & Kessler, R.C. (1990). Socioeconomic status differences in vulnerability to undesirable life events. *Journal of Health and Social Behavior, 31,* 162–172.

Miranda, J., & Green, B. L. (1999). The need for mental health services research focusing on poor young women. *Journal of Mental Health Policy and Economics, 2,* 73–80.

Mirowsky, J., & Ross, C. E. (2003). *Social causes of psychological distress.* New York: Walter de Gruyter.

Mittelman, M. (2002). Family caregiving for people with Alzheimer's disease: Results of the NYU spouse-caregiver intervention study. *Generations, 26*(1), 104–106.

Mittelman, M. (2004). The feeling of family caregivers: Dealing with emotional challenges of caring for an individual with Alzheimer's disease. Retrieved from http://rci.gsw.edu/expalzppt.htm.

Mittelman, M., Epstein, C., & Pierzchala, A. (2003). *Counseling the Alzheimer's caregiver: A resource for health care professionals.* Chicago, IL: American Medical Association Press.

Mittelman, M. S., Ferris, S. H., Shulman, E., Steinberg, G., Ambinder, A., Mackell, J. A., & Cohen, J. (1995). A comprehensive support program: Effect on depression in spouse-caregivers of AD patients. *Gerontologist, 35*(6), 792–802.

Mittelman, M. S., Ferris, S. H., Steinberg, G., Shulman, E., Mackell, J. A., Ambinder, A., & Cohen, J. (1993). An intervention that delays institutionalization of Alzheimer's disease patients: Treatment of spouse-caregivers. *Gerontologist, 33*(6), 730–740.

Mittelman, M. S., Ferris, S. H., Shulman, E., Steinberg, G., & Levin, B. (1996). A family intervention to delay nursing home placement of patients with Alzheimer disease: A randomized controlled trial. *JAMA, 276*(21), 1725–1731.

Mittelman, M. S., Roth, D. L., Coon, D. W., & Haley, W. E. (2004a). Sustained benefit of supportive intervention for depressive symptoms in caregivers of patients with Alzheimer's disease. *American Journal of Psychiatry, 161*(5), 850–856.

Mittelman, M. S., Roth, D. L., Haley, W. E., & Zarit, S. H. (2004b). Effects of a caregiver intervention on negative caregiver appraisals of behavior problems in patients with Alzheimer's disease: Results of a randomized trial. *Journals of Gerontology, Series B: Psychological Sciences and Social Sciences, 59*(1), P27-P34.

Murali, V., & Oyebode, F. (2004). Poverty, social inequality and mental health. *Advances in Psychiatric Treatment, 10,* 216–224.

Murrary, R. M., Jones, P. B., Susser, E., van Os, J., & Cannon, M. (Eds.). (2003). *The epidemiology of schizophrenia.* New York: Cambridge University Press.

National Alliance for Caregiving. (2004). *Caregiving in the U.S.* Retrieved from www.caregiving.org/4–6–04release.htm.

National Institute of Mental Health. (2009). *Older Adults: Depression and Suicide Facts (Fact Sheet).* Retrieved from www.nimh.nih.gov/health/publications/older-adults-depression-and-suicide-facts-fac...

National Registry of Evidence-based Programs and Practice. (2010). *New York University Caregiver Intervention (NYUCI).* Retrieved from www.nrepp.samsha.gov/listofprograms.asp?textsearch=Mary+Mittelman&ShowHid...

Northridge, M. E., Sclar, E. D., & Biswas, P. (2003). Sorting out the connections between the built environment and health: A conceptual framework for navigating pathways and planning healthy cities. *Journal of Urban Health, 80*(4), 556–568.

Ojeda, V. D., & McGuire, T.G. (2006). Gender and racial/ethnic differences in use of outpatient mental health and substance use services by depressed adults. *Psychiatric Quarterly, 77*(3), 211–222.

Oslin, D. W., Streim, J., Katz, I. R., Edell, W. S., & TenHave, T. (2000). Change in disability follows inpatient treatment for late life depression. *Journal of the American Geriatric Society, 48,* 357–362.

Ostbye, T., Yarnall, K. S., Krause, K. M., Pollak, K. I., Gradison, M., & Michener, J. L. (2005). Is there time for management of patients with chronic diseases in primary care? *Annals of Family Medicine, 3*(3), 209–214.

Ostir, G. V., Eschbach, K., Markides, K. S., & Goodwin, J. S. (2003). Neighbourhood composition and depressive symptoms among older Mexican Americans. *Journal Epidemiology and Community Health, 57*(12), 987–992.

Pearlin, L. (1999). Stress and mental health: A conceptual overview. In A. Horowitz and T. Scheid (Eds.), *A handbook for the study of mental health.* Cambridge, UK: Cambridge University Press.

Pedraza, O., Dotson, V. M., Willis, F. B., Graff-Radford, N. R., & Lucas, J. A. (2009). Internal consistency and test-retest stability of the geriatric depression scale-short form in African American older adults. *Journal of Psychopathology and Behavioral Assessment, 31*(4), 412–416.

Perlis, M. L., Smith, L.J., Lyness, J. M., Matteson, S. R., Pigeon, W. R., Jungquist, C. R., & Tu, X. (2006). Insomnia as a risk factor for onset of depression in the elderly. *Behavioral Sleep Medicine, 4*(2), 104–113.

Pfaff, J. J., & Almeida, O. P. (2005). Detecting suicidal ideation in older patients: Identifying risk factors within the general practice setting. *British Journal of General Practice, 55* (513), 269–273.

Phelan, E. A., Borson, S., Grothaus, L., Balch, S., & Larson, E. B. (2009). Hospitalizations and preventable hospitalizations in demented and non-demented older adults (preparing for resubmission). Unpublished paper abstract. *American Journal of Geriatric Psychiatry, 17*(3).

Pinquart, M., Duberstein, P. R., & Lyness, J. M. (2006). Treatments for later-life depressive conditions: A meta-analytic comparison of pharmacotherapy and psychotherapy. *American Journal of Psychiatry, 163*(9), 1493–1501.

Prigerson, H. G. (2003). Costs to society of family caregiving for patients with endstage Alzheimer's disease. *New England Journal of Medicine, 349,* 1891–1892.

Prohaska, T., Belansky, E., Belza, B., Buchner, D., Marshall, V., McTigue, K., et al. (2006). Physical activity, public health, and aging: Critical issues and research priorities. *Journals of Gerontology, Series B: Psychological Sciences and Social Sciences, 61*(5), S267–S273.

Rabins, P. V. (1996). Barriers to diagnosis and treatment of depression in elderly patients. *American Journal of Geriatric Psychiatry, 4,* S79–S83.

Rabins, P. V., Black, B. S., Roca, R., German, P., McGuire, M., Robbins, B., et al. (2000). Effectiveness of a nurse-based outreach program for identifying and treating psychiatric illness in the elderly. *JAMA, 21,* 2802–2809.

Raina, P., Santaguida, P., Ismaila, A., Patterson, C., Cowan, D., Levine, M., et al. (2008). Effectiveness of cholinesterase inhibitors and memantine for treating dementia: Evidence review for a clinical practice guideline. *Annals of Internal Medicine, 148*(5), 379–397.

Reijneveld, S. A. (1998). The impact of individual and area characteristics on urban socioeconomic differences in health and smoking. *International Journal of Epidemiology, 27*(1), 33–40.

Research!America. (2006). American speaks: Poll data summary (Vol. 7) (p. 25). Alexandria, VA; Research!America. Retrieved from www.researchamerica.org/uploads/AmericaSpeaksV7.pdf.

Russo, A., Hambrick, M., & Owens P. (2007). *Healthcare Cost and Utilization Project (HCUP)* (Statistical Brief No. 40). Rockville, MD: Agency for Healthcare Research and Quality. Retrieved from www.hcup-us.ahrq.gov/reports/statbriefs/sb40.jsp.

Sachs, G. A., Shega, J. W., & Cox-Hayley, D. (2004). Barriers to excellent end-of-life care for patients with dementia. *Journal of General Internal Medicine, 19*(10), 1057–1063.

Saddichha, S., & Pandey, V. (2008). Alzheimer's and non-Alzheimer's dementia: A critical review of pharmacological and nonpharmacological strategies. *American Journal Alzheimer's Disease and Other Dementia, 23*(2), 150–61.

Sadik, K., & Wilcock, G. (2003). The increasing burden of Alzheimer disease. *Alzheimer Disease and Associated Disorders, 17*(Suppl. 3), S75–S79.

Sands, L. P., Ferreira, P., Stewart, A. L., Brod, M., & Yaffe, K. (2004). What explains differences between dementia patients' and their caregivers' ratings of patients' quality of life? *American Journal of Geriatric Psychiatry, 12*(3), 272–280.

Satariano, W. A. (2006). *Epidemiology of aging: An ecological approach.* Sudbury, MA: Jones and Bartlett.

Schneider, L. S. (1995). Efficacy of clinical treatment for mental disorders among older persons. In M. Gatz (Ed.), *Emerging issues in mental health and aging* (pp. 19–71). Washington, DC: American Psychological Association.

Schoeni, R. F., House, J. S., Kaplan, G. A., & Pollack, H. (Eds.) (2008). *Making Americans healthier: Social and economic policy as health policy.* New York: Russell Sage Foundation.

Schubert, C. C., Boustani, M., Callahan, C. M., Perkins, A. J., Carney, C. P., Fox, C., et al. (2006). Comorbidity profile of dementia patients in primary care: Are they sicker? *Journal of the American Geriatric Society, 54*(1), 104–109.

Schubert, C. C., Boustani, M., Callahan, C. M., Perkins, A. J., Hui, S., & Hendrie, H. C. (2008). Acute care utilization by dementia caregivers within urban primary care practices. *Journal of General Internal Medicine, 23*(11), 1736–40.

Schulz, R., Burgio, L., Burns, R., Eisdorfer, C., Gallagher-Thompson, D., Gitlin, L. & Mahoney, D. (2003a). Resources for enhancing Alzheimer's caregiver health (REACH): Overview, site-specific outcomes, and future directions. *Gerontologist, 43*(4), 514–520.

Schulz, R., Mendelsohn, A. B., Haley, W. E., Mahoney, D., Allen, R. S., Zhang, S., et al. (2003b). Resources for enhancing Alzheimer's caregiver health investigators: End-of-life care and the effects of bereavement on family caregivers of persons with dementia. *New England Journal of Medicine, 349*, 1936–1943.

Seedat, S., Nyamai, C., Njenga, F., Vythilingum, B., & Stein, D. J. (2004). Trauma exposure and post-traumatic stress symptoms in urban African schools: Survey in Capetown and Nairobi. *British Journal of Psychiatry, 184*, 169–175.

Sharp, L. K., & Lipsky, M. S. (2002). Screening for depression across the lifespan: a review of measures for use in primary care settings. *American Family Physician, 66*(6), 1001–1008.

Shelley, D., Fahs, M., Yerneni, R., Das, D., Nguyen, N., Hung, D., et al. (2008). Effectiveness of tobacco control among Chinese Americans: A comparative analysis of policy approaches versus community-based programs. *Preventive Medicine, 47*(5), 530–536.

Sherrington, C., Whitney, J. C., Lord, S. R., Herbert, R. D., Cumming, R. G., & Close, J. C. (2008). Effective exercise for the prevention of falls: A systematic review and meta-analysis. *Journal of the American Geriatric Society*, 56(12), 2234–2243.

Sirey, J. A., Bruce, M. L., Alexopoulos, G. S., Perlick, D. A., Raue, P., Friedman, S. J., & Meyers, B. S. (2001). Perceived stigma as a predictor of treatment discontinuation in young and older outpatients with depression. *American Journal of Psychiatry*, 158(3), 479–481.

Sirey, J. A., Bruce, M. L., Carpenter, M., Booker, D., Reid, M. C., Newell, K., & Alexopoulos, G. S. (2008). Depressive symptoms and suicidal ideation among older adults receiving home delivered meals. *International Journal of Geriatric Psychiatry*, 23, 1306–1311.

Sloane, P. D., Zimmerman, S., Suchindran, C., Reed, P., Wang, L., Boustani, M., & Sudha, S. (2002). Impact of Alzheimer's disease, 2000–2050: Potential implication of treatment advances. *Annals of Review of Public Health*, 23, 213–331.

Small, G. W., Rabins, P. V., Barry, P. P., Buckholtz, N. S., DeKosky, S. T., Ferris, S. H., et al. (1997). Diagnosis and treatment of Alzheimer's disease and related disorders. Consensus statement of the American Association for Geriatric Psychiatry, the Alzheimer's Association, and the American Geriatrics Society. *JAMA*, 278, 1363–1371.

Smith, G. D., & Susser, E. (2002). Zena Stein, Mervyn Susser, and epidemiology: Observation, causation, and action. *International Journal of Epidemiology*, 31, 34–37.

Snowden, M., Steinman, L., & Frederick, J. (2008). Treating depression in older adults: Challenge to implementing the recommendation of an expert panel. *Preventing Chronic Disease*, 5(1), A26.

Spijker, A., Vernooij-Dassen, M., Vasse, E., Adang, E., Wollersheim, H., Grol, R., & Verhey, F. (2008). Effectiveness of nonpharmacological interventions in delaying the institutionalization of patients with dementia: A meta-analysis. *Journal of American Geriatric Society*, 56(6), 1116–1128.

Stuck, A. E., Walthert, J. M., Nikolaus, T., Büla, C. J., Hohmann, C., & Beck, J. C. (1999). Risk factors for functional status decline in community-living elderly people: A systematic literature review. *Social Science Medicine*, 48(4), 445–469.

Sundaram, V., Helweg-Larsen, K., Laursen, B., & Bjerregaard, P. (2004). Physical violence, self rated health, and morbidity: Is gender significant for victimisation. *Journal of Epidemiology and Community Health*, 58(1), 65–70.

Susser, E., Hoek, H. W., & Brown, A. (1998). Neurodevelopmental disorders after prenatal stage: The story of the Dutch Famine Study. *American Journal of Epidemiology*, 147(3), 213–216.

Thomson, J., Rankin, H., Ashcroft, G. W., Yates, C. M., McQueen, J. K., & Cummings, S. J. (1982). The treatment of depression in general practice: A comparison of L-tryptophan, amitriptyline, and a combination of L-tryptophan and amitriptyline with placebo. *Psychology of Medicine*, 12, 741–751.

Truong, K. D., & Ma, S. (2006). A systematic review of relations between neighborhoods and mental health. *Journal Mental Health Policy and Economics*, 9(3), 137–154.

United States Department of Health and Human Services [US DHHS]. (1999). *Mental health: A report of the Surgeon General*. Baltimore, MD: United States Public Health Service.

United States Department of Health and Human Services [US DHHS]. (2000). *Healthy people 2010*. Washington, DC: U. S. Government Printing Office.

Unützer, J., Patrick, D. L., Simon, G., Grembowski, D., Walker, E., Rutter, C., & Katon, W. (1997). Depressive symptoms and the cost of health services in HMO patients aged 65 years and older: A 4-year prospective study. *JAMA, 277*(20), 1618–1623.

Unverzagt, F. W., Gao, S., Baiyewu, O., Ogunniyi, A. O., Gureje, O., Perkins, A., et al. (2001). Prevalence of cognitive impairment: Data from the Indianapolis Study of Health and Aging. *Neurology, 57*(9), 1655–1662.

US Census Bureau. (2008). 2008 National Population Projections. Retrieved from www.census.gov/population/www/projections/summarytables.html.

US Preventive Services Task Force. (2009). Screening for depression in adults: U.S. preventive services task force recommendation statement. *Annals of Internal Medicine, 151*(11), 784–792.

Vickrey, B. G., Mittman, B. S., Connor, K. I., Pearson, M. L., Della Penna, R. D., Ganiats, T. G., et al. (2006). The effect of a disease management intervention on quality and outcomes of dementia care: A randomized, controlled trial. *Annals of Internal Medicine, 145*(10), 713–726.

Vlahov, F., Freudenberg, N., Proietti, F., Ompad, D., Quinn, A., Nandi, V., & Galea, S. (2007). Urban as a determinant of health. *Journal of Urban Health, 84*(1), i16–i26.

Wagner, E. H., Austin, B. T., & Von Korff, M. (1996). Organizing care for patients with chronic illness. *Milbank Quarterly, 74*(4), 511–544.

Wagner, E. H., Davis, C., Schaefer, J., Von Korf, M., & Austin, B. (2002). A survey of leading chronic disease management programs: Are they consistent with the literature? *Journal of Nursing Care, 16*(2), 67–80.

Wang, P. S., Lane, M., Olfson, M., Pincus, H. A., Wells, K. B., & Kessler, R. C. (2005). Twelve-month use of mental health services in the United States: Results from the National Comorbidity Survey Replication. *Archives of General Psychiatry, 62*(6), 629–640.

Warner, K.E. (2000). The need for, and value of, a multi-level approach to disease prevention: The case of tobacco control. In B.D. Smedley & S.L. Syme (Eds.), *Promoting health: Intervention strategies from social and behavioral research*, pp. 417–449. Washington, DC: National Academy Press.

Weinberger, M.I., Mateo, C., & Sirey, J. (2009). Perceived barriers to mental health care and goal setting among depressed, community-dwelling older adults. *Patient Prefer Adherence, 3*, 145–149.

Weisman, M. M., Bruce, M. L., Leaf, P. J., Florio, L.P., & Holzer, C.E. (1991). Affective disorders. In L. N. Robins & D. A. Regier (Eds.). *Psychiatric disorders in America: The Epidemiologic Catchment Area Study* (pp. 53–80). New York: The Free Press.

Wells, K. B., Rogers, W., Burnam, A., Greenfield, S., & Ware, J. E., Jr. (1991). How the medical comorbidity of depressed patients differs across health care settings: Results from the Medical Outcomes Study. *American Journal of Psychiatry, 148*(12), 1688–1696.

Wight, R. G., Cummings, J. R., Karlamangla, A. S., & Aneshensel, C. S. (2009). Urban neighborhood context and change in depressive symptoms in late life. *Journals of Gerontology, Series B: Psychological Sciences and Social Sciences, 64*(2), 247–251.

Williams, D. R. (1986). The epidemiology of mental illness in Afro-Americans *Hospital and Community Psychiatry*, *37*: 42–49.

Williams, D. R. (2002). Racial/ethnic variations in women's health: The social embeddedness of health. *American Journal of Public Health*, *92*(4), 588–597.

Williams, D. R., Yu, Y., Jackson, J. S., & Anderson, N. B. (1997). Racial differences in physical and mental health: Socioeconomic status, stress, and discrimination. *Journal of Health Psychology*, *2*(3), 335–351.

Wisniewski, S., Belle, S., Marcus, S., Burgio, L., Coon, D., Ory, M., et al. (2003). The resources for enhancing Alzheimer's caregiver health (REACH: Project design and baseline characteristics. *Psychology of Aging*, *18*(3), 375–384.

World Heath Organization. (2007). Global age friendly cities: A guide. Paris, France: World Health Organization.

Yen, I. H., & Kaplan, G. A. (1999). Poverty area residence and changes in depression and perceived health status: Evidence from the Alameda County Study. *International Journal of Epidemiology*, *28*(1), 90–94.

Zarit, S., & Femia, E. (2008). Behavioral and psychosocial interventions for family caregivers. *Journal of Social Work and Education*, *44*(3), S49–S57.

15 Protecting urban families from community violence

Neal Cohen

Introduction

Increasingly, the public health and mental health literature has taken notice of the environmental effects upon physical and mental well-being of living in poor inner-city neighborhoods (Freudenberg, Galea, & Vlahov, 2006). Among a multitude of stressors associated with urban life, especially in poor, disadvantaged neighborhoods, interpersonal violence is recognized as a traumatic stressor with many negative health and mental health outcomes for children and adults (Horowitz, McKay, & Marshall, 2005). This chapter examines the direct and indirect consequences of exposures to community violence for families struggling to cope with the challenges of life in poor inner-city neighborhoods and the evidence-base for developing a risk and protective factor framework for public mental health policy and program planning.

Through the lens of traumatic stress studies

The last two decades have seen a burgeoning body of research examining the deleterious health and mental health consequences associated with exposure to the stressors of community and domestic violence in impoverished inner-city neighborhoods. In large measure, this research focus was stimulated by advances in the conceptual models and empirical findings in the field of traumatic stress studies, which offered a framework for understanding the sequelae of living in an environment with ongoing threats to the safety to oneself and/or one's family.

The return from Vietnam in the late 1970s of hundreds of thousands of soldiers with combat exposure and a unique constellation of psychiatric symptomatology was the impetus for the introduction of posttraumatic stress disorder (PTSD) as a formal diagnostic category in the third edition of the *Diagnostic and Statistical Manual of Mental Disorders* (DSM-III) (American Psychiatric Association [APA], 1980). The essential features for a DSM-III diagnosis of PTSD focused on three categories of symptoms:

1   *reexperiencing* the traumatic event (through flashbacks, intrusive thoughts, nightmares, or dreams);
2   *numbing* of responsiveness or *avoidance* of stimuli associated with the event; and
3   *hyperarousal* (such as difficulty concentrating or problem sleeping).

Furthermore, the conceptualization of the PTSD diagnosis required exposure to a markedly distressing event outside the range of the usual experiences of everyday life. Consequently, the earliest investigations of PTSD phenomenology focused on population groups that experienced specific traumatic events, such as Vietnam War combat (Kulka, Schlenger, Fairbank, Hough, Jordan, & Marmar, 1990), criminal victimization (Kilpatrick, Saunders, Amick-McMullan, Best, Veronen, & Resnick, 1989), mass shootings (Schwartz & Kowalski, 1991), and natural disasters (Freedy, Kilpatrick, & Resnick, 1993; Pynoos, Goenjian, Tashjian, Karakashian, Manjikian, Manoukian et al., 1993).

While the initial diagnostic formulation of PTSD addressed the survivors of relatively circumscribed and short-lived traumatic events, clinicians and researchers recognized that the PTSD diagnosis did not capture the severe psychological harm that occurs with prolonged, repeated trauma (van der Kolk, Roth, Pelcovitz, Sunday, & Spinazzola, 2005). Herman (1992a; 1992b) proposed a new diagnosis, "Complex PTSD," to describe the symptoms of long-term trauma in which the victim is generally held in a state of captivity, either physically or emotionally, and is unable to flee. Groups identified as at-risk for complex posttraumatic syndrome due to prolonged, repeated victimization include survivors of concentration camps, prisoner of war camps, child sexual abuse, long-term severe physical abuse, and long-term domestic violence. In addition to expanding the definition of PTSD to include chronic trauma exposure, Herman's characterization of complex PTSD syndrome encompassed three broad areas of disturbance that transcend simple PTSD symptomatology. These include symptomatology that is more complex, diffuse, and long-lasting than in simple PTSD; characterology that manifests deformations of relatedness and identity; and vulnerability to repeated future harm, either self-inflicted or from others.

The 1990s saw significant research interest and reporting on complex clinical syndromes deriving from persistent and severe stress and abuse, often meeting the criteria for PTSD, but going well beyond it in affecting victims across many levels of functioning, including somatic, emotional, cognitive, behavioral, and characterological (e.g., Briere & Elliott, 1997; Dickinson, de Gruy, Dickinson, & Candib, 1998; Norris & Kaniasty, 1994; Pelcovitz, van der Kolk, Roth, Mandel, Kaplan, & Resick, 1997; Rahe, 1993; Roth, Newman, Pelcovitz, van der Kolk, & Mandel, 1997; van der Kolk, Pelcovitz, Roth, Mandel, McFarlane, & Herman, 1996). Field trials for the development of the DSM-IV included investigation of the psychopathology and diagnosis of long-term trauma exposure, which was tentatively labeled "disorders of extreme stress, not otherwise specified" (DESNOS). Results supported the categorization of a distinctly complex adaptation to chronic trauma and abuse in both children and adults, but the DESNOS symptomatology was incorporated into the DSM-IV as "associated and descriptive features" of PTSD, not as a distinct diagnosis (APA, 1994).

With the recognition that many different types of traumatic experiences lead to PTSD symptomatology, the introduction of the DSM-IV in 1994 replaced emphasis on the traumatic event itself with the subjective appraisal of the event. The DSM-IV definition embedded in Criterion A changed to:

> The personal experience of an event that involves actual or threatened death or serious injury, or other threat to one's physical integrity; or witnessing an event that involves death, injury, or a threat to the physical integrity of another person; or learning about unexpected or violent death, serious harm, or threat of death or injury experienced by a family member or other close associate. ... The person's response to the event must involve intense fear, helplessness, or horror.
>
> (APA, 1994, p. 424)

As the focus of PTSD diagnosis shifted from an extraordinary traumatic event to the quality of the response (intense fear, helplessness, or horror), great interest emerged in examining the interrelationship of trauma and PTSD in disadvantaged inner city communities (Breslau, Kessler, Chilcoat, Schultz, David, & Andreski, 1998; Kessler, Sonnega, Bromet, Hughes, & Nelson, 1995; Norris, 1992; Resnick, Kilpatrick, Danska, Saunders, & Best, 1993). The 1996 Detroit Area Survey of Trauma collected data on a wide range of traumas experienced by individuals in metropolitan Detroit neighborhoods in order to estimate their prevalence and the risk of a variety of traumatic stressors leading to PTSD (Breslau et al., 1998). The survey of 2,191 adults (ages 18 to 45) found that lifetime prevalence of exposure to trauma varied widely across traumatic events, with a mean number of 4.8 traumatic events reported by persons exposed to any trauma. While women were about half as likely as men to be exposed to assaultive violence (mugging or threatened with a weapon: 34% of men versus 16.4% of women; shot or stabbed: 8.2% of men versus 1.8% of women), they were more likely than men to be victims of sexual assault (rape: 9.4% of women versus 1.1% of men; other sexual assaults: 9.4% of women versus 2.8% of men).

The conditional probability of PTSD occurring in response to exposure to a traumatic event was assessed both for specific events and for exposure to any type of trauma. Overall, the probability of PTSD after exposure to a traumatic event was 9.2% (SE = 1.0) to 13.0% (SE = 1.6) in women and

6.2% (SE = 1.2) in men. Assaultive violence was responsible for 39.5% of PTSD cases and had the highest probability (20.9%) of PTSD occurring following exposure. When sociodemographic variables were controlled, gender was a significant risk factor for PTSD; women had a two-fold higher rate of PTSD than men, a finding that was unrelated to the number of traumas experienced by men and women. Furthermore, independent of the type of traumatic exposure, PTSD persisted longer among women, with a median duration of 48.1 months versus 12.0 months in men. The greater vulnerability of women to PTSD following exposure to trauma in the Detroit Area Survey is consistent with numerous reports in the literature, including the National Comorbidity Survey (NCS) (Kessler et al., 1995), which reports the female-to-male relative risk as 4.0, adjusted for trauma type.

Trauma in the community

The broadening of the DSM diagnosis of PTSD in both the stressor criterion (Part A) and the symptom response (Part B) that occurred in the mid-1990s created greater interest and opportunity for researchers to examine trauma associated with the threats to safety experienced by those living in low-income, inner-city neighborhoods with relatively greater risks of exposure to repeated traumatization and victimization. The DSM-IV field trials found consensus for a more complex constellation of symptomatology than seen in "simple" PTSD in response to exposure in early life to repeated and/or prolonged traumatic stressors:

> The following associated constellation of symptoms may occur and are more commonly seen in association with interpersonal stressors (e.g., childhood sexual or physical abuse, domestic battering...): impaired affect modulation; self-destructive and impulsive behavior; dissociative symptoms; somatic complaints; feelings of ineffectiveness, shame, despair, or hopelessness; feeling permanently damaged; a loss of previously sustained beliefs; hostility; social withdrawal; feeling constantly threatened; impaired relationships with others; or a change from the individual's previous personality characteristics.
>
> (APA, 1994, p. 425)

The complexity of the posttraumatic psychopathology recorded in the DSM-IV field trials (and incorporated into the "associated and descriptive features" of PTSD in the DSM-IV-R) was more likely to occur when the onset of trauma stressors was in the first decade of life. Although the trials did not analyze the number of separate stressor events across each participant's life span, van der Kolk, Roth, Pelcovitz, Sunday, and Spinazzola (2005) posit that repeated traumatic experiences in combination with early life exposure may be responsible for more pervasive impact. Further complicating the clinical presentation of traumatized persons is the finding that 84% of people with PTSD had another lifetime diagnosis, most frequently depression, phobias, anxiety, dissociative or somatoform disorders (Kessler et al., 1995). The variety of traumatic stressors and the multi-dimensional responses to exposure to trauma among community populations has propelled a heightened research focus on interpersonal traumatization among low-income, inner-city residents at greatest risk.

Violence in the community

Community violence is a term applied to a broad range of events occurring in neighborhoods, including actual crimes, threats of violence, or widespread sexual, physical, and emotional abuse (Hamblen & Goguen, 2010). Often characterized as "interpersonal violence," the clinical and research literature has tended to focus either on the abuse of children (e.g., sexual or physical abuse) or on the abuse of adults (e.g., domestic violence, rape, assaults). While the earlier research literature on PTSD focused largely on specific trauma events of limited duration (e.g., natural disasters, sexual assaults, mass shootings), interest in the examination of community violence through a "trauma lens" shifts the focus toward trauma that is prolonged, repeated, and associated with a perception of ongoing threat to one's safety.

While some traumas may affect only an individual, community violence often has effects on entire families and neighborhoods. For example, children and adults may be exposed to multiple types of community violence, such as abuse and/or violent events in the home along with violence directly or indirectly experienced in the community. Horowitz, Weine, and Jekel (1995) proposed the term "compounded community trauma" to denote this pattern of repeated exposure to multiple types of threats to safety and violence either through direct or indirect modalities of contact.

Risks to children and adolescents

There has been considerable interest in the way children respond to threats to safety in their homes and their community (Buka, Stichick, Birdthistle, & Earls, 2001; Lynch, 2003; Margolin & Gordis, 2000; Osofsky, 2003). The research literature most often relies upon child or parent reports of exposure to traumatic events – either through witnessing the victimization of another person or being victimized themselves. In low-income, inner-city neighborhoods the prevalence of experiencing (directly or indirectly) community violence among children is quite high; a majority of youth have witnessed violent events, and about one-third have been direct victims of violence (Sheehan, DiCara, LeBaily, & Christoffel, 1997).

Children witnessing and hearing about violent events in the community may also compromise the ability of their family members to provide a consistent sense of safety and security that would buffer the toxic stress associated with living in these threatening environments (Aisenberg & Herrenkohl, 2008; Linares, Heeren, Bronfman, Zuckerman, Augustyn, & Tronick, 2001). Consequently, longer-term exposure to community violence and direct victimization by violence places children at greater risk for a number of behavioral and psychological problems, including aggressive behavior, depression, distrust, fearfulness, and PTSD (Lynch, 2003; Schwab-Stone, Chen, Greenberger, Silver, Lichtman, & Voyce, 1999). Furthermore, children who experience greater levels of community violence manifest physiological markers of stress, including higher blood pressure, heart rate, and cortisol levels (Murali & Chen, 2005). Other reports link community violence to childhood morbidity of decreased lung function and elevated asthma rates (Suglia, Ryan, Laden, Dawson, & Wright, 2007; Wright, 2006).

Along with the emotional distress and expression of stress symptomatology, the exposure of children to violence in the home or in the community may alter many of the developmental processes that shape the formation of a cohesive self-identity, basic trust, and connectedness with others. Exposure to violence will affect children differently if involving a family member instead of a stranger (Lynch, 2003; Osofsky, 2003), with greater anxiety experienced when the victim or perpetrator is known to the child (Ward, Flisher, Zissis, Muller, & Lombard, 2001).

Exposure to community violence has been linked to aggressive anti-social behavior in children ranging from six to 15 years old (Miller, Wasserman, Neugebauer, Gorman-Smith, & Kamboukes, 1999; Plybon & Kliewer, 2001). Very young children may view violence as a means to assert control over chaotic and dangerous environments – that is, as a coping strategy. Jenkins and Bell (1997) studied 536 children in grades two, four, six, and eight and found a link between witnessing family violence and children's physical aggression, including carrying knives and guns, offensive fighting, and trouble in school. Bell (1995) describes the "intergenerational cycle of violence" that is propagated through experiencing violence in childhood as a way to resolve conflict and to assert control over other people, even in intimate relationships.

Among adolescents, response to community violence exposure is influenced by the nature and degree of exposure earlier in childhood as well as a range of individual, family, and community factors. DuRant, Pendergrast, and Cadenhead (1994) reported a study of 225 African American adolescents in which previous exposure to community violence and victimization were the strongest predictors of social and emotional disturbances. Exposure to violence explained 26% of the variation in adolescents' later use of violent behavior, as compared to only 3.8% for depression. Among 337 inner-city adolescents, Moses (1999) found that exposure to violence of all types was highly correlated with each other and associated with elevated hostility and depression. Moses (1999) posits an adaptive process by which inner-city adolescents become habituated to their environments and thereby desensitized to the great degree of violence occurring in their neighborhoods. However, in a meta-analytic review of 18 studies of the relationship between child violence exposure and adolescent anti-social behavior, Wilson, Stover, and Berkowitz (2009) found a stronger relationship when actual victimization, not just exposure, is assessed. Given the high co-occurrence of both domestic violence and child maltreatment (Osofsky, 2003), witnessing violence in the home and in the community is often associated with direct victimization and should be more consistently assessed in both research and clinical work.

Substance use and abuse, frequently in association with early aggressive and antisocial behavior, has been found to be elevated among adolescents exposed to community violence (Gilvarry, 2000; Kilpatrick, Aciero, Saunders, Resnick, Best, & Schnurr, 2000; Zinzow, 2009). The study of Kilpatrick and colleagues (2000) of more than 4,000 adolescents reported a three-fold increase in risk of abuse or dependency for all substances among those exposed to community violence.

Increasingly, researchers are discovering that children in low-income, inner-city neighborhoods often are exposed to co-existing community violence-related risk factors, such as elevated rates of violent neighborhood crime, child maltreatment/abuse, and domestic violence (Lynch, 2003; Lynch & Cicchetti, 1998). Margolin (1998) found that 45 to 70% of children exposed to domestic violence are also victims of physical abuse; consequently, it is extremely difficult to determine the unique effects of exposure to specific events of community violence on children's development (Lynch, 2003). Instead, we are left with a judgment of cumulative risk for children, which is associated with multiple exposures to a wide range of community violence events in disadvantaged urban communities.

A cumulative risk model must also recognize the protective factors that moderate children's responses to community violence. Consistently, clinical researchers have recognized the ameliorative effects that family support and cohesion have on the adverse consequences of community violence exposure among children (Buka et al., 2001; Horowitz et al., 2005; Plybon & Kliewer, 2001).With the risks associated with bullying, victimization, anti-social and violent peers, and substance use on older children, O'Donnell, Schwab-Stone, and Muyeed (2002) identified three key factors favoring children's resilience: parental support; school support; and peer support. Importantly, the expanding empirical research on characteristics of schools and neighborhoods that are linked with positive youth development has potential implications for health promotion interventions at the community level (Gershoff & Aber, 2006).

Risks to women

Despite a burgeoning research literature on the mental health consequences of community violence for young children and adolescents, much less attention had been paid to its impact on adults. The lack is especially notable for women, given their role in protecting their children from the consequences of violence. Data from primary healthcare settings in urban communities underscore the heightened utilization by low-income women of a wide range of stress-related health and mental health visits that are associated with the experience of neighborhood-based threats to safety (Clark, Ryan, Kawachi, Canner, Berkman, & Wright, 2007; Johnson, Solomon, Shields, McDonald, McKenzie, & Gielen, 2009). The National Women's Study found that 21% of urban women report witnessing serious injury or death, and there is a heightened risk for PTSD among those experiencing directly life-threatening traumatic events (Resnick et al., 1993; Ruggiero, Van Wynsbergh, Stevens, & Kilpatrick, 2006). While the greater risk of women for PTSD was reported in the NCS (Kessler et al., 1995), the specific effect of community violence on PTSD and other mental health problems (e.g., depression, anxiety) is not well known.

A study of a cohort of 1,000 city-dwelling, Latina mothers of very young children for their exposure to community violence found that 66% had witnessed significant community violence that increased their likelihood for clinically meaningful anxiety or depressive symptoms (Clark et al., 2007). These Latina mothers also had an increased likelihood for mental health symptoms from being victims of domestic violence, an effect that was independent of their exposure to violence in the community. However, this study, along with several others (Bogat, Leahy, Von Eye, Maxwell, Levendosky, & Davidson, 2005), recognizes the frequent co-occurrence of neighborhood violence with victimization by domestic violence. These findings highlight the need to address multiple sources of violence exposure as triggers for traumatic stress responses among women (and their families) living in urban neighborhoods with ongoing violence. Bogat and colleagues (2005) examined the relationship of community crime (using police reports of aggravated assault and disorderly conduct), mental health problems of women in those communities, and the severity of domestic violence victimization. They found that increasing severity of domestic violence victimization was consistently associated with worsening of mental health outcomes, but community violence alone did not influence measurements of these women's mental health.

Intimate partner violence

Increasingly over the past decade, research has been addressing the specific health and mental health consequences that low-income women living in inner-city neighborhoods face from direct domestic violence victimization, now generally referred to as intimate partner violence (IPV) (Bogat, Levendosky, Theran, von Eye, & Davidson, 2003; Bogat et al., 2005; Campbell, 2002; Dutton, Kaltman, Goodman, Weinfurt, & Vankos, 2005; Kessler, Molnar, Feurer, & Appelbaum, 2001; Sutherland, Bybee, & Sullivan,

2002). Collectively, these studies find that women who have experienced IPV have comparatively greater levels of psychological distress, including anxiety, depression, PTSD, substance use, and lowered self-esteem. IPV is clearly a serious health issue and public health challenge as it affects about 30% of adult women over a lifetime and between 2 and 10% of women annually (Rennison, 2001; Tjaden & Thoennes, 2000).

A number of studies underscore the unique and even greater impact that emotional and psychological abuse may have on women's mental well-being as compared to physical abuse (Martinez, Garcia-Linares, & Pico-Alfonso, 2004; O'Leary, 1999; Sackett & Saunders, 1999; Street & Arias, 2001). Controlling for physical and sexual abuse, emotional abuse has an independent effect on the development of PTSD (Dutton, Goodman, & Bennet, 2001; Hedin & Janson, 1999; Sutherland et al., 2002), and in some studies, emotional abuse is perceived by women as more harmful than physical abuse (O'Leary, 1999; Street & Arias, 2001).

Women reporting childhood abuse are at greater risk for IPV, both physical and emotional, in their adulthood (Bensley, Van Eenwyk, Wynkoop, & Simmons, 2003; Desai, Arias, Thompson, & Basile, 2002). Pico-Alfonso (2005) highlights the relational revictimization that occurs for women with histories of child abuse and adult IPV. Women previously victimized by child sexual abuse have a markedly increased risk for PTSD in adulthood, and IPV may be mediated by the PTSD symptomatology and other psychological sequelae of the childhood trauma. Rowan, Foy, Rod-riguez, and Ryan (1994) found that childhood sexual abuse is a more fre-quent antecedent to PTSD than physical abuse. Despite efforts to separate the components of abuse in childhood and in adulthood (physical, sexual, emotional), most often a pattern of co-occurring, repeated, and cumulative abuse experiences places children and adults at great risk for revictimiza-tion and significant adverse health and mental health outcomes.

An extensive report on IPV against women in New York City found that from 2003 to 2005, nearly half of fatal violence against women (44%) was confirmed to be the result of IPV, with black and Hispanic women more than twice as likely as women of other racial/ethnic groups to be killed or injured by an intimate partner (Stayton, Olson, Thorpe, Kerker, Henning, & Wilt, 2008). Only 15% of women killed by an intimate partner had a court-issued Order of Protection. Additionally, in 2005, nearly 4,000 New York City women were treated in emergency depart-ments from injuries that they acknowledged were due to IPV. Many more were treated for assault injuries of unknown origin. Overall, women living in neighborhoods with very low median household income had at least twice the IPV-related death, hospitalization, and emergency department visit rates compared to women living in higher income neighborhoods.

There is growing awareness of the public health challenge of IPV as a serious and disturbingly prevalent risk to the health and mental health of women, especially those in low-income, inner-city neighborhoods; it is equally important to recognize the harm to the physical and mental well-being of their exposed children. In the U.S., more than 15 million children are living in families where IPV occurred during the previous year (McDonald, Jouriles, Ramisett-Mikler, Caetano, & Green, 2006). Physical and psychological aggression in IPV each have direct and indirect influences on the emergence of child behavior problems. Several studies have found that the adverse effects of psychological aggression on children's externalizing and internalizing behavior problems are mediated by maternal distress and are beyond the effects of physical aggression alone (Clarke, Koenen, Taft, Street, King, & King, 2007; Levendosky & Graham-Bermann, 2001; Panuzio, Taft, Black, Koenen, & Murphy, 2007).

The interrelationship of maternal distress with dysfunctional parenting behavior can be synergistic in promoting emotional and behavioral problems among children in trauma-exposed families. Parenting behavior influences young children's attachment style and behavior, which is developmentally associated with children's social and emotional functioning (Levendosky, Leahy, Bogat, Davidson, & von Eye, 2006). Maternal distress undermines a mother's ability to be sensitively attuned to her children's emotional needs and their subsequent ability to self-regulate emotions (Little & Carter, 2005). A number of research studies describe the adverse effects of IPV on the social and emotional development of infants and toddlers. DeJonghe, Bogat, Levendosky, von Eye, and Davidson (2005) report that infants exposed to IPV show greater distress reactions to other adult conflict than those not living in homes with IPV. Levendosky and colleagues (2006) found that even experiences of IPV during pregnancy are associated with infant externalizing behavior at age one. The authors posit that stress-induced physiological changes occurring *in utero* and ongoing parenting behavior may mediate these infant behavioral problems.

Taken together, the studies on families affected by IPV are consistent with the large body of literature that links maternal mental health and parenting behavior to critical outcomes of child health and development. Child-rearing in inner-city neighborhoods, with ongoing exposure to community violence and threats to safety, is burdened with multiple parenting-related stressors that require considerable social, financial, and health care resources (Mistry, Stevens, Sareen, DeVogli, & Halfon, 2007).

Resilience resources in inner-city communities

Stress and coping process research in the last two decades has increasingly focused on the adaptive strengths and capacity for resilience at the individual, family, and community levels (Holahan & Moos, 1994; King, King, Fairbank, Keane, & Adams, 1998; Norris & Kaniasty, 1996; Wandersman & Nation, 1998). Psychosocial resources are widely recognized as central to current conceptualizations of stress and coping processes, and resource losses are associated with negative life events and declines in mental health (Hobfoll, Johnson, Ennis, & Jackson, 2003; Holahan, Moos, Holahan, & Cronkite, 1999). A number of cross-sectional studies of natural disasters (e.g., Hurricane Hugo; Hurricane Andrew; Sierra Madre earthquake) discovered that material and psychosocial resource losses are associated with increased levels of psychological distress, including depression and PTSD (Freedy, Shaw, Jarrell, & Masters, 1992; Freedy, Saladin, Kilpatrick, Resnick, & Saunders, 1994; Ironson, Wymings, Schneiderman, Baum, Rodriguez, Greenwood, et al., 1997). Additionally, resource loss was identified in some studies as mediating the worsening psychological sequelae of negative life events (King et al., 1998; Norris & Kaniasty, 1996).

Hobfoll and Vaux (1993); and Hobfoll, Freedy, Green, and Solomon (1996) proposed a conservation of resources (COR) theory that has been applied to the onset and persistence of both PTSD and depression among traumatized inner-city women (Hobfoll & Vaux, 2003; Walter & Hobfoll, 2009). In the COR formulation, people are driven to obtain and protect their valued resources and to act to minimize loss and maximize resource gain. Traumatic stressors (e.g., exposure directly or indirectly to community violence or IPV) are thought to weaken traumatized women's ability to maintain material and psychosocial resources, leading to elevated rates of PTSD and depression and a further downward resource spiral. Therefore, trauma triggers a rapid decline of available resources, which in turn further undermines recovery processes (Hobfoll et al., 2003). Interrupting this cycle of resource depletion and associated loss spirals can potentially stabilize and even reverse the persistence of stress responses and weakened capacity for recovery among inner-city families. In a 10-year longitudinal study, depression persisted for adults who continued to experience resource loss, while those who gained resources across the 10 years were likely to recover from depression (Holahan et al., 1999).

Walter and Hobfoll (2009) followed 102 inner-city women who initially met diagnostic criteria for PTSD over a six-month period without psychological treatment. Women who recovered from their PTSD diagnosis had significantly less resource loss at the six-month follow up than did women whose symptoms did not improve. The study highlights some possible naturalistic processes that may enable people to recover from their stress-induced mental disorder. Additionally, it recognizes resilience resources as changing and variable as individuals attempt to cope and recover from their psychological distress.

Given the value of maintaining material and psychosocial resources in promoting resistance to trauma, further study of the dynamics underlying both "resource protection" and "resource recovery" will further our ability to support families regularly exposed to these stressors. The relationship of social support and mental health has received wide attention (Cohen, 2004; Kawachi & Berkman, 2001), and Alim, Feder, Adriana, Graves,

Wang, Weaver, et al. (2008) examined psychosocial factors associated with resistance to traumatic stressors, providing insight into the processes of resilience and recovery. In a study of 259 high-risk, African American adults exposed to a range of severe traumas, a sense of "purpose in life" was strongly associated with both resilient and recovered status. However, sense of mastery and active coping strategies were associated with recovery (past DSM-IV disorder, but none currently) but not resilience (absence of any lifetime DSM-IV disorder). Resilient individuals manifested a dispositional trait of optimism and were more likely to be attendees of religious services. The authors posit that recovery reflects a more active and "effortful" process than the experience of resilient individuals, who have access to more stable and stress-resistant psychosocial supports.

Recovery from cumulative and severe trauma exposure can also provide insight regarding intervention models for affected families. In a large retrospective study of 777 women, those who reported either child abuse or adult rape were at greater risk for major depression (three times greater) and PTSD (six to seven times greater) than women without trauma histories (Schumm, Briggs-Phillips, & Hobfall, 2006). Furthermore, child abuse was a significant risk factor for adult rape, and when women reported trauma during both periods, their risk for PTSD was increased by a factor of 17. The compounding of PTSD symptoms by cumulative trauma across developmental stages underscores the interwoven nature of exposure to trauma. Schumm and colleagues (2006) found significantly lower rates of PTSD and depression among women who had been exposed to cumulative trauma in both childhood and adult life but who also reported high degrees of social support. These findings suggest a potentially critical phase for interventions with young adult urban women whose abuse histories in childhood place them at further risk for revictimization in their interpersonal relationships and undermine their capacity to maintain supportive psychosocial resources.

Strengthening 'at-risk' families

The consensus from the research literature regarding the mental and physical well-being of families living in highly stressful, inner-city neighborhoods points to the balance among complex risk and protective factors that children and parents encounter in their daily lives. For young children and adolescents, exposure to family and community violence has been linked with a number of internalizing and externalizing psychological and behavioral problems; nevertheless, some who are exposed will adapt well. This highlights the need to develop service delivery models that proactively screen "at-risk" families with very young children for signs of psychological distress and promote interventions that provide relationship-based treatment for parents and young children affected by traumatic or toxic stress.

At the community level, significant progress in developing family-focused service delivery has been made for women and children victimized by IPV. Shelter-based care has been the model most adapted to protect women and children from violent domestic partners. To a degree, domestic violence policy makers have resisted the involvement of mental health professionals in order not to pathologize the victims of domestic violence. Nevertheless, partnerships of community, religious, educational, health, mental health, and social service leadership are needed to develop violence prevention and victim assistance programs that reflect and build upon the strengths of communities.

Children and families in inner-city settings who are identified, often by school authorities, as needing evaluation for psychological symptoms or behavioral problems face barriers to mental health care. Indeed, there is a low rate of follow-up with mental health professionals. In a study of high-risk, inner-city youth referred for mental health services, McKay, Lynn, and Bannon (2005) found that service use for youth and their families had no relationship to the number of mental health issues, stressors, or level of identified trauma exposure. In the study, 28% of youth accepted for services were never seen for an initial appointment. Research on the factors prompting parents to link their children with mental health services is minimal (Landsverk, Madsen, Litrownki, Ganger, & Newton, 1998). Thus, we have little information on how parenting-related stressors, parental mental health problems, and access to material and psychosocial resources influence the ability of inner-city families to address child-identified mental health needs.

Mistry and colleagues (2007) used data from the 2000 National Survey of Early Childhood Health (NSECH), a cross-sectional telephone survey of parents of more than 2,000 infants and toddlers, to examine associations between maternal mental health, parenting stressors, social and financial resources, and child health care access. Parenting stressors related to social and financial factors are disproportionately prevalent among low-income families and increased the risk of poor maternal health. Building on the work of Waddell, Shannon, and Durr (2001), the authors advocate at the community level for family resource centers that can provide "a single portal for families to access a network of community support services" (p. 1265).

Family-focused service delivery requires identifying "at-risk" parents and their young children in order to screen for stress-related mental health problems and provide linkage with a network of services that can address material and psychosocial supports and resources. Services that are components of a continuum that supports family strengths and resilient functioning may better allow parents to meet their children's developmental needs (Conroy & Brown, 2004). Such services could be initiated in multiple health care settings that engage children and families, including "well-baby", other pediatric, and family practice settings that offer a two-generation model that is family-focused, culturally informed, and accessible to vulnerable populations (Institute of Medicine, 2009).

However, developing family-focused care that integrates health, mental health, and social service systems will require demonstration projects at the community, state, and federal levels to test the efficiency and efficacy of new service delivery models and must also address existing systemic, work-force, and fiscal barriers.

Exposure to traumatic stressors does not lead to psychopathology and impairments in most people; thus, a research agenda to better understand resilience in the face of adversity at the level of individuals, families, and communities is needed. A strong consensus has emerged from a burgeoning literature that violence in our inner-city neighborhoods and communities with its variety and range of behaviors, intensity, and perceived threat to safety has wide-ranging influences on children and their families, Such studies provide an empirical basis for prevention and intervention programs for children and families that can help neutralize the consequences of these exposures and strengthen resilience mechanisms over time and across generations.

References

Aisenberg, E., & Herrenkoh, T. (2008). Community violence in context: Risk and resilience in children and families. *Journal of Interpersonal Violence, 23*(3), 296–315.

Alim, T. N., Feder, A. F., Graves, R. E., Wang, Y., Weaver, J., et al. (2008). Trauma, resilience, and recovery in a high-risk African American population. *American Journal of Psychiatry, 165*(12), 1566–1575.

American Psychiatric Association. (1980). *Diagnostic and statistical manual of mental disorders (DSM-III)* (3rd ed.). Washington, DC: American Psychiatric Press.

American Psychiatric Association. (1994). *Diagnostic and statistical manual of mental disorders (DSM-IV)* (4th ed.). Washington, DC: American Psychiatric Press.

Bell, C. (1995). Exposure to violence distresses children and may lead to their becoming violent. *Psychiatric News, 30*, 6–18.

Bensley, L., Van Eenwyk, J., & Wynkoop, K. W., & Simmons, K. (2003). Childhood family violence history and women's risk for intimate partner violence and poor health. *American Journal of Preventive Medicine, 25*, 38–44.

Bogat, G. A., Leahy, L., Von Eye, A., Maxwell, C., Levendosky, A. A., & Davidson, W. S. (2005). The influence of community violence on the functioning of women experiencing domestic violence. *American Journal of Community Psychology, 36*, 123–132.

Bogat, G. A., Levendosky, A. A., Theran, S., von Eye, A., & Davidson, W. S. (2003). Predicting the psychosocial effects of interpersonal partner violence (IPV): How much does a woman's history of IPV matter? *Journal of Interpersonal Violence, 18*, 121–142.

Breslau, N., Kessler, R. C., Chilcoat, H. D., Schultz, L. R., David, G. C., & Andreski, P. (1998). Trauma and posttraumatic stress disorder in the community: The 1996 Detroit area survey of trauma. *Archives of General Psychiatry, 55*, 626–632.

Briere, J., & Elliott, D. M. (1997). Psychological assessment of interpersonal victimization effects in adults and children. *Psychiatry: Theory, Research and Practice, 34*, 353–364.

Brown, J. R., Hill, H. M., & Lambert, S. F. (2005). Traumatic stress symptoms in women exposed to community and partner violence. *Journal of Interpersonal Violence, 20*, 1478–1494.

Buka, S. L., Stichick, T. L., Birdthistle, I., & Earls, F. J. (2001). Youth exposure to violence: Prevalence, risks, and consequences. *American Journal of Orthopsychiatry, 71*, 298–310.

Campbell, J. C. (2002). Health consequences of intimate partner violence. *Lancet, 359*, 1331–1336.

Clark, C., Ryan, L., Kawachi, I., Canner, M. J., Berkman, L., & Wright, R. J. (2007). Witnessing community violence in residential neighborhoods: A mental health hazard for urban women. *Journal of Urban Health, 85*, 22–38.

Clarke, S. B., Koenen, K. C., Taft, C. T., Street, A. E., King, L. A., & King, D. W. (2007). Intimate partner psychological aggression and child behavior problems. *Journal of Traumatic Stress, 20*(1), 97–101.

Cohen, S. (2004). Social relationships and health. *American Psychologist, 59*, 676–684.

Conroy, M. A., & Brown, W. H. (2004). Early identification, prevention, and early intervention with young children at risk for emotional or behavioral disorders: Issues, trends, and a call to action. *Behavioral Disorders, 29*, 224–236.

DeJonghe, E., Bogat, G. A., Levendosky, A. A., von Eye, A., & Davidson, W. S. (2005). Infant exposure to domestic violence predicts heightened sensitivity to adult verbal conflict. *Infant Mental Health Journal, 26*, 268–281.

Desai, S., Arias, I., Thompson, M. P., & Basile, K. C. (2002). Childhood victimization and subsequent adult re-victimization assessed in a nationally representative sample of women and men. *Violence Victims, 17*, 639–653.

Dickinson, L. M., de Gruy, F. V., Dickinson, W. P., & Candib, L. M. (1998). Complex posttraumatic stress disorder: Evidence from the primary care setting. *General Hospital Psychiatry, 20*, 214–224.

DuRant, R. H., Pendergrast, R. A., & Cadenhead, C. (1994). Exposure to violence and victimization and fighting behavior by urban black adolescents. *Journal of Adolescent Health, 15*, 311–318.

Dutton, M. A., Goodman, L. A., & Bennet, L. (2001). Court-involved battered women's responses to violence: The role of psychological, physical and sexual abuse. In K. D. O'Leary & R. D. Mairuro (Eds.), *Psychological abuse in violent and domestic relations* (pp. 177–196). New York: Springer Publishing Company.

Dutton, M. A., Kaltman, S., Goodman, L. A., Weinfurt, K., & Vankos, N. (2005). Patterns of intimate partner violence: Correlates and outcomes. *Violence and Victims, 20*, 483–497.

Freedy, J. R., Kilpatrick, D. G., & Resnick, H. S. (1993). Natural disaster and mental health: Theory, assessment, and intervention. *Journal of Social Behavior and Personality, 8*(5), 49–103.

Freedy, J. R., Saladin, M. E., Kilpatrick, D. G., Resnick, H. S., & Saunders, B. E. (1994). Understanding acute psychological distress following natural disaster. *Journal of Traumatic Stress, 7*, 257–73.

Freedy, J. R., Shaw, D., Jarrell, M. P., & Masters, C. (1992). Towards an understanding of the psychological impact of natural disaster: An application of the conservation resources stress model. *Journal of Traumatic Stress, 5*, 441–454.

Freudenberg, N., Galea, S., & Vlahov, D. (Eds.). (2006). *Cities and the health of the public*. Nashville, TN: Vanderbilt University Press.

Gershoff, E. T., & Aber, J. L. (2006). Neighborhoods and schools: Contexts and consequences for the mental health and risk behaviors of children and youth. In L. Balter & C. Tamis-LeMonda (Eds.), *Child psychology: A handbook of contemporary issues* (2nd Ed.) (pp. 611–645). New York: Psychology Press/Taylor & Francis.

Gilvarry, E. (2000). Substance abuse in young people. *Journal of Child Psychology and Psychiatry, 41*, 55–80.

Hamblen, J., & Goguen, C. (2010). *Community Violence Online Fact Sheet of the National Center for PTSD*. Retrieved from www.ptsd.va.gov/professional/pages/community-violence.asp.

Hedin, L. W., & Janson, P. O. (1999). The invisible wounds: The occurrence of psychological abuse and anxiety compared with previous experience of physical abuse during the childbearing year. *Journal of Psychosomatic Obstetric Gynecology, 20*, 136–144.

Herman, J. L. (1992a). Complex PTSD: A syndrome in survivors of prolonged and repeated trauma. *Journal of Traumatic Stress, 3*(1), 377–391.

Herman, J. L. (1992b). *Trauma and recovery*. New York, NY: Basic Books.

Hobfoll, S. E., Freedy, J. R., Green, B. L., & Solomon, S. D. (1996). Coping in reaction to extreme stress: The roles of resource loss and resource availability. In M. Zeidner and N. Endler (Eds.), *Handbook of coping: Research, theory, and application* (pp. 322–349). New York: Wiley.

Hobfoll, S. E., Johnson, R. J., Ennis, N. E., & Jackson, A. P. (2003). Resource loss, resource gain, and emotional outcomes among inner-city women. *Journal of Personality and Social Psychology, 84*, 632–643.

Hobfoll, S. E., & Vaux, A. (1993). Social support: Social resources and social context. In L. Goldberger & S. Breznitz (Eds.), *Handbook of stress: Theoretical and clinical aspects* (pp. 685–705). New York: Free Press.

Holahan, C. J., & Moos, R. H. (1994). Life stressors and mental health: Advances in conceptualizing stress resistance. In W. R. Avison & I. H. Gotlib (Eds.), *Stress and mental health: Contemporary issues and prospects for the future* (pp. 213–238). New York: Plenum.

Holahan, C. J., Moos, R. H., Holahan, C. K., & Cronkite, R. C. (1999). Resource loss, resource gain, and emotional outcomes among inner-city women. *Journal of Personality and Social Psychology, 77*, 620–629.

Horowitz, K., Weine, S.M., & Jekel, J. (1995). PTSD symptoms in urban adolescent girls: Compounded community trauma. *Journal of the American Academy of Child and Adolescent Psychiatry, 34*, 1353–1361.

Horowitz, K., McKay, M., & Marshall, R. (2005). Community violence and urban families: Experiences, effects, and directions for intervention. *American Journal of Orthopsychiatry, 75*(3), 356–368.

Institute of Medicine (IOM) (2009). *Depression in parents, parenting, and children: Opportunities to improve identification, treatment, and prevention*. Washington, DC: National Academies Press.

Ironson, G., Wymings, C., Schneiderman, N., Baum, A., Rodriguez, M., Greenwood, et al. (1997). Posttraumatic stress symptoms, intrusive thoughts, loss, and immune function after Hurricane Andrew. *Psychosomatic Medicine, 59*, 128–141.

Jenkins, E. J., & Bell, C. C. (1997). Exposure and response to community violence among children and adolescents. In J. Osofsky (Ed.), *Children in a violent society* (pp. 9–31). New York: Guilford Press.

Johnson, S. L., Solomon, B. S., Shields, W. C., McDonald, E. M., McKenzie, L. B., & Gielen, A. C. (2009). Neighborhood violence and its association with mothers' health: Assessing the relative importance of perceived safety and exposure to violence. *Journal of Urban Health, 86*, 538–550.

Kawachi, I., & Berkman, L. F. (2001). Social ties and mental health. *Journal of Urban Health, 78*, 458–467.

Kessler, R. C., Molnar, B. E., Feurer, I. D., & Appelbaum, M. (2001). Patterns and mental health predictors of domestic violence in the United States: Results from the National Comorbidity Survey. *International Journal of Law and Psychiatry, 24*, 487–508.

Kessler, R. C., Sonnega, A., Bromet, E., Hughes, M., & Nelson, C. B. (1995). Post-traumatic stress disorder in the national comorbidity survey. *Archives of General Psychiatry, 52*, 1048–1060.

Kilpatrick, D. G., Aciero, R., Saunders, B., Resnick, H., Best, C., & Schnurr, P. P. (2000). Risk factors for adolescent substance abuse and dependence: Data from a national sample. *Journal of Consulting and Clinical Psychology, 68*, 19–30.

Kilpatrick, D. G., Saunders, B. E., Amick-McMullan, A., Best, C. L., Veronen, L. J., & Resnick, H. S. (1989). Victim and crime factors associated with the development of crime-related post-traumatic stress disorder. *Behavior Therapy, 20*, 199–214.

King, L. A., King, D. W., Fairbank, J. A., Keane, T. M., & Adams, G. A. (1998). Resilience-recovery factors in post-traumatic stress disorder among female and male Vietnam veterans: Hardiness, postwar social support, and additional stressful life events. *Journal of Personality and Social Psychology, 74*, 420–434.

Kulka, R. A., Schlenger, W. E., Fairbank, J. A., Hough, R. L., Jordan, B. K., & Marmar, C. R. (1990). *Trauma and the Vietnam War generation: Report of findings from the National Vietnam Veterans Readjustment Study*. New York: Brunner/Mazel.

Landsverk, J., Madsen, J., Litrownik, A., Ganger, W., & Newton, R. (1998). Mental health problems of foster children. *Journal of Child and Family Studies, 7*, 283–296.

Levendosky, A. A., & Graham-Bermann, S. A. (2001). Parenting in battered women: The effects of domestic violence on women and their children. *Journal of Family Violence, 16*, 171–192.

Levendosky, A. A., Leahy, K. L., Bogat, A., Davidson, W. S., & von Eye, A. (2006). Domestic violence, maternal parenting, maternal mental health, and infant externalizing behavior. *Journal of Family Psychology, 20*, 544–552.

Linares, L. O., Heeren, T., Bronfman, E., Zuckerman, B., Augustyn, M., & Tronick, E. (2001). A mediational model for the impact of exposure to community violence on early child behavior problems. *Child Development, 72*(2), 639–652.

Little, C., & Carter, A. S. (2005). Negative emotional reactivity and regulation in 12-month olds following emotional challenge: Contributions of maternal-infant emotional availability in a low-income sample. *Infant Mental Health Journal, 26*, 354–388.

Lynch, M. (2003). Consequences of children's exposure to community violence. *Clinical Child & Family Psychology Review, 6*, 187–194.

Lynch, M., & Cicchetti, D. (1998). An ecological-transactional analysis of children and contexts: The longitudinal interplay among child maltreatment, community violence, and children's symptomatology. *Developmental Psychopathology, 10*(2), 235–257.

Margolin, G. (1998). Effects of witnessing violence on children. In P. K. Trickett & C. J. Schellenbach (Eds.), *Violence against children in the family and the community* (pp. 57–102). Washington, DC: American Psychological Association.

Margolin, G., & Gordis, E. B. (2000). The effects of family and community violence on children. *Annual Review of Psychology, 51*, 445–479.

Martinez, M., Garcia-Linares, M. I., & Pico-Alfonso, M. A. (2004). Women victims of domestic violence: Consequences for their health and the role of the health system. In R. Klein & B. Wallner (Eds.), *Conflict, gender, and violence* (pp. 127–155). Vienna: Studien-Verlag.

McDonald, R., Jouriles, E. N., Ramisetty-Mikler, S., Caetano, R., & Green, C. E. (2006). Estimating the number of American children living in partner-violent families. *Journal of Family Psychology, 20*, 137–142.

McKay, M. M., Lynn, C. J., & Bannon, W. M. (2005). Understanding inner city child mental health need and trauma exposure: Implications for preparing urban service providers. *American Journal of Orthopsychiatry, 75*(2), 201–210.

Miller, L. S., Wasserman, G. A., Neugebauer, R., Gorman-Smith, D., & Kamboukos, D. (1999). Witnessed community violence and anti-social behavior in high-risk urban boys. *Journal of Clinical and Child Psychology, 28*, 2–11.

Mistry, R., Stevens, G. D., Sareen, H., DeVogli, R., & Halfon, N. (2007). Parenting-related stressors and self-reported mental health of mothers with young children. *American Journal of Public Health, 97*(7), 1261–1268.

Moses, A. (1999). Exposure to violence, depression, and hostility in a sample of inner city high school youth. *Journal of Adolescence, 22*, 21–32.

Murali, R., & Chen, E. (2005). Exposure to violence and cardiovascular and neuroendocrine measures in adolescents. *Annals of Behavioral Medicine, 30*, 155–163.

Norris, F. H. (1992). Epidemiology of trauma: Frequency and impact of different potentially traumatic events on different demographic groups. *Journal of Consulting Clinical Psychology, 60*, 409–418.

Norris, F. H., & Kaniasty, K. (1994). Psychological distress following criminal victimization in the general population: Cross-sectional, longitudinal, and prospective analyses. *Journal of Consulting and Clinical Psychology, 62*, 111–123.

Norris, F. H., & Kaniasaty, K. (1996). Received and perceived social support in times of stress: A test of the social support deterioration deterrence model. *Journal of Personality and Social Psychology, 71*, 498–511.

O'Donnell, D. A., Schwab-Stone, M. E., & Muyeed, A. Z. (2002). Multidimensional resilience in urban children exposed to community violence. *Child Development, 73*, 1265–1282.

O'Leary, K. D. (1999). Psychological abuse: A variable deserving critical attention in domestic violence. *Violence Victims, 14*, 3–23.

Osofsky, J. (2003). Prevalence of children's exposure to domestic violence and child maltreatment: Implications for prevention and intervention. *Clinical Child and Family Psychology Review, 6*, 161–170.

Panuzio, J., Taft, C. T., Black, D. A., Koenen, K. C., & Murphy, C. M. (2007). Relationship abuse and victim's posttraumatic stress disorder symptoms: Associations with child behavior problems. *Journal of Family Violence, 22*, 177–185.

Pelcovitz, D., van der Kolk, B., Roth, S., Mandel, F., Kaplan, S., & Resick, P. (1997). Development of a criteria set and a structured interview for disorders of extreme stress (SIDES). *Journal of Traumatic Stress, 10*, 3–16.

Pico-Alfonso, M. A. (2005). Psychological intimate partner violence: The major predictor of posttraumatic stress disorder in abused women. *Neuroscience and Biobehavioral Reviews, 29*, 181–193.

Plybon, L., & Kliewer, W. (2001). Neighborhood types and externalizing behavior in urban school-age children: Tests of direct, mediated, and moderated effects. *Journal of Child and Family Studies, 10*, 429–437.

Pynoos, R. S., Goenjian, A., Tashjian, M., Karakashian, M., Manjikian, R., Manoukian, G., et al. (1993). Posttraumatic stress reactions in children after the 1988 Armenian earthquake. *British Journal of Psychiatry, 163*, 239–247.

Rahe, R. H. (1993). Acute versus chronic post-traumatic stress disorder. *Integral Physiological Behavioral Science, 28*, 46–56.

Rennison, C. M. *Intimate Partner Violence and Age of Victim, 1993–99* (2001). Washington, D.C.: Bureau of Justice Statistics, U.S. Department of Justice.

Resnick, H. S., Kilpatrick, D. G., Dansky, B. S., Saunders, B. F., & Best, C. L. (1993). *Journal of Consulting and Clinical Psychology, 61*, 984–991.

Roth, S., Newman, E., Pelcovitz, D., van der Kolk, B., & Mandel, F. S. (1997). Complex PTSD in victims exposed to sexual and physical abuse: Results from the DSM-IV field trial for posttraumatic stress disorder. *Journal of Traumatic Stress, 10*, 539–555.

Rowan, A. B., Foy, D. W., Rodriguez, N., & Ryan, S. (1994). Posttraumatic stress disorder in a clinical sample of adults sexually abused as children. *Child Abuse Neglect, 18*, 51–61.

Ruggiero, K. J., Van Wynsbergh, A., Stevens, T., & Kilpatrick, D. G. (2006). Traumatic stressors in urban settings: Consequences and implications. In N. Freudenberg, S. Galea, & D. Vlahov (Eds.), *Cities and the health of the public* (pp. 225–246). Nashville, TN: Vanderbilt University Press.

Sackett, L. A., & Saunders, D. G. (1999). The impact of different forms of psychological abuse on battered women. *Violence Victims, 14*, 105–17.

Schumm, J. A., Briggs-Phillips, M., & Hobfoll, S. E. (2006). Cumulative interpersonal traumas and social support as risk and resiliency factors in predicting PTSD and depression among inner-city women. *Journal of Traumatic Stress, 19*, 825–836.

Schwab-Stone, M., Chen, C., Greenberger, E., Silver, D., Lichtman, J., & Voyce, C. (1999). No safe haven: The effects of violence exposure on urban youth. *Journal of the American Academy of Child and Adolescent Psychiatry, 38*, 359–367.

Schwartz, E. D., & Kowalski, J. M. (1991). Malignant memories: PTSD in children and adults after a school shooting. *Journal of the American Academy of Child and Adolescent Psychiatry, 30*, 936–944.

Sheehan, D., DiCara, J., LeBaily, S., & Christoffel, K. (1997). Children's exposure to violence in an urban setting. *Archives of Pediatrics and Adolescent Medicine, 151*, 502–504.

Stayton, C., Olson, C., Thorpe, I., Kerker, B., Henning, K., & Wilt, S. (2008). *Intimate partner violence against women in New York City, 2008*. Report from the New York City Department of Health and Mental Hygiene, New York.

Street, A. E., & Arias, I. (2001). Psychological abuse and posttraumatic stress disorder in battered women: Examining the roles of shame and guilt. *Violence Victims, 16*, 65–78.

Suglia, S. F., Ryan, L., Laden, F., Dawson, J., & Wright, R. J. (2008). Violence exposure, a chronic psychosocial stressor, and childhood lung function. *Psychosomatic Medicine, 70*, 160–169.

Sutherland, C. A., Bybee, D. I., & Sullivan, C. M. (2002). Beyond bruises and broken bones: The joint effects of stress and injuries on battered women's health. *American Journal of Community Psychology, 30*, 609–636.

Tjaden, P. G., & Thoennes, N. (2000). *Full report of the prevalence, incidence, and consequences of violence against women: Findings from the national violence against women survey.* Washington, D.C.: U.S. Department of Justice, Office of Justice Programs, National Institute of Justice.

van der Kolk, B., Pelcovitz, D., Roth, S., Mandel, F., McFarlane, A., & Herman, J. L. (1996). Dissociation, affect dysregulation, and somatization: The complexity of adaptation trauma. *American Journal of Psychiatry, 153*(7 Suppl.), 83–89.

van der Kolk, B., Roth, S., Pelcovitz, D., Sunday, S., & Spinazzola, J. (2005). Disorders of extreme stress: The empirical foundation of a complex adaptation to trauma. *Journal of Traumatic Stress, 18*, 389–399.

Waddell, B., Shannon, M., & Durr, R. (2001). *Using family resource centers to support California's young children and their families.* Center for Healthier Children, Families, and Community. Los Angeles, CA: University of California.

Walter, K. H., & Hobfoll, S. E. (2009). Resource loss and naturalistic reduction of PTSD among inner-city women. *Journal of Interpersonal Violence, 24*(3), 482–498.

Wandersman, A., & Nation, M. (1998). Urban neighborhoods and mental health: Psychological contributions to understanding toxicity, resilience, and interventions. *American Psychologist, 53*(6), 647–656.

Ward, C. L., Flisher, A. J., Zissis, C., Muller, M., & Lombard, C. (2001). Exposure to violence and its relationship to psychopathology in adolescents. *Injury Prevention, 7*, 297–301.

Wilson, H. W., Stover, C. S., & Berkowitz, S. J. (2009). The relationship between childhood violence exposure and juvenile antisocial behavior: A meta-analytic review. *Journal of Child Psychology and Psychiatry, 60*, 769–779.

Zinzow, H. M., Ruggiero, K. J., Hanson, R. F., Smith, D. W., Saunders B. E., & Kilpatrick, D. G. (2009). Witnessed community and parental violence in relation to substance use and delinquency in a national sample of adolescents. *Journal of Traumatic Stress, 22*, 525–533.

16 Public health and population approaches for suicide prevention

Eric D. Caine, Kerry L. Knox, and Yeates Conwell

Introduction

Now at the beginning of the second decade of the 21st century, the US is entering a critical developmental time in the field of suicide research and prevention. More than two decades have passed since the Centers for Disease Control and Prevention (CDC) began to highlight the burden of suicide as a critical public health concern (Centers for Disease Control and Prevention [CDC], 1992; Rosenberg, Gelles, Holinger, Zahn, Stark, Conn et al., 1987) and more than a decade since the World Health Organization (WHO) issued its pivotal report (World Health Organization [WHO], 1996). Governmental and nongovernmental efforts to prevent suicide have grown rapidly, inspired by resolutions in the Senate (SRes. 84; May 6, 1997) and the House (HRes. 212; October 10, 1998), by the Surgeon General's *Call to Action to Prevent Suicide* (Satcher, 1999), by the *National Strategy for Suicide Prevention* (Satcher, 2001), and by reports from the Institute of Medicine (Goldsmith, Pellmar, Kleinman, & Bunney, 2002; New Freedom Commission on Mental Health, 2003), the WHO (Krug, Mercy, Dahlberg, & Zwi, 2002). These also were followed in 2003 by a report from the President's New Freedom Commission on Mental Health (New Freedom Commission on Mental Health, 2003). Thus far, funding of more than $100 million through the Garrett Lee Smith Memorial Act has provided many states, tribes, universities, and schools with the resources to build suicide prevention programs for young people.

However, the vast bulk of suicide prevention activities have not been informed by any substantive evidence base (Brown, Wyman, Brinales, & Gibbons, 2007). With the exception of a few initiatives (Wyman, Brown, Inman, Cross, Schmeelk-Cone, Guo, & Pena, 2008), programs have not been promulgated using rigorously developed research designs. More systematic evaluations are underway, but these have yet to be published. Furthermore, most research efforts funded by the National Institutes of Health have focused on mechanisms for suicidal thoughts or behaviors (both biological and psychological) and therapeutics for suicidal individuals that are, by implication, mechanism-oriented. Too often suicidal behaviors have been viewed as epiphenomena of core psychiatric conditions, where attention to the presumed fundamental diagnostic state has been considered the primary focus for research and for therapeutic interventions. Now there is attention to proposed "endophenotypes" (Mann, Arango, Avenevoli, Brent, Champagne, Clayton, et al., 2009), described as more fundamental "proto-presentations" (our characterization), manifestations of fundamental, neurobiologically mediated behavioral constellations. Viewing suicide and attempted suicide as derivative targets for treatment also may have had the unintended consequence of closing off many mental health researchers and clinicians from exploring the benefits of public health and preventive interventions (Knox, Conwell, & Caine, 2004).

Thus, to date, most research has been grounded largely in a medical or clinical model, individual-focused, and primarily conducted inside the clinic or the therapy room. While this has great value, it does not provide knowledge suited to implementing large-scale suicide prevention efforts. In addition to treating acutely ill individuals, broad-based suicide prevention activities must have a community and a population focus, given that most people who have died by suicide either have not seen mental health providers or did not see them close to their time of death (Conwell et al., 1996; Luoma, Martin, & Pearson, 2002).

In this chapter, we review public health approaches to the prevention of suicide, focusing on a range of measures directed at

1   broader population groups where it is difficult to identify those who are suicidal or bear greater apparent risk and where the goals of intervention include culture and attitude change, as well as influence on individual behavior;
2   service-based selective interventions for vulnerable groups known to bear high risk – where some but not all of the members have the potential for suicide; and
3   indicated or clinical interventions for those individuals who have exhibited suicidal behaviors or, for example, for those experiencing inadequately treated depressive disorders or substance abuse.

We argue that these prevention strategies must have a two-fold purpose. They should strive to reduce the burden caused by an array of risk factors – family turmoil, school and work disruption, and substantial social pathology (e.g., violence in homes and communities), which are known to contribute to the development of psychopathology or to worsening psychiatric conditions and distress. Just as important, they must buttress protective factors that promote broader community, family, and individual health. Such protective factors buffer the effects of traumatic life events, psychopathology, and adverse environmental exposures. At its heart, we view suicide prevention as the "entry key" to the potentially much larger (though minimally developed) field of public health and preventive psychiatry.

The perspective from 2010

Worldwide, suicide accounts for more deaths annually than war and homicide combined (Krug, Mercy, Dahlberg, & Zwi, 2002). In the Epidemiologic Catchment Area (ECA) Study, 2.9% of subjects age 18 years and over reported having attempted suicide at some time in their lives (Moscicki, O'Carroll, Rae, Locke, Roy, & Regier, 1988), while the National Comorbidity Study (NCS) (1990–1992) and the National Comorbidity Study Replication (NCS-R) (2001–2003) found a 12-month reported prevalence of attempts among adults of 0.4% and 0.6%, respectively (Kessler, Berglund, Borges, Nock, & Wang, 2005). Of those who attempt suicide, 10 to 20% will make an additional attempt within one year; 1 to 2% will kill themselves within the year of an attempt; and approximately 10 to 15 % of suicide attempters will eventually die by their own hand (Fremouw, dePerczel, & Ellis, 1990).

Given current demographics, the greatest suicide-related social burden in terms of potential years of life lost involves men aged 20 to 54 years old and is often associated with chronic alcohol or substance misuse and its ravaging effects, including domestic violence, problems with parenting, and lost effectiveness in the workplace. Suicide and suicidal behaviors account for a major portion of the mortality and morbidity experienced by people suffering from mental and substance use disorders. In the US, these disorders collectively are associated with greater disease burden than either cardiovascular diseases or cancer (WHO, 2009).

Suicide was the 11th leading cause of death in the US in 2007, accounting for 34,598 deaths – surpassing more publically noted causes of mortality, such as homicide (18,381) or HIV (11,295) (CDC, 2010). Suicide is the third leading cause of death for 15 to 24 year olds, after unintentional injury and homicide, and it is second for 25 to 34 year olds, with unintentional injury and homicide as first and third, respectively. For those aged 35 to 44 years old, suicide is the fourth leading cause of death, after accidental death, malignant neoplasms, and cardiac diseases (CDC, 2010).

Data from the CDC point to a subtle but important change in the method for those in the middle years of life, with greater use of poisoning and a reduction in firearm suicides (CDC, 2007). Given the marked difference in case-fatality ratios between these methods (Elnour, 2008), this finding suggests that attempts very likely have increased. Recent data demonstrate that rates for both men and women in their middle years (aged 35 to 64) rose significantly from 1999 to 2007 (CDC, 2010). In 1999, the crude suicide rate in the US was 10.46 per 100,000 people; it hovered at or slightly above 11.0 from 2004 to 2006, and climbed to 11.48 in 2007. For those 34 years old or younger, rates decreased overall, except for a one-year increase among youth aged 15 to 24 years old in 2004, and a rise in 2007 among those 25 to 34 years old. The suicide rate for persons aged 65 years and older also declined during this period. However, increases in rates for middle-aged persons far outweighed the decreases in the younger and older populations. For those aged 35 to 64 years, there were steady annual increases from 1999 to 2007: Men climbed from 21.50 to 25.11 and women from 6.18 to 7.85, for a total change in those ages from 13.70 to 16.35 per 100,000. This 21st century increase followed a decade of decline in the 1990s, which started with rates in excess of 12 per 100,000 and experienced steady decreases to lows in 1999 and 2000, before the upward inflection.

Thus, there is an urgent need for public health-oriented research to prevent suicide.

The declines among youth and those over age 65 years are encouraging, but the factors that may explain them are most uncertain. While the comparison of NCS and NCS-R data found that "treatment increased dramatically" for "ideators who made a gesture" and for "ideators who made an attempt" (Kessler et al., 2005), this change has not translated into declines in deaths. Nor have death rates declined in any fashion that is proportionate to the substantial increase in national trends for outpatient treatment of depression (Baldessarini, Tondo, Strombom, Dominguez, Fawcett, Licinio, et al., 2007; Olfson & Marcus, 2009; Olfson, Marcus, Druss, Elinson, Tanielian, & Pincus, 2002).

The Suicide Prevention Resource Center (SPRC) is an engine to disseminate knowledge of best practices, as well as provide consultation to interested entities. Review of the SPRC's Best Practices Registry (BPR) For Suicide Prevention (www.sprc.org/featured_resources/bpr/index.asp), finds 11 "prevention initiatives" and three "treatment modalities." Of those, nine target youth specifically; two involve youth-oriented social skills curricula, one for high-risk youth and the other for Zuni Indian youth. Seven depend upon identifying high-risk youth in need of treatment. One effort researched the effect of psychotherapeutic interventions in primary care settings with elders (largely women, who have a very low suicide rate), and another focused on women with borderline personality disorder. One involved training for emergency rooms and another for hotlines.

Collectively, these screening or clinical approaches often are analogous to what we have described as "trying to catch people at the edge of the cliff," or if not at the edge, not far from it! Compounding this dilemma, no tool or measure has yet been designed that successfully identifies individuals at risk for suicide with sufficient sensitivity and specificity to be clinically useful (Pena & Caine, 2006; Pokorny, 1983). As we discuss later, the use of "risk factors" in current discussions about individually-oriented suicide prevention efforts fundamentally misunderstands their derivation or utility. Notably, the SPRC website lists the United States Air Force (USAF) as one of the programmatic efforts that is "evidence-based." While we have assessed the USAF initiative, and discuss it further below, it remains uncertain whether its lessons can be transported effectively to other settings, given that its effectiveness depended centrally on creating a cohesive strategic vision and having sufficient political will to drive the process forward in a concerted and sustained fashion.

There is considerable tension in the field between the need for action *now* to prevent suicide and the need for more evidence about what works (or not) in real-world settings, among populations, and among individuals at imminent risk. There also is tension within the research arena, involving long-held traditions of clinical research and the burgeoning demand for public health initiatives. It is essential to unify these seemingly disparate objectives through the development of novel, community-integrated research methods that lead to carefully constructed trials addressing the pressing needs of communities. These efforts also must be integrated with novel approaches to identifying and enrolling traditionally difficult-to-engage individuals, many of whom personally carry great risks for future adverse outcomes.

However, it remains difficult in the US to focus on broader population issues, given the mindset of policy makers and the public. For example, after the Food and Drug Administration required a "black box warning" for pediatric (and, subsequently, for young adult) use of antidepressants, many argued that such use was not truly associated with increased suicide and that the ruling paradoxically could lead to increased youth suicide rates (Gibbons, Hur, Bhaumik, & Mann, 2005; Libby, Brent, Morrato, Orton, Allen, & Valuck, 2007; Libby, Orton, & Valuck, 2009; Morrato, Libby, Orton, Degruy, Brent, Allen, & Valuck, 2008; Nemeroff, Kalali, Keller, Charney, Lenderts, & Cascade, 2007; Olfson, Marcus, & Druss, 2008; Rosack, 2005; Valuck, Libby, Orton, Morrato, Allen, & Baldessarini, 2007). Indeed, some asserted that it did, citing 2004 data (Gibbons, Brown, Hur, Marcus, Bhaumik, & Mann, 2007). However, CDC data since has shown a decline in youth suicide rates from 2005 to 2007 (CDC, 2010).

This simmering debate, by focusing on clinical treatment and speculation about a relatively smaller number of deaths, may have inadvertently downplayed the importance of developing new methods and interventions aimed at higher-risk populations that largely reside outside clinical treatment settings. It is highly probable that any increase in deaths due to medication-related, adverse events – if any – is far outweighed by the failure to effectively identify those in greatest need, given their numbers and lack of engagement. Put another way, the universe of unrecognized, unengaged, unassessed, and untreated is far larger than the pool of treated or might-be-treated, among which current therapeutic fluctuations occur.

The promise for suicide prevention in 2004

We view the year 2004 as a departure point, or reasonable "base year," for assessing national progress in suicide prevention. By then all of the major national proclamations and calls to action had been promulgated, the last major declaration having come in mid-2003 with publication of the report from the President's New Freedom Commission (New Freedom Commission on Mental Health, 2003). This report listed as Goal 1.1 "Advance and implement a national campaign to reduce the stigma of seeking care and a national strategy for suicide prevention." Two papers by our group (Knox et al., 2004; Knox, Litts, Talcott, Feig, & Caine, 2003) highlighted apparent significant progress in the field. The first, in December 2003, described the impact of the suicide prevention efforts of the United States Air Force, and the second, in January 2004, laid out in greater detail the potential structure for public health approaches to and charting the progress of suicide prevention, modeled after heart disease prevention efforts. July 2004 saw collaborative funding from the National Institute of Mental Health (NIMH), the National Institute on Drug Abuse, (NIDA), and the National Institute for Alcohol Abuse and Alcoholism (NIAAA) for three "developing centers" at Columbia University, the University of Pennsylvania, and the University of Rochester to research prevention and clinical intervention approach for suicide. The latter was public health and population oriented, while the first two targeted high-risk individuals. (Later changes in NIMH priorities led to a subsequent decision to discontinue funding for these programs.) The year also saw the opening of the National Suicide Prevention Lifeline (1–800–273-TALK), which was funded by SAMHSA, and in October 2004, Congress passed the Garrett Lee Smith (GLS) Memorial Act (Public Law 108–355, 118 Stat. 1404–1415), which authorized funding through SAMHSA for diverse state, tribal, and campus-based prevention initiatives. The legislation also assured further funding of the SPRC. Appropriations for GLS sponsored programs have continued since. Thus, one could argue that in 2004 the US was sufficiently prepared to make a dent in the relatively stable overall level of suicide-related mortality.

In our January 2004 paper (Knox et al., 2004), we compared high-risk and population-oriented approaches for preventing death or other adverse cardiovascular disease (CVD) outcomes (Gordon & Kannel, 1971; Gordon, Kannel, Dawber, & McGee, 1975; Gordon & Thom, 1975; Kannel & Gordon, 1982; Kannel, Gordon, & Castelli, 1981; Pearson, 2000; Wong, Black, & Gardin, 2000). For example, the high-risk approach to blood pressure control would entail identifying the relatively small number of individuals who constitute the 2.5% of the population occupying the upper end of the normally distributed blood pressure curve; intensive treatments aim to move them to the middle of the curve. Most cases of CVD, however, do not arise among these high-risk subjects but rather from the relatively "normal" blood pressure group (Rose, 1992). This phenomenon is in accord with what is called Rose's theorem: "a large number of people at small risk may give rise to more cases of disease than a small number who are at high risk" (Rose, 1985). Alone, the high-risk strategy identifies a minority of those individuals who die from cardiac disease and stroke and is palliative for those already identified as symptomatic, usually with temporary benefit. Only an alternative, radical approach aimed at shifting the entire population distribution of risk has resulted in significant reductions of CVD-related morbidity and mortality (Wong & Gardin, 2000).

With this framework in mind, preventive cardiology – our model for the prevention of suicide and attempted suicide – deployed a progression of universal, selective, and indicated prevention efforts (Pearson, 2000). These included broad population and clinical smoking cessation programs during the 1970s, community-based programs for hypertension during the 1980s, and standardized risk assessment during the 1990s (Rose, 1992; Wong et al., 2000; Wong & Gardin, 2000). Thus, modern prevention strategies for CVD target very early risk factors of diet and exercise for heart disease, seeking to change the trajectory of health and illness years before the overt expression of symptoms.

In this context, we recommended adapting the framework proposed by Gordon (Gordon, 1983) and elaborated in 1994 by a seminal report from the Institute of Medicine (Mrazek & Haggerty, 1994) to develop universal, selective, and indicated approaches to preventing suicide (see Table 16.1).

This framework acknowledges the ultimate need for "multilayered" approaches, in that one level of preventive intervention is not sufficient. Fundamentally, it reaches beyond clinical settings to engage

1 broad swaths of the general population,
2 groups where the "average" level of risk of its members is elevated (even though each member may not share in the overall risk), and
3 symptomatic individuals needing active treatment.

Such public health approaches may well include clinical or therapeutic interventions. The key element, much as in response to sexually transmitted diseases or influenza, is not to wait until affected individuals come to the clinic but to reach into diverse community and social settings to affirmatively involve them where they live, work, or can be identified in higher frequencies. The latter may be considered "points of capture" or, in perhaps less coercive language, sites of engagement.

The review of Mann and colleagues (2005), while not published until 2005, noted two approaches to prevention that had supporting evidence: (1) Means (or methods) control and (2) education of primary care physicians to detect and treat depressed patients prior to developing life-ending plans or actions. Nearly all published suicide prevention efforts that have shown a measurable impact on deaths have employed population-oriented approaches, such as the replacement of coal gas with less toxic North Sea gas in the United Kingdom (Kreitman, 1976; Kreitman & Platt, 1984) or more recent changes in the packaging of paracetamol (acetaminophen) and salicylates in the UK (Hawton, Townsend, Deeks, Appleby, Gunnell,

Table 16.1 The language of prevention applied to suicide and attempted suicide

Intervention terminology	Approach	Target	Objectives	Examples of potential prevention efforts
Universal Prevention Interventions ("Distal" Prevention Efforts)	Population	Implement sweeping, broadly directed initiatives in entire populations or communities; not based upon individual risk Develop programs that reach asymptomatic individuals	Prevent disease through reducing risk and enhancing protective or mitigating factors across broad groups of people	1. Restrict means of suicide (e.g., firearm safety, pill packaging, bridge barriers) 2. Widely deploy alcohol & substance use prevention programs & control access 3. Support community-level violence reduction programs among men, ages 16–34 years 4. Offer crisis call lines to enhance social connection & access to care 5. Broadly apply "gatekeeper" training, supported with rehearsal and booster tools, to identify at-risk individuals and refer them to care 6. Support prevention-oriented health insurance – not dependent on "episodes" of illness
Selective Prevention Interventions	High Risk	Identify of groups that collectively bear a significantly higher-than-average risk of developing mental disorders, substance use disorders, and adverse outcomes	Prevent disease through addressing population-specific characteristics that place individuals at higher-than-average risk	1. Promote community programs to contact isolated elders 2. Deploy court based programs • Provide therapeutic support to victims of domestic violence • Deploy 'engagement' interventions for criminal defendants with substance use disorders

Indicated Preventive Interventions ("Proximal" Prevention Efforts)	High Risk	Identify high-risk individuals with detectable symptoms Future: Include asymptomatic individuals bearing defined risk markers related to "mechanism of disease"	Treat individuals with precursor or prodromal signs and symptoms to prevent emergence of full-blown disorder: Treat people with psychiatric disorders to reduce risk of suicide attempts	1. Increase screening and treatment for depressed elders in primary care settings 2. Vigorously treat elders with chronic pain syndromes and functional limitations 3. Enhance lithium maintenance for persons with recurrent bipolar disorder 4. Use targeted psychotherapy to treat suicidal thoughts and behaviors 5. Contact-engage suicidal patients who are 'lost' to care

Bennewith, & Cooper, 2001). The use of jumping barriers on iconic sites serves as another example of means control (Beautrais, Gibb, Fergusson, Horwood, & Larkin, 2009).

In a widely cited intervention implemented on the Swedish island of Gotland, primary care physicians were trained to recognize and treat depression (Rihmer, 2001; Rihmer, Rutz, & Pihlgren, 1995) and reduction in depression-related morbidity was observed. Although suicide was not the original target, the researchers also found a transient, statistically significant reduction in the suicide rate based solely on fewer deaths among women. Some have argued that this outcome was attributable to the intervention (Rutz, 2001; Rutz, von Knorrring, & Walinder, 1992), while others have viewed the result as a statistical fluctuation. Efforts at replication have been intriguing but not definitive (Szanto, Kalmar, Hendin, Rihmer, & Mann, 2007).

Several other leads were apparent in 2004. One of the more intriguing and well-known findings came from the work of Motto and Bostrom (2001). The researchers demonstrated a reduction in suicides after hospitalization with follow-up postcard contact. Although this has yet to be replicated specifically in other work, Carter, Clover, Whyte, Dawson, & D'Este (2005; 2007) found encouraging, similar results from contact in emergency rooms.

During 2004 to 2005 in the US, most suicide-prevention resources focused on acute interventions for suicidal or high-risk youth, including school-based screening programs (Gould, Greenberg, Velting, & Shaffer, 2003; Pena & Caine, 2006; Shaffer, Scott, Wilcox, Maslow, Hicks, Lucas, et al., 2004), brief training of "gatekeepers" to identify and refer high-risk youth to treatment (Quinnett, 2005), and treatments for youth having thoughts or plans or suicide or for patients shortly after a non-fatal suicidal attempt. There are few data to support the notion that these efforts are effective at preventing suicide, even as it is clear that systematic screening identifies many distressed youth who potentially may benefit from services (Scott, Wilcox, Schonfeld, Davies, Hicks, Turner, & Shaffer, 2009). The sole randomized trial of the widely used Question-Persuade-Refer (QPR) gatekeeper program demonstrated no effect for high school students and only a minute effect for middle-school children (Wyman et al., 2008).

Against this background, the experience of the US Air Force (USAF) served as a touchstone for policy makers and advocates committed to suicide prevention. Faced with a daunting increase in suicide rates during the early 1990s, the Vice Chief of Staff of the USAF ordered his Surgeon General and all other component members of the service's leadership to develop a comprehensive program. Rather than view it as medically based, they developed a community-oriented approach (Knox, Litts, Talcott, Feig, & Caine, 2003). The initiative had 11 core elements, including attention to individual and family needs; workplace performance; education for command and non-commissioned officers, for all personnel and for members of the broader community; attention to mental health and inordinate alcohol use; reformulation of confidentiality policies; continuing surveillance; and, perhaps most central to any programmatic effort, defined accountability.

In evaluating the USAF Suicide Prevention Program, it was evident that the whole was greater than the sum of its parts – at the heart of the program was an unequivocal change in culture that espoused and implemented programs offering help while seeking to remove the stigma of accepting help ("strong men can ask for help"). The cohesive nature of the service, long-standing values affirming "the Air Force family," and a sustained commitment that transcended the rotation of top leadership all contributed to the effective implementation of such a radical undertaking. The program led to a sustained decline in suicide and, just as important, in violent deaths and violence behaviors. What had been deployed as a suicide prevention program was, in fact, a program that broadly promoted social health and violence prevention. (See Table 16.2.)

With 2004 as a pivotal benchmark, we and others thought that the ensuing years would see a decline in suicide rates in the US, driven by expanding prevention efforts. Unfortunately, this has not been the case.

Moving toward effective public health approaches

Suicide rates have risen and fallen in the US over the course of decades. An honest appraisal would argue that we do not yet understand the mechanisms that underpin these temporal transitions. Nonetheless, these rates must serve as the benchmark for our public health and prevention efforts.

As noted earlier, suicide rates climbed overall between 1999 and 2007, driven by increases among those in the middle years of life. We anticipate that this trend will continue for 2008 to 2010 and perhaps beyond, due to the extraordinary economic crisis that began in 2007, accelerated in 2008,

Table 16.2 Comparison of effects of risk for suicide and related adverse outcomes in US Air Force population before (1990–1996) and after implementation of program (1997–2002)

Outcome	Relative risk (95% CI)	Risk reduction (1-relative risk)	Excess risk (relative risk-1)
Suicide	0.67 (0.57 to 0.80)	33%	–
Homicide	0.48 (0.33 to 0.74)	51%	–
Accidental death	0.82 (0.73 to 0.93)	18%	–
Severe family violence	0.46 (0.43 to 0.51)	54%	–
Moderate family violence	0.70 (0.69 to 0.73)	30%	–
Mild family violence	1.18 (1.16 to 1.20)	–	18%

and continues for many at present. Changes in suicide rates are robustly associated with changes in unemployment rates, a pattern that has been found in many countries (Platt & Hawton, 2000). Thus, we expect that the suicide rate will continue to creep upward, with an increasingly heavy burden on those of working age. Indeed, it would be quite unusual if there were no increase in suicide rates during this time of economic displacement and distress.

Though overall suicide rates have been increasing, the national picture is not uniform (CDC, 2010). Rates have trended downward substantially among elders since the early 1990s. The rate among this group had increased steadily throughout the 1980s, peaking during the last years of the decade (with 6,464 deaths in 1987; 21.82 per 100,000), before beginning a clear descent in 1991 to current, relatively stable levels (e.g., 5,421 deaths in 2007; 14.29 per 100,000). Among youth, ages 10 to 19 years old, the observed decline of the new century has been small but intriguing: There were 1,857 deaths in 1999 (4.61 per 100,000), which increased to 1,921 in 2000, began to drop before climbing for one year to 1,983 in 2004 (4.75 per 100,000), and declined to 1,661 (3.98 per 100,000) in 2007.

There are no published definitive findings to explain such declines. For elders we suspect that improved overall health status and access to health services, together with better economic and social circumstances, may have served to mitigate longer-term factors that underpin the development of distress and depression during the later years. Enhanced protective factors may be showing their effect, but these are difficult to demonstrate empirically. Relative to youth, there are no evaluation studies that tie the extensive development of youth-oriented screening or prevention programs to the recent decline in rates, so any conclusions are premature.

This is a young science where results are preliminary and definitive evidence is lacking. Thus, at this point in their development, suicide prevention efforts must grapple with five fundamental challenges in order to reduce the burdens of related mortality and mortality and to move the field forward.

Challenge 1: Identifying "true cases"

The first challenge is the inability to discriminate the relatively few "true cases" from the large numbers of "false positive" cases of psychiatrically ill or emotionally distressed individuals who describe many of the same thoughts and plans as those who seriously injure or kill themselves. This failure to discriminate reflects the low base of suicide in the general population and the commonality of complaints, symptoms, and signs of psychopathology. To date, available data reveal virtually no clinical characteristics that can be used at the individual level to distinguish those who will go on to die by suicide from those who will not.

This situation ties directly to how researchers, preventionists, clinicians, and policy makers use the notion of "risk factors for suicide" as they develop tools and programs, particularly screening programs and gate-keeper programs. For example, Kraemer (2003) wrote a pointed critique of our work and that of others gleaning "risk factors" from retrospective psychological autopsy studies. She was absolutely correct!

In heart disease studies, risk factors are defined prospectively and then tested to assess their predictive validity (Clayton, Lubsen, Pocock, Voko, Kirwan, Fox, & Poole-Wilson, 2005). However, psychopathological studies seeking to discriminate suicides, as well as those interested in social factors, have compared either deceased people with community controls, or attempters with controls or comparison psychiatric subjects. In these static, cross-sectional studies, investigators determine "statistically significant" differences between the involved study groups. Derived "risk factors" (i.e., differences at the $p < 0.05$ level) are extraordinarily common phenomena – psychopathological disorders, substance misuse, family turmoil, and job disruption, but suicide is a rare outcome. Thus, the predictive validity of such risk factors is extremely low (Pena & Caine, 2006; Pokorny, 1983). Moreover, a strongly associated risk factor for a population-level outcome does not provide a basis for prediction for individuals (Ware, 2006).

Screening programs used in public health initiatives build directly on the predictive utility of risk factors. When broadly applied for cardiovascular risk factors – blood lipid levels and triglycerides or, more recently, blood indices of inflammation – such markers are used to initiate treatment with agents that have demonstrated population-level benefits of reducing future cardiovascular events, even as they cannot be predictive of individual level effects. This is not the case for suicide; nonetheless, policy makers and researchers have invoked similar strategies for suicide prevention. Many resources now are devoted in secondary schools, universities (Gould, Klomek, & Batejan, 2009), and in the US Army to screen for suicide potential based on "risk factor profiles." While there is a growing literature supporting the effectiveness for screening programs to detect and refer "high-risk youth" (Gould et al., 2009), no studies have demonstrated an impact on suicide rates, and therefore the cost-effectiveness of such programs remains uncertain. In great measure, this results from the commonness of the retrospectively defined differences separating suicides from case-controls – depression, substance use, or even psychosis – as compared to the uncommon outcome of suicide (a needle-in-the-haystack problem).

This is especially true in the nation's secondary schools, where overall suicide rates remain low despite the common occurrence of suicide ideation on the Youth Risk Survey. In 2007, 14.5% of students reported seriously considering suicide during the year prior to the survey, 11.3% made a plan, 6.9% attempted, and 2% made a suicide attempt that required medical attention for an injury, poisoning, or overdose (CDC, 2008). One

can argue that youth who are "false positives" desperately require therapeutic intervention even when their conditions never would have proceeded to death. While this is doubtless true, it only may be tangentially
related to preventing suicide. Also, many of the most distressed youth leave
school before graduating, and are therefore beyond reach of school-based
programs. Further, the heaviest contributions to the national suicide
burden arise from other populations; thus, this becomes an issue for establishing funding priorities. The cost of screening programs is not inconse-
quential – when measured on a per person level it is relatively low, but
when measured in terms of lives saved, these costs become quite high.
Should these resources instead be used for general population screening or
perhaps for direct services, which are in dire shortage for many youth?

While understanding its limitations, use of screening tools – as compared to screening programs – may offer other practical benefits that ultimately contribute to suicide prevention efforts. For example, Lang, Uttaro,
Caine, Carpinello, and Felton (2009a; 2009b) focused on groups already
known to suffer elevated suicide rates (i.e., selective preventive intervention) and who populate many longer-term care outpatient settings. The
participants in this preliminary study were outpatients of state-supported
community mental health clinics who were suffering severe, persistent
mental disorders. The investigators used screening as a discriminating
method among a group people who, if assessed with a standard list of
"risks," would be positive; indeed, many of the participants reported persistent or regularly recurring suicidal ideation. The approach involved a
brief interviewer-rated list to identify recent significant life changes, stressful events, changes in hopefulness or future perspectives, and in turn,
changes in the intensity or quality of suicidal thinking if that had been
noted previously. Among the 471 participants, assessed a total of 1,671
times, 43 (9%) screened positive one or more times, leading to 69 positive
assessments and 62 further in-depth evaluations. Concerning responses
detected by the interviewers among the screen-negative participants
prompted another 62 evaluations. Thirty-four of the 69 positive screens
(49%) led to changes in clinical care; ultimately, only 84 of the 1,598
negative screening interviews (5%) were associated with changes in care.
While this type of work is exploratory, it suggests that embedding screening tools into already extant clinical programs may have a useful niche
when applied to selected populations (that is, applying the tool to a much
smaller haystack). This requires rigorous testing.

Even among the most psychiatrically impaired individuals, where suicide
rates are highest (e.g., people suffering bipolar disorder, major depression
with a past history of a suicide attempt, or schizophrenia), the vast majority of individuals will live many years and not die by their own hand,
despite their highly elevated levels of discerned risk. As noted by Lewis,
Hawton, and Jones (1997), even dramatic reductions in suicide among
defined high-risk groups will have relatively little impact on overall suicide

rates, in light of the dramatically smaller sizes of these groups relative to the general population (which, in turn, explains the relatively smaller contribution made to the overall suicide burden by "high risk deaths"). However, there is no doubt this population requires care, and clinical interventions can make a great difference in the lives of those involved, even as they may not greatly influence the overall national picture.

In sum, screening programs have been widely disseminated, premised on the effectiveness of detecting "high-risk" individuals in order to prevent suicide. Whether such methods save lives remains highly uncertain. They can lead to needed clinical referrals, which is gratifying, but in these economically distressed times, when there are many uninsured and when states, counties, and cities have been reducing funding for publically financed mental health services, one could argue for a different use of the resources. Such considerations underscore the intertwined nature of public health and political discussions when establishing spending priorities.

Challenge 2: The large number of "false negatives"

Unfortunately, a large number of individuals escape preventive detection by family, physicians, or other professionals, and proceed to kill themselves. This reflects a multiplicity of factors; for example, the rapidity of some deaths without warning (often called "impulsive"); the emergence of desperation and determination-to-die among lonely, isolated people, frequently following disruptions that have driven them apart from others; the calculated unwillingness of many to express their intent; the fatigue and demoralization of people with severe, persisting mental disorders, too often coincident with the "burnout" of family members and care providers; or the smoldering depression and decline of elders who carefully lay the foundation for their life-ending acts.

A large-scale approach to prevention, "gatekeeper training" has been widely deployed across the US. While there are many versions, the general format involves providing an educational program to individuals who then function as sentinels in schools, communities, and large organizations. Their job is to detect people who fit high-risk profiles and engage these individuals in conversations that will lead to a rapid referral to a mental health professional for further evaluation. The success of this approach ultimately depends upon imparting new knowledge and helping attitudes, as well as the skills needed to carry out the necessary engagement, negotiation, and referral tasks.

QPR is one of the most widely distributed, commercial approaches (Quinnett, 2005), though a variety of other similar methods abound. QPR involves a one-hour lecture format, while others involve lecture and modest rehearsal, and one model uses a two-day format. Once trained, QPR implementers are expected to identify and engage (question and persuade) potentially at-risk individuals and facilitate their entry into care (refer).

QPR is described as a "behavioral activation" program involving inter-
vener and target. The only large-scale, randomized trial published to date
showed that the training led to a sustained increase in knowledge and an
abiding change in attitudes, but it was not associated with substantial
reported changes in trainee behavior or in subsequent referrals (Wyman et
al., 2008). Thus, while trained gatekeepers may know more, it was not
evident that they see more or do more. Moreover, individuals with significant intent may avoid these potential guardians. The authors found that
"results from 2,059 8th and 10th graders surveyed showing that fewer students with prior suicide attempts endorsed talking to adults about distress." This observation is consistent with ample literature that shows that,
among elders who kill themselves, many see their primary care providers
very soon before death and neither signal their distress nor seek solace
(Luoma et al., 2002).

The apparent face validity of gatekeeper training together with its ease
of dissemination to large audiences has made it appealing. Its apparent
lack of impact underscores that the field is desperate for interventions yet
insufficiently patient to develop the types of training and the needed evaluation methods to rigorously assess whether we actually are making a difference in the lives of those whom we intend to reach. The well-intended,
widespread promulgation of gatekeeper methods, and of screening as well,
points to the desperation to save lives that is shared by all, even as outcome
evaluations have been lacking to date.

Like screening, gatekeeper training may hold promise. Discovering its
potential will require attention of "implementation scientists" (Madon,
Hofman, Kupfer, & Glass, 2007) to discern which methods promote
maximal development and use of essential skills and how to boost these
repeatedly over time. At the same time, new models of communication are
needed to foster greater interactions with those "unrecognized" who might
allow themselves to be detected.

Challenge 3: The inability of clinical and social services to reach many potentially lethal individuals

Most persons who are suicidal do not seek care or regularly attend clinical
settings. Instead, they must be identified and engaged in settings not
designed at this time for preventive or treatment interventions (e.g., the
courts, schools); thus, prevention efforts must be integrated into their
ecology, and suicide prevention for many populations of interest will
depend on deploying resources at potential "points of engagement." Prevention, if it is to be inclusive of targeted groups who collectively bear
greater risk, will need to "go where the action is."

To date, geography has not served as a major consideration for suicide
prevention. However, rates differ dramatically among major sectors of the
country, and rural areas here and in other countries have a higher burden

of death in comparison to cities and their immediate surround. Populations worthy of selective interventions are densely concentrated in many settings that are nearly devoid of prevention programs, and extensive programs are arrayed in many settings where the relative rates are low. As we will discuss further in Challenge 4, distribution of efforts based on geographic risk profiles can serve as an essential method of implementing ecologic-informed preventive interventions.

One way of relating ecologic thinking and risk perspectives involves mapping communities and considering where to identify and engage target populations, groups, and individuals. Every setting has its distinctive sample biases, which are at once advantageous when seeking to connect with specific groups and a limitation in terms of those who are missed. (See Table 16.3.)

Considering a site- (or setting-) based method, it is readily apparent that programs based in secondary schools will miss those who have dropped out or who already have become involved in gangs and legal entanglements. Similarly, university or college programs do not reach young adults who are not pursuing higher education. Digging deeper, one might explore the differences in the potential for engaging students who attend a school that primarily has a residential campus versus those in settings with substantial numbers of commuter-students, or four-year institutions as compared to community colleges. Each of these variants invites or requires adjustments that will not be easily apparent unless one examines a consideration of local geography-ecology.

A community's institutions can play an important role; county- and state-run social service agencies attend to family needs and can provide entrée for a variety of family-focused prevention initiatives. Similarly, the courts are a venue for identifying and engaging many individuals in the midst of great distress. Indeed, many men in their middle years with a history of domestic violence prior to suicide (Conner, Duberstein, & Conwell, 2000) or attempted suicide (Conner, Cerulli, & Caine, 2002) pass through court settings. Often it is just such disruptive distress that is observed in the weeks before suicide (Duberstein, Conwell, & Caine, 1993).

Conversely, one can map the community paths of groups of interest – particularly those composed of higher-risk individuals – as another method of planning engagement and intervention efforts. Such mapping complements the site-population approach; these methods can yield differing views of where resources might best be placed. (See Table 16.4.)

The CDC's Web-based Injury Statistics Query and Reporting System (WISQAR S™) offers another approach to geo-mapping (CDC, 2010), which invites consideration of ecological factors. This tool displays national maps at county levels to reveal the burden of suicide and other causes of violent death. Over time, this can lend itself to other forms of mapping to examine the relationship between the state and local policies,

Table 16.3 Site – population approaches

Sites	Populations potentially captured	Populations likely to be missed	Comments
Middle and High Schools	Adolescents attending school	School dropouts; youth in legal trouble	Useful for social skills education, enhancing protective factors, but tends to miss many high risk youths
Universities	Vulnerable individuals with new onset or recurrent mental disorders	Young adults not pursuing higher education, especially those who are unemployed or incarcerated	Requires distinctive programs for undergraduates and graduate students; potential for use of Internet and other computer assisted interactive tools
Organized Work Sites	Those employed in organized work sites; men and women in the middle years	Workers in small businesses, union hiring halls, day labor, unemployed workers, immigrant and migrant labor, underground workers	Potentially suitable for prevention-oriented employee assistance programs; depression and substance use are important targets for enhancing productivity
Medical Settings	Those with health insurance; those that are willing to access traditional medical settings	Un- & under-insured; low "utilizers" (men and young adults); users of alternative health care	Potentially suitable for screening of disability, pain, and depression; dependent on 'traffic-through-the-door'
Community NGOs (e.g., United Way)	Those targeted for service by the NGO funding source; those in private homeless shelters or coming to food banks	Anyone outside of perceived scope of agency	Potential to educate local NGOs about common risks for suicide and other form of premature death, violence and injury

Religious/Faith Organizations	Those who attend on a regular basis	Non-participants and those that drop out	Generally untapped resource that views suicide prevention as outside the scope of activities
Courts/Criminal Justice/Jails	Perpetrators and victims of domestic violence, probationers, prisoners	Failure to gain access for mental health and chemical dependency services for those identified through CJ settings	Major potential for integrating mental health and CJ services in a prevention and early intervention web of care
Local Government Agencies	Recipients from County-level social service and health departments; those in homeless shelters, county supervised housing	Those who do not access services from local departments of health or social service	Potential for integration into a comprehensive community system tuned to high risk service recipients
State Government Agencies, Medicaid	Unemployed workers seeking services; those with mentally disorders in state supported housing; state operated mental health centers and clinics, including high risk populations such as SMI and CD patients in clinics; Medicaid recipients	Chronically unemployed, migrants not eligible for services	Potential for integration into a comprehensive system tuned to high risk recipients
Federal Agencies, Medicare, Social Security Offices, in collaboration with States	Elders and those on disability, and Medicaid recipients	Broad swaths of the general population	New uses of Federal Government information sources would rouse confidentiality concerns

Table 16.4 High-Risk Groups and Sites to Contact Them

High-risk Groups	Sites	Potential Interventions	Comments
High-Risk Youth – school drop-outs, violent youth, & repeatedly transferred foster care youth	Community centers, police, jails, foster services; alternative schools	Comprehensive family and youth services integrated across community, school, social service, and criminal justice systems	Often missed in schools; requires careful integration and coordination not evident in most communities; leadership and funding issues are central. Later accrued "indirect" costs for non-intervention may be higher!
Patients with severe, persisting mental disorders	Mental health treatment settings	Fostering of early interventions; assertive community treatments; linkages to courts, supervised housing, and other agencies for integrated care.	Currently many encountered in the "alternate mental health system," i.e., local jails and state prison. Available medication interventions must be embedded into comprehensive systems of care and assertive community follow-up.
Men with alcohol and substance (CD) disorders; perpetrators of domestic violence; victims of DV	Chemical dependency (CD) treatment settings; courts	Integration of mental health and prevention services into CD programs; need for court integrated mental health and CD services	Dependent on development of integrated MICA services; rapid access to care for those in need crucial; insurance barriers remain major obstacle to services
Depressed Women and Men	Primary care settings	Enhanced detection, treatment, and follow-up of emerging symptoms	Requires education of care providers re: recognition and treatment; subsyndromal conditions important
Elders with Pain, Disability, Depression	Primary care offices, residential settings; Agency on Aging outreach programs	Pre-emptive treatment of pain and increasing medically related disability	Can miss socially isolated elders, who fail to come to PCP offices, and elders who do not express their needs openly
Attempters of suicide (may be counted as well among other groups); frequently involve comorbidities, including mood and personality disorders and CD problems	ERs, ICUs, inpatient psychiatry, and medical services – need for novel approaches to case identification, engagement, and follow-up	Community outreach for contacting "no-shows," reminder cards, assertive case management; surveillance as case identification	Those high in ideation and attempts in the context of personality disorders often are 'frequent fliers' to ERs, who challenge traditional care systems of care; major ethical and social questions involved with active surveillance and outreach intiatives

the expenditure of resources for social benefits, and in the future, the availability of health and educational resources. Together with an understanding of local ecological factors, of the needs of broad and specific population groups, and of how to track populations bearing risks of concern, it may be possible to develop the guidance needed to deploy integrated suicide prevention programs. Such knowledge is one key to developing successful suicide reducing programs. Other essential elements, as we learned from studying the Air Force, involve vision, leadership, and political-social will.

Challenge 3, together with Challenge 2, also reminds that the most effective forms of prevention demonstrated to date involve means control or restriction. As a broadly applied public health method, this depends not upon identifying an "at risk" person, but upon building protection into social structures or the social fabric, using such methods as bridge barriers, changes in packaging, substituting the sale of less lethal pesticides for early-generation products that were more lethal, or changing the composition of cooking gas. In the US, this would involve firearms, particularly handguns. While the Supreme Court has affirmed the individual right to bear arms, few efforts have been made to engage organizations such as the National Rifle Association in discussions of firearm safety and suicide prevention. This would likely involve extensive education – of families, physicians and other care providers, and potentially, individuals at risk. Past data showed that the three-day gun-waiting period required by the "Brady Bill" before the full-scale national implementation of a computer-based security-check system was associated with lowered handgun associated suicide rates among people older than 55 years (Ludwig & Cook, 2000). Notably, the USAF, given the nature of a military organization, did not seek to specifically control its most prevalent means of suicide – firearms – but imposed other safety measures to restrict personnel at risk. How, in civilian society, can we develop methods of having people "think twice" before pulling the trigger?

Challenge 4: A continuing paucity of knowledge regarding the fundamental biological, psychological, social, and cultural factors that contribute to suicide risk among diverse populations

There remains a limited understanding about how best to define and mobilize protective factors that may diminish the impact of risk factors that may vary according to age, race, gender and sexual orientation, residential geography, and socio-cultural and economic status. Risks are common; suicide is relatively rare. What keeps the vast majority of people alive even when faced by adversity or when long-burdened by severe or recurrent mental disorders?

A developmental perspective suggests that prevention and pre-emptive therapeutic interventions should be conceived of and implemented mindful of the *accumulating* nature of risk. While a full array of risk factors may be evident at death, they amass over time and across social contexts. It is through multilevel growth models that we can best track the course of increasing risk. Early interventions must account for these accumulating burdens, using methods and measurement schema that are distinctive from those that are appropriate later in the course of risk progression. For those people who bear the greatest pathology and attendant risk, treatment of psychiatric symptoms and signs is an essential element of care, including initiation of psychotropic medications, appropriate psychotherapies, and careful care planning. However, if clinicians fail to deal with the collective impact of aggravating factors that either preceded or accompanied the emergence of psychiatry symptoms and signs – i.e., long-term exposure to social turmoil and to the interpersonal, vocational, and functional consequences that contribute to and derive from severe psychopathology and substance misuse – there will be a continuing, heightened probability of clinical recurrence or relapse and an increased likelihood of suicide. Treating symptomatic psychopathology is necessary but not sufficient. This may provide one potential explanation for the increase in suicide rates among psychiatric patients during the first months following discharge from inpatient care (Qin & Nordentoft, 2005), even as many do not manifest suicidal thinking immediately prior to discharge (Hunt, Kapur, Webb, Robinson, Burns, Shaw, & Appleby, 2009).

Addressing these issues requires cohesive conceptual frameworks. While there are several theoretical constructs that focus studies of individual suicide and suicidal behaviors, no single unifying theoretical approach guides public health and population-oriented efforts. There do exist two general conceptual models for informing public health approaches to preventing suicide and attempted suicide. Neither is yet a testable theory; rather, they serve to organize approaches into more coherent frameworks for systematic testing and practical application.

Each of the conceptual frames has limitations as well as utility. The broadest – an ecological developmental model (or frame) – serves as an umbrella that organizes risk and potential protective factors into levels of analysis and links them to development, broadly defined (Bronfenbrenner, 1979; Krug et al., 2002). The ecologic (systems) model can be tied closely to the current language of prevention – language that invokes universal, selective, and indicated interventions – to serve as the foundation for systematically developing a comprehensive array of programmatic efforts. Within this context, a suicide-specific developmental framework complements the broader ecological frame. It presents a dynamic view that can depict accumulating risk, and it also may serve as a basis for organizing exploration of protective factors more specifically. This more specific developmental view can be considered for both populations and individuals. (See Figure 16.1.)

As noted above, we seek to integrate these perspectives, in part by mapping the community geography (agency/site) of contacts with populations of interest. This is accomplished both by defining sites and

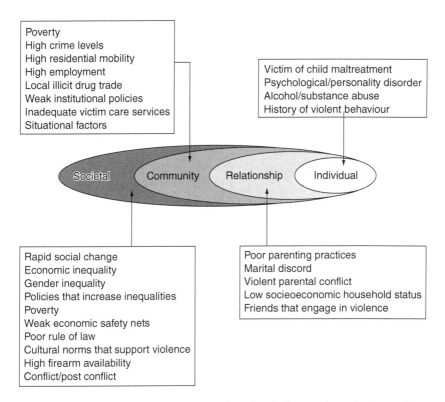

Figure 16.1 Ecological model showing shared risk factors for sub-times of inter-personal violence (source: From: "Preventing Violence: A guide to implementing the recommendations of the *World Report on Violence and Health*." WHO, 2004).

understanding their potential sampling biases-opportunities and by identifying target groups and examining the settings where they may be encountered. Such mapping activities give potential substance to the notion of multilevel interventions, which can be seen in both practical as well as conceptual terms.

Ultimately, to be successful at a "macro" level as well as for specific individuals in distress, suicide prevention efforts must involve the development of complementary initiatives that build a mosaic of programs – that is, programs that reach horizontally within and vertically across levels of potential change. Violence in general, and suicide in particular, must be understood as both individual and social phenomena – transactions within and across levels of analysis. While it remains daunting to truly integrate perspectives that examine large, social- and community-level forces with individual outcomes, this realm is the future of larger-scale public health suicide prevention efforts.

An example may serve to illustrate the challenges involved. Suicide rates are robustly correlated with unemployment rates; however, unemployment itself only serves as a modest risk factor among those who kill themselves, certainly far less than the population attributable risk of depression (Platt, 1984; 1986; Platt & Hawton, 2000; Platt & Kreitman, 1985). Recent data from Hong Kong showed the typical relationship between unemployment rates and suicide rates; however, the majority of the increase in deaths that occurred during recession was derived from the large pool of employed individuals rather than the much smaller pool of unemployed persons (Yip & Caine, 2010). Such findings invite consideration of macro-, meso-, and individual-level factors. The general literature has, to date, conflated population level indices and individual employment status. Disentangling such factors may enhance understanding about contributors to suicide and, hopefully, inform novel approaches to prevention.

Neither the language used in the 1994 Institute of Medicine report (Mrazek & Haggerty, 1994) nor our adaptation of this framework to population approaches for preventing suicide fully captures the dynamic nature of accumulating risks. This invites the addition of an individual-level developmental frame to the broader systems view provided by the ecologic model. There has been little work to date that considers the potentially distinctive effects of timing-dependent interventions that seek to alter developmental (life course) trajectories. In our work, we have depicted these based on risk information for stratified groups – e.g., younger men, men and women in the middle years of life, elders (typically men) – with the aim of establishing greater understanding of where in the trajectory toward suicide a specific program is deployed. The utility of such an approach is limited, however, by the paucity of specific risk and protective information for many groups – e.g., young and middle-aged black men, including both African-American and Afro-Caribbean males; American Indian and Alaskan Native youth and young adults; and adolescent girls and women, particularly white and Asian-American women, where the female suicide burden is highest.

Figure 16.2 depicts a model for adult men (especially white men) and adult women in the middle years of life. While this type of depiction lends itself to targeting distal risk factors in an effort to alter suicide outcomes, it also identifies factors that may be viewed as specifically "therapeutic" when dealing with individual needs. The model also underscores the previously noted dilemma that treating psychiatric symptoms alone, in the absence of mitigating other risks, leaves an individual vulnerable to relapse.

Challenge 5: The lack of coordinated strategies among myriad local, regional, state, and national agencies and organizations

Suicide prevention requires the development and sustained implementation of a highly coordinated plan, appreciating that no single measure will

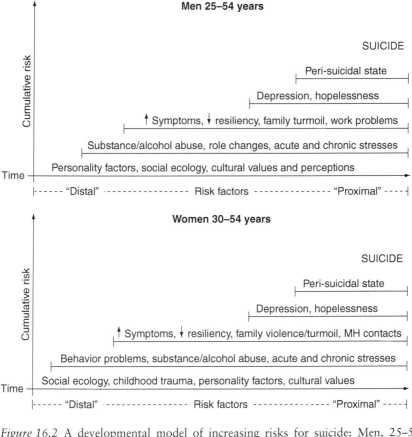

Figure 16.2 A developmental model of increasing risks for suicide: Men, 25–54 years (source: Caine & Conwell).

suffice. At this early juncture of the 21st century, the greatest impediment to implementing programs that can positively mitigate the adverse social, psychological, and behavioral factors that contribute to suicide – and ultimately to other forms of untimely, preventable death – is the lack of coordinated strategies among myriad local, regional, state, and national agencies and organizations that could, in theory, play a role in preventing suicide. Public health interventions must work at multiple levels – from major swaths of the general population, to communities or smaller (selective) risk-bearing groups, and to individuals who are in need. Prevention efforts must include community-based programs, as well as interventions implemented across health systems and in clinical practice.

Most public health and prevention initiatives are shaped around a definition of the burden of disease. In 2007, there were 1,661 suicides among those 10 to 19 years old, 2,659 among those 20 to 24 years old, 24,847 among those 25 to 64 years old, and 5,421 among those over 65 years old. Earlier in the chapter we demonstrated that the bulk of years of potential life lost is among those in the 20 to 54 year old age range (Knox & Caine, 2005), involving 22,437 lives in 2007. In the context of the Garrett Lee Smith Memorial Act, the majority of resources in the US are being spent on high school programs for in-school youth, ages 14 to 18 years, or on college-attending populations where the rate is approximately half of the level of non-college attending peers (Schwartz, 2006a; 2006b). Current spending priorities ignore the national burden of suicide and thus have little probability of changing national death rates. While policy makers may follow their hearts, and respond to the anguish of parents who have lost their children, such efforts may not best serve the needs of the nation as a whole.

Over-focus on one population is common when prevention efforts begin. The CVD prevention model, for example, at first focused almost exclusively on one group – middle-aged white men. This is much akin to the current preoccupation for suicide prevention among students in high schools and colleges or universities. As we have noted, most suicide prevention efforts have relied heavily on identifying and treating psychiatric symptoms and pathological psychology as "risk factors" for individuals, which is reminiscent of early, exclusive attention on elevated serum cholesterol levels and advocacy in the 1960s to substitute transfat-filled margarine for butter.

Over-emphasizing one domain of risk may obscure the importance of other areas that play important or formative roles far distal to the adverse outcome. Surely, psychiatric symptoms and signs are critical but not exclusive elements of risk; repeatedly they have been shown to hold the greatest amount of "population attributable risk" at the time of suicide attempt (Beautrais, 1998; 2000; Beautrais, Joyce, & Mulder, 1998). Garrett Lee Smith funding notwithstanding, most potential resources for suicide prevention are embedded in the traditional mental health system and devoted to reactive therapeutics – treating symptoms – rather than prevention. Little attention has been paid to understanding the impacts of a variety of other interacting factors, including how non-modifiable factors (e.g., age, gender, and area of residence) interact with individual level factors (e.g., psychological status and substance use, adverse life experiences) and with family and immediate social settings. These latter factors may be protective or risk enhancing, and socioeconomic and local ecological forces may influence them further.

Conclusion

How shall we move forward? Changing broadly defined behaviors depends upon societal and cultural imperatives and norms (e.g., attitudes regarding heavy alcohol use; approaches to firearm safety). Such changes are conveyed through available social networks – both formal and informal groups and processes (e.g., transforming perceptions of depression and suicide in the USAF). The explosive growth of "social networking" media potentially offers vibrant new methods for conveying important prevention messages and influencing critical social and personal health decisions. These media also offer important new venues for creative research. On the other hand, educating and training clinicians in order to deliver care to identified "high-risk" (i.e., highly symptomatic) individuals remains the most promising method of treating those with blatantly manifest psychiatric-biomedical risk factors. Community interventions usually are embraced by "early adopters" (e.g., those who change their lifestyles when new information becomes available), while targeted clinical approaches are necessary to engage "late adopters," who require their physician's strong encouragement to treat their symptoms (Pearson, 2000; Pearson & Lewis, 1998).

The fundamental premise for broadly applied public health approaches is straightforward: A population-oriented approach is potentially beneficial because it effects so-called "distal risk factors"; that is, it prevents or minimizes the likelihood that more people will develop a greater number of severe risk factors (e.g., effectively treating alcoholism before someone develops a progressively downhill course unto death). For example, a broad-based preventive intervention aimed at reducing aggressive-impulsive behavior in first grade reduces suicide ideation, and perhaps attempts, among young adults years later (Kellam et al., 2008; Wilcox et al., 2008). This is an example of a strategy built upon developmental theories (Bronfenbrenner, 1979), and when considering Rose's theorem, the bulk of the "death savings" would come from the broader (i.e., non-psychiatric) population, outside of clinical care settings. This position is reinforced, in part, by the conclusions of Lewis and colleagues (1997) that exclusive attention to defined high-risk patient groups would have a relatively small impact on overall national rates of suicide.

However, prospective studies are needed to test whether population-oriented approaches have relevance for suicide prevention. There also is a lingering controversy that we expect too much from Rose's theorem, sparked in part by several population-based CVD prevention programs that resulted in little or no effect (Carleton, Lasater, Assaf, Feldman, & McKinlay, 1995; Farquhar et al., 1990; Luepker et al., 1994). At the same time, these differences in efficacy, effectiveness, and broader service implementation may be due to inappropriate identification of populations for interventions, lack of a theoretical framework when developing an intervention, or inadequate evaluation methodology to detect appropriate outcomes (Pearson & Lewis, 1998). We also would argue that a key failure in the translation of research to effective widespread application relates to inadequate attention to the "how to" aspects that now fall under implementation science. Addressing "how to" cannot be divorced from content (e.g., "risk factors"); for example, our critique of gatekeeper training involves "how to" and "to whom" as well as "what."

Another apparent obstacle to moving forward derives from the historically limited range of research designs and analytic methods available to studying the low base rate for suicide and even suicide attempts for some studies (Brown & Liao, 1999; Brown et al., 2007; 2008; 2009; Brown, Wyman, Guo, & Pena, 2006). In addition, studies of diverse populations in real world settings (complex organizations, communities, regions, or states) may not lend themselves to randomized controlled trial designs that seek to reduce as much population and environmental heterogeneity as possible. Only now are potential designs and measurement methods emerging that might enable effectiveness studies in real world settings involving so-called "messy" populations of "multiply-morbid" subjects in scientifically rigorous fashion (Brown et al., 2007).

Beyond these concerns, the field also needs to heed one of the core principles of the *National Strategy for Suicide Prevention* (Satcher, 2001), that suicide prevention involves an array of community-focused interventions that require diligent planning, coordination, careful implementation, and rigorous evaluation of "benchmark" outcomes that are identified at the outset. This involves collecting critical outcome information contemporaneously, rather than struggling retrospectively and in a piecemeal fashion. Moreover, no program – however well planned – will have a demonstrable impact on suicide rates unless it includes those segments of the population and groups who bear the greatest burden of mortality and antecedent morbidity.

Related, the suicide prevention field must step beyond "suicide" and combat more fundamental risk behaviors and distal indicators, such as heavy alcohol use and illicit drug consumption among youth or pain among elders. Can suicide prevention advocates ally with Mothers Against Drunk Driving or organizations that seek to protect victims of intimate partner violence? The goals of all would benefit from curtailing binge drinking among youth and young adults and chronic alcohol consumption among adults in the middle years of their lives. Such alliances make sense at the community level, but whether diverse organizations can galvanize their efforts around common risks is uncertain. These are issues that reach beyond practical importance to fundamental questions of "equifinality" and "multifinality" – that multiple causes can lead to a single outcome and that multiple outcomes can arise from different effects of the same component depending on the organization of the particular system in which it operates (Cicchetti & Rogosch, 1996). Among youth and young adults, for example, there is substantial overlap involving factors that contribute to death from motor vehicle accidents, suicide, homicide, and accidental poisoning (including overdoses of illicit drugs). Indeed, while many recognize that alcohol and drugs play a heavy role in accidents and homicides, what is less commonly understood is that these substances independently and powerfully add to the risk for suicide (Wilcox, Conner, & Caine, 2004). Figure 16.3 illustrates the potential overlaps of suicide with other forms of premature death among youth and young adults and points to the potential for "common risk" approaches to intervention.

Ultimately, achieving success in preventing suicide and attempted suicide, while mitigating the effects of their antecedents, will depend upon visionary and sustained leadership. A central lesson from the USAF was the importance of leaders who set dramatic change into motion and institutions that develop the culture and infrastructures to sustain self-scrutiny and continuous improvement. Many more people are involved now in the nation's suicide prevention initiatives, as compared to two decades ago, and the change is remarkable. With the passage of the Garrett Lee Smith Memorial Act, substantial funds have flowed into states, tribes, and universities. There remains great potential to positively affect suicide – as it occurs at a national level – if communities, committed organizations, and leaders frankly consider and respond to the challenges. However, while we have described in this chapter concepts and elements necessary for building potentially effective public health prevention efforts, we are not yet certain that the necessary leadership or political will exist to transform such thinking into action. Without these forces, we may continue to observe that 2004 was a year of great optimism followed by relatively few positive outcomes. Thus, the second decade of the 21st century is a time of decision, and we hope, cohesive and sustained action that works to fully realize the vision of the Surgeon General's *Call to Action* and *National Strategy*.

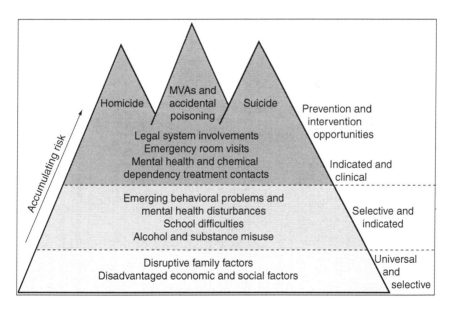

Figure 16.3 Diverse fatal outcomes in early adulthood: Premature death in early adulthood, common developmental contexts for different adverse outcomes.

Acknowledgments

Supported in part by grants P20 MH071897 (E.D. Caine, PI) and R25 MH68564 (E.D. Caine, PI) to the Center for the Study and Prevention of Suicide, R01 MH075017 (K.L. Knox, PI), and the Josh Locker Memorial Fund of the Department of Psychiatry.

References

Baldessarini, R. J., Tondo, L., Strombom, I. M., Dominguez, S., Fawcett, J., Licinio, J., et al. (2007). Ecological studies of antidepressant treatment and suicidal risks. *Harvard Review of Psychiatry, 15*(4), 133–145.

Beautrais, A. L. (1998). *Risk factors for suicide over the life course.* Washington, D.C.

Beautrais, A. L. (2000). Risk factors for suicide and attempted suicide among young people. [Review] [206 refs]. *Australian & New Zealand Journal of Psychiatry, 34*(3), 420–436.

Beautrais, A. L., Gibb, S. J., Fergusson, D. M., Horwood, L. J., & Larkin, G. L. (2009). Removing bridge barriers stimulates suicides: an unfortunate natural experiment. *Australian & New Zealand Journal of Psychiatry, 43*(6), 495–497.

Beautrais, A. L., Joyce, P. R., & Mulder, R. T. (1998). Unemployment and serious suicide attempts. *Psychological Medicine, 28*(1), 209–218.

Bronfenbrenner, U. (1979). *The ecology of human development.* Cambridge, MA: Harvard University Press.

Brown, C. H., & Liao, J. (1999). Principles for designing randomized preventive trials in mental health: an emerging developmental epidemiology paradigm [Review]. *American Journal of Community Psychology, 27*(5), 673–710.

Brown, C. H., Ten Have, T. R., Jo, B., Dagne, G., Wyman, P. A., Muthén, B., & Gibbons, R. D. (2009). Adaptive designs for randomized trials in public health. *Annual Review of Public Health, 30*, 1–25.

Brown, C. H., Wang, W., Kellam, S. G., Muthen, B. O., Petras, H., Toyinbo, P., et al. (2008). Methods for testing theory and evaluating impact in randomized field trials: intent-to-treat analyses for integrating the perspectives of person, place, and time. *Drug & Alcohol Dependence, 95*(Suppl 1), S74–S104.

Brown, C. H., Wyman, P. A., Brinales, J. M., & Gibbons, R. D. (2007). The role of randomized trials in testing interventions for the prevention of youth suicide. *International Review of Psychiatry, 19*(6), 617–631.

Brown, C. H., Wyman, P. A., Guo, J., & Pena, J. (2006). Dynamic wait-listed designs for randomized trials: New designs for prevention of youth suicide. *Clinical Trials, 3*(3), 259–271.

Carleton, R., Lasater, T., Assaf, A., Feldman, H., & McKinlay, S. (1995). The Pawtucket Heart Health Program: Community changes in cardiovascular risk factors and projected disease risk. *American Journal of Public Health, 85*(6), 777–785.

Carter, G., Clover, K., Whyte, I., Dawson, A., & D'Este, C. (2005). Postcards from the EDge project: Randomised controlled trial of an intervention using postcards to reduce repetition of hospital treated deliberate self poisoning. *BMJ,* doi:10.1136/bmj.38579.455266EO.

Carter, G. L., Clover, K., Whyte, I. M., Dawson, A. H., & D'Este, C. (2007). Post-cards from the EDge: 24-month outcomes of a randomised controlled trial for hospital-treated self-poisoning. *British Journal of Psychiatry, 191,* 548–553.

Centers for Disease Control and Prevention. (1992). *Youth suicide prevention programs: A resource guide.* Retrieved from http://wonder.cdc.gov/wonder/prevguid/p0000024/p0000024.asp

Centers for Disease Control and Prevention. (2007). *Suicide trends among youths and young adults aged 10–24 years – United States 1990–2004.* Retrieved from http://www.cdc.gov/mmwr/preview/mmwrhtml/mm5635a2.htm

Centers for Disease Control and Prevention. (2008). *Youth Risk Behavior Surveillance – 2007.* Retrieved from http://www.cdc.gov/mmwr/preview/mmwrhtml/ss5704a1.htm

Centers for Disease Control and Prevention. (2010). Web-based Injury Statistics Query and Reporting System (WISQARS™). Retrieved from Centers for Disease Control and Prevention: www.cdc.gov/ncipc/wisqars/default.htm.

Cicchetti, D., & Rogosch, F. A. (1996). Equifinality and multifinality in developmental psychopathology. *Development and Psychopathology, 8,* 597–600.

Clayton, T. C., Lubsen, J., Pocock, S. J., Voko, Z., Kirwan, B.-A., Fox, K. A., & Poole-Wilson, P. A. (2005). Risk score for predicting death, myocardial infarction, and stroke in patients with stable angina, based on a large randomised trial cohort of patients. *BMJ, 331*(7521), 869.

Conner, K., Cerulli, C., & Caine, E. (2002). Threatened and attempted suicide by partner-violent male respondents petitioned to family violence court. *Violence & Victims, 17*(2), 115–125.

Conner, K., Duberstein, P., & Conwell, Y. (2000). Domestic violence, separation, and suicide in young men with early onset alcoholism: Reanalyses of Murphy's data. *Suicide & Life-Threatening Behavior, 30*(4), 354–359.

Conwell, Y., Duberstein, P. R., Cox, C., Herrmann, J. H., Forbes, N. T., & Caine, E. D. (1996). Relationships of age and axis I diagnoses in victims of completed suicide: A psychological autopsy study. *American Journal of Psychiatry, 153*(8), 1001–1008.

Duberstein, P. R., Conwell, Y., & Caine, E. D. (1993). Interpersonal stressors, substance abuse, and suicide. *Journal of Nervous & Mental Disease, 181*(2), 80–85.

Elnour, A. A. H. J. (2008). Lethality of suicide methods. *Injury Prevention, 14,* 39–45.

Farquhar, J. W., Fortmann, S. P., Flora, J. A., Taylor, C. B., Haskell, W. L., Williams, P. T., et al. (1990). Effects of Communitywide Education on Cardiovascular Disease Risk Factors: The Stanford Five-City Project. *JAMA, 264*(3), 359–365.

Fremouw, W. J., dePerczel, M., & Ellis, T. E. (1990). *Suicide Risk: Assessment and Response Guidelines.* New York: Pergamon Press.

Gibbons, R., Brown, C., Hur, K., Marcus, S., Bhaumik, D., & Mann, J. (2007). Relationship between antidepressants and suicide attempts: An analysis of the Veterans Health Administration data sets. *American Journal of Psychiatry, 164*(7), 1044–1049.

Gibbons, R. D., Hur, K., Bhaumik, D. K., & Mann, J. J. (2005). The relationship between antidepressant medication use and rate of suicide. *Archives of General Psychiatry, 62*(2), 165–172.

Goldsmith, S. K., Pellmar, T. C., Kleinman, A. M., & Bunney, W. E. (Eds.). (2002). *Reducing suicide: A national imperative*. Washington, D.C.: Institute of Medicine: National Academy Press.

Gordon, R. (1983). An operational classification of disease prevention. *Public Health Reports, 98*(2), 107–109.

Gordon, T., & Kannel, W. B. (1971). Premature mortality from coronary heart disease: The Framingham study. *JAMA, 215*(10), 1617–1625.

Gordon, T., Kannel, W. B., Dawber, T. R., & McGee, D. (1975). Changes associated with quitting cigarette smoking: the Framingham Study. *American Heart Journal, 90*(3), 322–328.

Gordon, T., & Thom, T. (1975). The recent decrease in CHD mortality. *Preventive Medicine, 4*(2), 115–125.

Gould, M., Klomek, A., & Batejan, K. (2009). The role of schools, colleges and universities in suicide prevention. In C. Wasserman & D. Wasserman (Eds.), *Oxford Textbook of Suicidology and Suicide Prevention: A global perspective* (pp. 551–560). New York: Oxford University Press.

Gould, M. S., Greenberg, T., Velting, D. M., & Shaffer, D. (2003). Youth suicide risk and preventive interventions: A review of the past 10 years [Review]. *Journal of the American Academy of Child & Adolescent Psychiatry, 42*(4), 386–405.

Hawton, K., Townsend, E., Deeks, J., Appleby, L., Gunnell, D., Bennewith, O., & Cooper, J. (2001). Effects of legislation restricting pack sizes of paracetamol and salicylate on self poisoning in the United Kingdom: before and after study. *BMJ, 322*(7296), 1203–1207.

Hunt, I. M., Kapur, N., Webb, R., Robinson, J., Burns, J., Shaw, J., & Appleby, L. (2009). Suicide in recently discharged psychiatric patients: A case-control study. *Psychological Medicine, 39*(3), 443–449.

Kannel, W. B., & Gordon, T. (1982). The search for an optimum serum cholesterol. *Lancet, 2*(8294), 374–375.

Kannel, W. B., Gordon, T., & Castelli, W. P. (1981). Role of lipids and lipoprotein fractions in atherogenesis: The Framingham study. *Progress in Lipid Research, 20*, 339–348.

Kellam, S. G., Brown, C. H., Poduska, J. M., Ialongo, N. S., Wang, W., Toyinbo, P., et al. (2008). Effects of a universal classroom behavior management program in first and second grades on young adult behavioral, psychiatric, and social outcomes. *Drug & Alcohol Dependence, 95*(Suppl 1), S5–S28.

Kessler, R. C., Berglund, P., Borges, G., Nock, M., & Wang, P. S. (2005). Trends in suicide ideation, plans, gestures, and attempts in the United States, 1990–1992 to 2001–2003. *JAMA, 293*(20), 2487–2495.

Knox, K., & Caine, E. (2005). Establishing Priorities for Reducing Suicide and Its Antecedents in the United States. *American Journal of Public Health, 95*(11), 1898–1903.

Knox, K., Conwell, Y., & Caine, E. (2004). If suicide is a public health problem, what are we doing to prevent it? *American Journal of Public Health, 94*(1), 37–45.

Knox, K. L., Litts, D. A., Talcott, G. W., Feig, J. C., & Caine, E. D. (2003). Risk of suicide and related adverse outcomes after exposure to a suicide prevention programme in the US Air Force: cohort study. *BMJ, 327*(7428), 1376.

Kraemer, H. (2003). Current concepts of risk in psychiatric disorders. *Current Opinion in Psychiatry, 16*, 421–430.

Kreitman, N. (1976). The coal gas story. United Kingdom suicide rates, 1960–71. *British Journal of Preventive & Social Medicine, 30*(2), 86–93.

Kreitman, N., & Platt, S. (1984). Suicide, unemployment, and domestic gas detoxi-fication in Britain. *Journal of Epidemiology & Community Health, 38*(1), 1–6.

Krug, E. G., Mercy, J. A., Dahlberg, L. L., & Zwi, A. B. (2002). *World report on violence and health.* Retrieved from www.ncbi.nlm.nih.gov/entrez/query.fcgi?cmd=Retrieve&db=PubMed&dopt=Citation&list_uids=12596453.

Lang, M., Uttaro, T., Caine, E., Carpinello, S., & Felton, C. (2009a). Implementing routine suicide risk screening for psychiatric outpatients with serious mental dis-orders: I. Qualitative results. *Archives of Suicide Research, 13*(2), 160–168.

Lang, M., Uttaro, T., Caine, E., Carpinello, S., & Felton, C. (2009b). Implement-ing routine suicide risk screening for psychiatric outpatients with serious mental disorders: II. Quantitative results. *Archives of Suicide Research, 13*(2), 169–177.

Lewis, G., Hawton, K., & Jones, P. (1997). Strategies for preventing suicide. *British Journal of Psychiatry, 171*, 351–354.

Libby, A. M., Brent, D. A., Morrato, E. H., Orton, H. D., Allen, R., & Valuck, R. J. (2007). Decline in treatment of pediatric depression after FDA advisory on risk of suicidality with SSRIs. *American Journal of Psychiatry, 164*(6), 884–891.

Libby, A. M., Orton, H. D., & Valuck, R. J. (2009). Persisting decline in depression treatment after FDA warnings. *Archives of General Psychiatry, 66*(6), 633–639.

Ludwig, J., & Cook, P. J. (2000). Homicide and suicide rates associated with imple-mentation of the Brady Handgun Violence Prevention Act. *JAMA, 284*(5), 585–591.

Luepker, R. V., Murray, D. M., Jacobs, D. R., Mittelmark, M. B., Bracht, N., Carlaw, R., et al. (1994). Community education for cardiovascular disease pre-vention: Risk factor changes in the Minnesota Heart Health Program. *American Journal of Public Health, 84*(9), 1383–1393.

Luoma, J. B., Martin, C. E., & Pearson, J. L. (2002). Contact with mental health and primary care providers before suicide: a review of the evidence. *American Journal of Psychiatry, 159*(6), 909–916.

Madon, T., Hofman, K. J., Kupfer, L., & Glass, R. I. (2007). Public health. Imple-mentation science. *Science, 318*(5857), 1728–1729.

Mann, J., Apter, A., Bertolote, J., Beautrais, A., Currier, D., Haas, A., et al. (2005). Suicide prevention strategies: A systematic review. *JAMA, 294*(16), 2064–2074.

Mann, J., Arango, V., Avenevoli, S., Brent, D., Champagne, F., Clayton, P., et al. (2009). Candidate endophenotypes for genetic studies of suicidal behavior. *Bio-logical Psychiatry, 65*(7), 556–563.

Morrato, E. H., Libby, A. M., Orton, H. D., Degruy, F. V., Brent, D. A., Allen, R., & Valuck, R. J. (2008). Frequency of provider contact after FDA advisory on risk of pediatric suicidality with SSRIs. *American Journal of Psychiatry, 165*(1), 42–50.

Moscicki, E. K., O'Carroll, P., Rae, D. S., Locke, B. Z., Roy, A., & Regier, D. A. (1988). Suicide attempts in the Epidemiologic Catchment Area Study. *Yale Journal of Biology and Medicine, 61*, 259–268.

Motto, J. A., & Bostrom, A. G. (2001). A randomized controlled trial of postcrisis suicide prevention. *Psychiatric Services, 52*(6), 828–833.

Mrazek, P. J., & Haggerty, R. J. (Eds.). (1994). *Reducing risks for mental dis-orders: Frontiers for preventive intervention research.* Washington, D.C.: Insti-tute of Medicine: National Academy Press.

Nemeroff, C. B., Kalali, A., Keller, M. B., Charney, D. S., Lenderts, S. E., Cascade, E. F., et al. (2007). Impact of publicity concerning pediatric suicidality data on physician practice patterns in the United States. *Archives of General Psychiatry, 64*(4), 466–472.

New Freedom Commission on Mental Health. (2003). *Achieving the Promise: Transforming Mental Health Care in America.* Rockville, MD: New Freedom Commission on Mental Health.

Olfson, M., & Marcus, S. C. (2009). National patterns in antidepressant medication treatment. *Archives of General Psychiatry, 66*(8), 848–856.

Olfson, M., Marcus, S. C., Druss, B., Elinson, L., Tanielian, T., & Pincus, H. A. (2002). National trends in the outpatient treatment of depression. *JAMA, 287*(2), 203–209.

Olfson, M., Marcus, S. C., & Druss, B. G. (2008). Effects of Food and Drug Administration warnings on antidepressant use in a national sample. *Archives of General Psychiatry, 65*(1), 94–101.

Pearson, T. A. (2000). Primary prevention. In B. H. Wong ND, Gardin JM (Eds.), *Preventive Cardiology* (pp. 539–556). McGraw-Hill: McGraw-Hill.

Pearson, T. A., & Lewis, C. (1998). Rural epidemiology: Insights from a rural population laboratory. *American Journal of Epidemiology, 148*(10), 949–957.

Pena, J. B., & Caine, E. D. (2006). Screening as an approach for adolescent suicide prevention. *Suicide & Life-Threatening Behavior, 36*(6), 614–637.

Platt, S. (1984). Unemployment and suicidal behaviour: A review of the literature. *Social Science & Medicine, 19*(2), 93–115.

Platt, S. (1986). Parasuicide and unemployment. *British Journal of Psychiatry, 149*, 401–405.

Platt, S., & Hawton, K. (2000). Suicidal behaviour and the labour market. In K. Hawton, & K. van Heerigen (Eds.), *The international handbook of suicide and attempted suicide* (pp. 310–384). New York: Wiley.

Platt, S., & Kreitman, N. (1985). Is unemployment a cause of parasuicide? *British Medical Journal Clinical Research Education, 290*(6462), 161.

Pokorny, A. D. (1983). Prediction of suicide in psychiatric patients. Report of a prospective study. *Archives of General Psychiatry, 40*(3), 249–257.

Qin, P., & Nordentoft, M. (2005). Suicide risk in relation to psychiatric hospitalization: Evidence based on longitudinal registers 1. *Archives of General Psychiatry, 62*(4), 427–432.

Quinnett, P. (2005). *QPR: Ask a Question, Save a Life. Certified QPR Gatekeeper's Instructor's Manual.* Spokane, WA: QPR Institute.

Rihmer, Z. (2001). Can better recognition and treatment of depression reduce suicide rates? A brief review. *European Psychiatry, 16*(7), 406–409.

Rihmer, Z., Rutz, W., & Pihlgren, H. (1995). Depression and suicide on Gotland. An intensive study of all suicides before and after a depression-training programme for general practitioners. *Journal of Affective Disorders, 35*(4), 147–152.

Rosack, J. (2005). New data show declines in antidepressant prescribing. *Psychiatric News*, 1–6.

Rose, G. (1985). Sick individuals and sick populations. *International Journal of Epidemiology, 14*(1), 32–38.

Rose, G. (1992). *The strategy of preventive medicine.* Oxford, England: Oxford University Press.

Rosenberg, M. L., Gelles, R. J., Holinger, P. C., Zahn, M. A., Stark, E., Conn J. M., et al. (1987). Violence: Homicide, assault and suicide. In R. W. Amler & H. B. Dull (Eds.), *Closing the gap: the burden of unnecessary illness*. New York: Oxford University Press.

Rutz, W. (2001). Preventing suicide and premature death by education and treatment. *Journal of Affective Disorders, 62*(1–2), 123–129.

Rutz, W., von Knorrring, L., & Walinder, J. (1992). Long-term effects of an educational program for general practitioners given by the Swedish Committee for the Prevention and Treatment of Depression. *Acta Pscyhiatrica Scandinavica, 85*, 414–418.

Satcher, D. (1999). *The Surgeon General's Call to Action to Prevent Suicide*. Washington, DC: US Public Health Service.

Satcher, D. (2001). *National Strategy for Suicide Prevention: Goals and Objectives for Action*. Rockville, MD: US Department of Health and Human Services.

Schwartz, A. J. (2006a). College student suicide in the United States: 1990–1991 through 2003–2004. *Journal of American College Health, 54*(6), 341–352.

Schwartz, A. J. (2006b). Four eras of study of college student suicide in the United States: 1920–2004.[Erratum appears in J Am Coll Health. 2006 Sep-Oct;55(2):98]. *Journal of American College Health, 54*(6), 353–366.

Scott, M. A., Wilcox, H. C., Schonfeld, I. S., Davies, M., Hicks, R. C., Turner, J. B., & Shaffer, D. (2009). School-based screening to identify at-risk students not already known to school professionals: the Columbia suicide screen. *American Journal of Public Health, 99*(2), 334–339.

Shaffer, D., Scott, M., Wilcox, H., Maslow, C., Hicks, R., Lucas, C. P., et al. (2004). The Columbia Suicide Screen: validity and reliability of a screen for youth suicide and depression. *Journal of the American Academy of Child & Adolescent Psychiatry, 43*(1), 71–79.

Szanto, K., Kalmar, S., Hendin, H., Rihmer, Z., & Mann, J. J. (2007). A suicide prevention program in a region with a very high suicide rate. *Archives of General Psychiatry, 64*(8), 914–920.

Valuck, R. J., Libby, A. M., Orton, H. D., Morrato, E. H., Allen, R., & Baldessarini, R. J. (2007). Spillover effects on treatment of adult depression in primary care after FDA advisory on risk of pediatric suicidality with SSRIs. *American Journal of Psychiatry, 164*(8), 1198–1205.

Ware, J. H. (2006). The limitations of risk factors as prognostic tools. *New England Journal of Medicine, 355*(25), 2615–2617.

Wilcox, H. C., Conner, K. R., & Caine, E. D. (2004). Association of alcohol and drug use disorders and completed suicide: an empirical review of cohort studies. *Drug & Alcohol Dependence, 76*(Suppl), S11–S19.

Wilcox, H. C., Kellam, S. G., Brown, C. H., Poduska, J. M., Ialongo, N. S., Wang, W., Anthony, J. C. (2008). The impact of two universal randomized first- and second-grade classroom interventions on young adult suicide ideation and attempts. *Drug & Alcohol Dependence, 95*(Suppl 1), S60–S73.

Wong, N., Black, H., & Gardin, J. (2000). *Preventive Cardiology: A Practical Approach*. New York, NY: McGraw-Hill.

World Health Organization. (1996). *Prevention of suicide: Guidelines for the formulation and implementation of national strategies*. New York, New York; United Nations.

World Health Organization. (2009). The Global Burden of Disease: 2004 Update. Disease and injury country estimates. Retrieved from www.who.int/healthinfo/ global_burden_disease/estimates_country/en/index.html.

Wyman, P. A., Brown, C. H., Inman, J., Cross, W., Schmeelk-Cone, K., Guo, J., & Pena, J. B. (2008). Randomized trial of a gatekeeper program for suicide prevention: 1-year impact on secondary school staff. *Journal of Consulting & Clinical Psychology, 76*(1), 104–115.

Yip, P. S., & Caine, E. D. (2010). Employment status and suicide: The complex relationships between changing unemployment rates and death rates. *Journal of Epidemiology and Community Health*. 2010.

Conclusion

17 Twenty-first century public health practice

Preventing mental illness and promoting mental health

Neal Cohen and Sandro Galea

Mental health is public health

A framework for a preventive science approach to mental disorders was launched in 1994 with the publication of two reports, prepared by the National Institute of Mental Health (NIMH) and by the Institute of Medicine (IOM), both in response to Congressional requests. The NIMH report, *The Prevention of Mental Disorders: A National Research Agenda* (NIMH, 1994), underscored the components of a prevention science approach that would undertake risk and protective factor studies, controlled preventive intervention trials, and evidence-based implementation efforts. The groundbreaking IOM report, *Reducing Risks for Mental Disorders: Frontiers for Preventive Intervention Research* (IOM, 1994), reaffirmed the distinct parameters of treatment and prevention within a risk and protective factor framework for interventions prior to the onset of illness. The report advanced a typology for the pathways through which prevention-oriented interventions are targeted.

1 "Universal" preventive interventions are directed at a population base without specific knowledge of their health and mental well-being.
2 "Selective" preventive interventions are directed at those who are deemed to be at elevated risk for mental health problems.
3 "Indicated" preventive interventions are directed at individuals already manifesting psychological symptoms suggesting high risk for mental illness.

Since 1994, progress in advancing a prevention/health promotion research agenda for mental disorders has accelerated further. Using a new metric for calculating the disabling aspects of 107 diseases in a comparative framework, the Global Burden of Disease Study expanded the traditional focus of public health concerns, drawing greater attention to healthy life (Murray & Lopez, 1996). Consequently, for the first time, mental disorders were recognized as among the leading causes of diminished human productivity, with impairments of social functioning contributing years of disability comparable to cardiovascular and respiratory diseases and surpassing all cancers and HIV. Furthermore, five of the 10 leading causes of disability worldwide were recognized as mental health-related problems, including major depression, schizophrenia, bipolar disorders, alcohol use, and obsessive-compulsive disorders.

The evidence for the enormous burden of mental disorders in terms of both human suffering and economic hardship underscored the need to apply the tools and strategies of public health practice in an integrated health and mental health agenda. An eminent public health leader, Surgeon General David Satcher, became a leading voice for the mainstreaming of mental health into the larger public health landscape with the publication of *Mental Health: A Report of the Surgeon General* (U.S. Public Health Service, 1999a), in which he stated:

> Through much of this era of great challenge and greater achievement, however, concerns regarding mental illness and mental health too often were relegated to the rear of our national consciousness. Tragic and devastating disorders such as schizophrenia, depression and bipolar disorder, Alzheimer's disease, the mental and behavioral disorders suffered by children, and a range of other mental disorders affect nearly one in five Americans in any year, yet continue too frequently to be spoken of in whispers and shame.
>
> (Preface)

Dr. Satcher noted that over the previous two decades a revolution in science and service delivery had deepened our understanding of mental health and illness and improved the way in which mental health care is provided. While encouraging individuals to seek treatment when experiencing disturbances to their mental well-being, the Surgeon General's message also advocated moving the mental health/mental illness focus into the core priorities of our nation's public health agenda. As a follow-up to the message of this first report, additional reports on suicide prevention (U.S. Public Health Service, 1999b) and cultural perspectives (U.S. Public Health Service, 2000) further developed the framework for applying the tools and strategies of public health practice to the challenges of mental illness prevention and mental health promotion.

The challenge of mainstreaming mental health requires a broad-based public health research agenda with more advanced epidemiologic data providing the basis for a population-based risk and protective factor framework for preventive interventions. The findings of the National Comorbidity Study Replication (NCS-R) on the age of onsets of mental disorders have provided an opportunity for a 21st century focus on prevention and mental health promotion (Kessler, Berglund, Demler, Jin, Merikangas, & Walters 2005a). The NCS-R found that half of adult respondents with *Diagnostic and Statistical Manual of Mental Disorders,*

Fourth Edition (DSM-IV) diagnosable conditions had onsets by age 14 and three-fourths by age 24 years. The early-life onset of mental disorders supports a major thrust for prevention and mental health promotion in childhood and early adolescence and involvement of child serving settings such as schools and primary pediatric healthcare.

The NCS-R also found significant delays in detection of mental disorders from the age of onset when symptoms were first manifest. Depressive illness was found to have delays of eight to 13 years from onset to diagnosis; anxiety disorders had even longer delays, nine to 15 years from onset to diagnosis. These findings give further evidence for a "window of opportunity" to implement portals of screening for symptomatology during childhood and adolescence in order to intervene (indicated prevention) before the onset of a full-blown DSM-IV diagnosable mental disorder.

The last decade has seen the shift toward an era of "risk factor" epidemiology (Susser & Morabia, 2006), which has identified individual, family, and community-level factors at which to target interventions to mitigate the onset and progression of mental disorders. The prevention field has increasingly recognized the cumulative risk associated with exposure to a multitude of factors often present in disadvantaged inner-city neighborhoods. Consequently, the aim of lowering or eliminating risks and bolstering strengths and external supports underpins 21st century policies, programs, and practices intended to reduce the burden of mental disorders.

The 2009 IOM Report, *Preventing Mental, Emotional, and Behavioral Disorders Among Young People: Progress and Possibilities* (IOM, 2009a), underscores that the risk and protective factor framework for intervention must recognize the influences that experiences at younger ages may have on outcomes at later stages. Thus, the report endorses a perspective in which developmental and contextual factors are understood and addressed through interventions that aim to prevent or mitigate the progression of mental health problems. These factors can be influenced at many levels: individual, biological, psychological, family, community, and cultural. While some risk factors are fixed and cannot be changed (e.g., gender, ethnicity), other risk factors may be modified by interventions taking place at "downstream" (e.g., individuals, families) or "upstream" (e.g., public policies) levels of influence. The last decade has seen a growing literature on the association between risk factors and a number of mental health problems and disorders (Biglan, Brennan, Foster, & Holder, 2004; Garber, 2006; Luthar, 2003). Multilevel assessment can identify those high-risk groups that are most likely to benefit from targeted preventive interventions, which can be developed both to reduce risk factors and to bolster protective factors to disrupt the causal processes and pathways involved in negative outcomes.

Kraemaer, Stice, Kazdin, Offord, and Kupfer (2001) caution that a risk approach to understanding the complex etiologic processes leading to mental health disorders requires a careful analysis of how risk factors work together. They underscore that merely counting or scoring the multitude of risk factors associated with mental health outcomes does little to promote development of interventions that are optimally timed or delivered for the prevention of negative outcomes. Furthermore, when there are chains of risk factors that mediate outcomes in a sequential manner, targeting only one link in that chain may produce effects of minor clinical or policy significance. Consequently, elucidating the multiple causal paths of risk factors leading to mental disorders provides the best opportunity for developing a strategic plan with meaningful preventive interventions.

In particular, the cumulative risk associated with exposure to multiple adversities in disadvantaged inner-city neighborhoods suggests the need for interventions that can address multiple risk and protective factors in these communities. Risk factors are commonly positively correlated with each other and negatively correlated with protective factors (IOM, 2009a). Pollard and colleagues (Pollard, Hawkins, & Arthur, 1999) found that among students in sixth to twelfth grade, those who were in the highest quintile on a cumulative measure of risk factors were likely to be in the lowest quintile in the measure of protective factors. Further, multiple risk factors are strongly associated with poor mental health outcomes. Sameroff and colleagues (Sameroff, Gutman, & Peck, 2003) found that youth with eight or more risk factors were at much greater risk of displaying problem behavior and mental health problems than youth with three or fewer risk factors.

Further research is required to understand the relationship of risk factors to each other and to protective factors. For example, a "mediational model" of influence suggests risk and protective factors affect another set of factors that in turn affects the development of mental, emotional, and behavioral problems. In support of this model, a number of researchers have found that parenting difficulties have been a mediator of the effects of multiple risk factors on youth outcomes including poverty, parental mental health problems, and family violence (Grant, Compas, Stuhlmacher, Thurm, McMahon, & Halpert, 2003; Kwok, Haine, Sandler, Ayers, & Wolchik, 2005; Wolchik, Wilcox, Tein, & Sandler, 2000). A "moderational model" places greater emphasis on the influence of protective factors in disrupting the pathways between risk factors and mental disorders. For example, researchers have recognized the importance of parents in buffering the exposure of children to community violence in disadvantaged inner-city neighborhoods (Grant et al., 2003). In addition, neighborhood-level characteristics (e.g., socioeconomic status, assaultive crime, gang presence) can affect the mental well-being of families living with an ongoing sense of threat to their safety. Maternal depression has been associated with community/neighborhood factors (IOM, 2009b) and may result in direct and indirect (mediation and moderation models) influences on a mother's ability to parent effectively and to buffer the severe stress that will be experienced by her children across ages and developmental stages.

The "power problem"

The emerging field of prevention research is uniquely challenged by a limited knowledge of the bio-psychosocial pathways that lead to mental disorders and the low specificity of most known risk factors. Cuijpers (2003) highlights the difficulty in demonstrating actual reductions in the incidence of new cases of mental disorder according to diagnostic criteria by prevention programs and researchers. Among the barriers, Cuijpers cites the "power problem" (the need for very large numbers of subjects to statistically identify potential effects of interventions), the need to use intensive diagnostic interviews, and the subsequent high costs of such studies.

To date, research studies have generally focused on reducing the prevalence and adverse influences of some of the known risk factors for mental disorders. The difficulty with this approach is that no single risk factor for mental disorders has heretofore been found to account for more than 15% of the onset of cases of mental illness (McGuire & Troisi, 1997). In a meta-analytic review of thirteen prevention studies meeting rigorous inclusion criteria for pretest-posttest randomized controlled design, Cuijpers, Van Straten and Smit (2005) found a statistically significant and clinically relevant reduction in the incidence of new cases of mental disorders. When separating the effects of "selective" prevention, aimed at high-risk groups, and "indicated" prevention, targeting those with evidence of symptoms of mental disorder but not meeting diagnostic criteria, indicated prevention did show statistical significance of risk reduction, though selective prevention did not. However, these results may not refute the potential benefits of selective prevention with groups at elevated risk, as they may reflect the "power problem." That is, greater incidence rates may occur among groups with elevated risk associated with multiple risk factors and evidence of subclinical signs and symptoms.

An example: Targeting depression for a prevention focus

The interest in prevention approaches to mental disorders undoubtedly has been enhanced over the past decade by the Global Burden of Disease study (Lopez, Mathers, Ezzati, Jamison, & Murray, 2006), which established mental disorders as among the most debilitating health conditions worldwide. Major depressive disorder, as a single diagnostic entity, emerged in these studies as the leading cause of disability worldwide. Additionally, the epidemiologic findings of the NCS-R in the US found a lifetime prevalence of major depression among adults to be 16.2%, with another 4.1% meeting the diagnostic criteria for dysthymic disorder, a milder but still disabling and chronic form of depression (Kessler, Berglund, Demler, Jin, Koretz, Merikangas, et al., 2003). The high incidence rate for depression in the general population and the potential for further targeting of preventive interventions to "at-risk" subgroups provides an opportunity for both meaningful clinical benefit and the needed statistical power to support research investigations.

Depression, along with other mental disorders, has been associated with a number of non-specific risk factors including poverty, exposure to violence, social isolation, child maltreatment, and family breakup (Gladstone & Beardslee, 2009). Additionally, there are specific risk factors that elevate depression risk, including earlier history of depression, an extensive family history of depression, a "depressogenic" cognitive style, and symptoms of depression that do not fully meet diagnostic criteria. Gladstone and Beardslee (2009) propose a youth prevention approach to depression that targets both non-specific and specific risk factors in view of the research on the additive effects of childhood risk factors.

The high rates of depression and early age of onset has stimulated greater attention to the influences of adverse family environments as a major risk factor for adolescent depression and other mental disorders (Evans et al., 2005). Along with determining lifetime prevalence rates for a number of mental health disorders, the NCS-R also collected data on the exposure of respondents to twelve different major childhood adversities (CAs) prior to the age of 18 years. Factor analysis grouped a number of CAs into those reflecting maladaptive family functioning (MFF), including parental mental illness, parental substance abuse, criminal behavior, domestic violence, physical abuse, sexual abuse, and neglect. Among those with exposure to at least one CA within the MFF factor, multiple CAs were the norm (Green et al., 2010). Green and colleagues (2010) examined the association between these CAs and the later onset of a number of DSM-IV disorders and found an increase in onsets with a higher count of CA exposures; MFF category childhood adversities were associated with a number of later mental disorders. In a further analysis of the NCS-R data by the same research team, McLaughlin, Green, Gruber, Sampson, Zaslavsky, and Kessler (2010) found that, compared to other CAs, MFF-related CAs were more strongly associated with persistent mental disorders, especially adult mood disorders. In a commentary on these studies and the adult mental health consequences of childhood adversity, Scott, Varghese, and McGrath (2010) identified a need for preventive interventions that address MFF "in a more holistic perspective rather than one CA at a time" (p. 111).

While we require greater understanding of the pathways linking CAs to negative mental health outcomes in later life, we have good evidence for the frequent transgenerational transmission of childhood adversity; adults whose own mental health problems are associated with childhood adversity are at greater risk to expose their children to similar adversities (Dixon, Browne, & Hamilton-Giachritsis, 2005; Sroufe, 2005). These findings underscore the potential benefit of family-focused preventive intervention models that can target the dysfunction in family environments that are most toxic to the next generation.

Parental depression and two generation family-based interventions

The 2009 Institute of Medicine report, *Depression in Parents, Parenting, and Children: Opportunities to Improve Identification, Treatment, and Prevention* (IOM, 2009b), describes a large clinical and epidemiologic literature that has found associations between parental depression and impairments in children's health and development. Children of depressed parents are about four times more likely to experience an episode of major depression than children of non-ill controls and two times more likely compared to children of parents with other psychiatric or medical conditions (Rice, Harold, & Thaper, 2002). Prospective high-risk family studies have reported the risk for depression among children of depressed parents compared to children of non-ill control families increases throughout childhood ages and stages (Beardslee, Keller, Lavori, Staley, & Sacks, 1993; Weissman, Warner, Wickramaratne, Moreau, & Olfson, 1997). In a review by Avenevoli and Merikangas (2006), multiple family environmental factors (e.g., parenting skills, stress, marital discord) have been recognized as mediating or moderating the association between parental depression and children's development of depression.

The greater risk for depressive disorders among women and the usual primary caretaking role of mothers for infants, toddlers, and young children underscores the risks associated with maternal depression. Skills in parenting are widely regarded as instrumental in facilitating healthy development in children and must be adaptable to the developmental needs of young children at different ages and stages (IOM, 2009b). Cole, Martin, and Dennis (2004) highlight the importance of providing age-appropriate levels of warmth and structure to promote healthy regulation of emotions and overall well-being. Consequently, parenting practices that are unresponsive to very young children's needs are seen as mediating the adverse influences of maternal depression on their children's healthy development.

Using direct observations of parents and children in families with depressed mothers, there is consistent evidence directly linking maternal depression with problematic parenting practices, including less maternal responsiveness, less verbal and visual interaction, and more intrusiveness (Campbell et al., 2004; Civic & Holt, 2000; Horwitz, Briggs-Gowan, Storger-Isser, & Carter, 2007, NICHD Early Child Care Research Network, 1999). Although most studies of the nature of parent-child interactions have been limited to elevated depression symptom levels and not formal diagnoses, the findings provide consistent support for associations between maternal depression and parenting styles that are withdrawn/disengaged or intrusive/harsh, with significant risks to the development of infants and toddlers.

Older children and adolescents are also affected by parenting behaviors of their depressed parents. Depressed parents of older children may exhibit a similar range of dysfunctional behaviors as depressed parents of very young children, including more negative and unpredictable parental behaviors (e.g., irritability, inconsistent discipline), less supportive parental responses, and heightened marital discord (Cummings, Keller, & Davies, 2005). Studies of older children have also reported these parenting styles to at least partially mediate the associations between parental depression and the development of behavioral or emotional problems in their older children (DuRocher Schuldlich & Cummings, 2007; Elgar, Mills, McGrath, Waschbusch, & Brownridge, 2007; Jaser et al. 2008).

With an estimated 15.6 million children under age 18 living with a parent who had major depression in the past year (IOM, 2009b), family-focused interventions that offer prevention and treatment services to parents and children and that also enhance the parenting practices of a depressed parent can offer significant individual, family, and societal benefits. Despite the plethora of clinical and epidemiologic studies of depression in individuals and families, few studies have explicitly examined the association of parenting-related stressors to the expression of depression, anxiety, and other behavioral health problems. Consequently, there is little information on the influences of parenting-related stressors, parental mental health problems, and access to material and psychosocial resources on the ability of families to address child mental health needs.

Using data from the 2000 National Survey of Early Childhood Health (NSECH), Mistry and colleagues (Mistry, Stevens, Sareen, DeVogli, & Halfon, 2007) found social and financial parenting stressors disproportionately prevalent among low-income families and associated with increased risk of poor maternal health. Building on the work of Waddell, Shannon, and Durr (2001), the authors propose that community-level family resource centers be developed so that families can access a network of community support services. Community-based and family-focused, these resource centers can strengthen and support resilient family functioning, reduce parenting stressors, and promote better parental response to their children's developmental needs. Services could be initiated in a variety of health care settings that engage children and families, including "well-baby" and other pediatric and family practice settings, and can offer a two-generation model that is family-focused, culturally informed, and accessible to vulnerable populations (IOM, 2009a). Developing family-focused care that integrates the health, mental health, and social service systems will require demonstration projects at the community, state, and federal levels to evaluate the efficiency and efficacy of new service delivery models and will need to address existing systemic, workforce, and fiscal barriers.

Preventive interventions targeting children of depressed parents and the interruption of intergenerational transmission of risk for poor health and mental health outcomes must be recognized as a major focus for community-level activity. Beardslee and colleagues (Beardslee & Gladstone, 2001; Beardslee, Gladstone, Wright, & Cooper, 2003) have devised a series of family-based preventive interventions to enhance the family environment and to mitigate the transmission of elevated risk for depression among the children of parents affected by depressive disorders. The interventions include a clinician-facilitated six to ten-session psychoeducational program delivered to parents and children; another intervention is comprised of a two-session lecture format delivered to the parents only. In a two and a half year follow-up, children in both interventions reported a decrease in internalizing symptoms (Beardslee et al., 2003).

Primary care screening

The National Comorbidity Survey-Replication (NCS-R), conducted between 2001 and 2003, documented the expansion of primary healthcare as the main provider of psychiatric treatment, compared to the specialty mental health sector (Kessler et al., 2005b). As the emergence of serotonin specific reuptake inhibitor drugs was associated with fewer adverse drug reactions and health risks than the previous generation of tricyclic antidepressant medications, primary care physicians became increasingly willing to treat depression in their office-based practices. Nevertheless, screening of patients for mental health problems in primary care settings has had limited implementation outside of academic and research-oriented program services. This issue has been the focus of a good deal of debate. Critics of wider use of mental health screens have argued that the costs, time, and outcomes associated with screening do not warrant its wide-scale use in general practice. (Coyne, Palmer, & Sullivan, 2003; Valenstein, Vijan, Zeber, Boehm, & Buttar, 2001), while advocates cite the relatively high prevalence of depression and associated morbidity as problematic if undetected and untreated.

Weissman, Neria, Gameroff, Pilowsky, Wickramaratne, Lantigua, Shea, and Olfson (2010) followed 519 low-income primary care patients who were screened for depression. Those who screened positive reported significantly poorer mental and social functioning and worse general health at the four year follow-up interview. These patients were also more likely to use emergency psychiatric services in the year prior to the follow-up interview. These findings of adverse outcomes after four years of clinically unrecognized and untreated depression were also evident in screens for other disorders, including generalized anxiety disorder, panic disorder, and alcohol or drug use disorder. For this population of low-income patients, simple screening procedures for depression and other mental health symptomatology identified a cohort that would experience persistent and increasingly disruptive mental health problems over time. Thus, screening appears likely to be a valuable tool for the secondary prevention of mental disorders.

Promoting resilience

The risk and protective factor framework has offered the field of prevention research a conceptual approach to maximizing positive outcomes in response to stress and adversities. While we have limited ability to predict outcomes from any set of specific and known risk and protective factors, the concept of "resilience" informs a number of relevant research areas. Using a consensus definition of resilience as "the process of, capacity for, or outcome of successful adaptation after trauma or severe stress," Norris, Tracy, and Galea (2009, p. 2190) describe the unique characteristics of the trajectory toward good mental health following exposure to traumatic events among resilient individuals. The authors posit that different response trajectories can be measured and studied across stressors and settings, allowing for the potential implementation of relevant interventions to enhance resiliency and recovery.

In their review of the mechanisms of resilience among families at different levels of risk, Vanderbilt-Adriance and Shaw (2008a) found resilience to be a dynamic process that fluctuates within and across developmental stages and is better conceptualized as limited to specific outcomes at specific time points. Masten and colleagues (2004) underscored the dynamic nature of resilience across developmental stages, highlighting the positive influence of protective factors in adolescence even subsequent to the circumstances of childhood adversity. Luthar and Cicchetti (2000) emphasize the need to understand the overall context that allows protective factors to emerge, develop, and mitigate risk; they caution against trying to change individual protective factors when the environmental context will not change, instead advocating for interventions to enhance multiple protective factors across domains, including child, family, and the larger community. Similarly, in order to facilitate resilience, decreasing overall exposure to risk increases the benefit of protective factors (Vanderbilt-Adriance & Shaw, 2008b).

Although research has examined factors associated with both positive and negative outcomes, there has been minimal focus on the processes by which these factors overcome adversity. Recognizing the dynamic processes associated with resilience should facilitate the translational research agenda needed for a new era of preventive interventions in high-risk neighborhoods and communities.

Mental health promotion

> We know more today about how to treat mental illness effectively and appropriately than we know with certainty about how to prevent mental illness and promote mental health. Common sense and respect for our fellow humans tells us that a focus on the positive aspects of mental health demands our immediate attention.
>
> (U.S. Public Health Service, 1999a, Preface)

While mental health prevention work has advanced substantially since the 1994 IOM report, promoting positive mental health at the population level has received scant attention. Distinguishing mental health promotion from illness prevention can be difficult given the general overlap in the field of practice, but it is helpful to establishing a set of principles underlying health and mental health promotion that uniquely contribute to physical and mental well-being. Key to the conceptualization of mental health promotion as distinct from prevention activities is a definition of mental health that is not solely the absence of signs and symptoms of mental disorder.

The 2009 IOM Report (2009a) adopted a definition of mental health promotion compatible with recent international efforts (Jane-Llopis & Anderson, 2005; Substance Abuse and Mental Health Services Administration, 2007; World Health Organization (WHO), 2004): "Mental health promotion includes efforts to enhance individuals' ability to achieve developmentally appropriate tasks (developmental competence) and a positive sense of self-esteem, mastery, well-being, and social inclusion and to strengthen their ability to cope with adversity" (p. 67). With a focus on healthy outcomes and positive aspects of mental well-being and greater distinction from illness prevention activities, the IOM committee (2009a) proposed that mental health promotion be recognized as a significant component of the mental health intervention spectrum, which can serve as a foundation for both prevention and treatment of disorders.

Over the past several decades, clinical medicine has increasingly addressed health promoting activities and behaviors as a component of routine care. Public health and medical science have identified numerous biological, behavioral, and environmental risk factors for illnesses, leading to recommendations for lifestyle choices (e.g., diet, exercise, tobacco, drugs and alcohol) that are empirically linked to improved health. Building upon this model, the goal of mental health promotion would be the attainment of an optimal state of mental well-being, but the relative lack of consensus on how to define and measure positive mental health has impeded progress in developing an evidence base for mental health promotion. The greater clarity of definitions and goals for promotion and prevention should create opportunities to more rigorously test mental health promoting activities in a less stigmatizing field of 21st century mental health practice.

Looking forward

With the publication of two major IOM reports in 2009 (2009a; 2009b), the field of practice for the prevention of mental disorders has received critical support as a mainstream public health priority. Over the past few decades, significant advances in mental health epidemiology have provided opportunities to recognize the associated factors that place people at risk for illness and those that confer some protection against those risks. With multiple risk factors affecting both physical and mental well-being, 21st century public health practice is discovering models of integrated health and mental health focus that promise to synergistically extend the reach of preventive interventions toward a more holistic conceptualization of health.

In the past 10 years, a scientific consensus has recognized that many adult health problems have their origins in early childhood exposures to stressors and adversities (Green et al., 2010; National Research Council, & Institute of Medicine, 2000; Repetti, Taylor, & Seeman, 2002; Shonkoff, Boyce, & McEwen, 2009). Shonkoff and colleagues (2009) posit that negative health consequences may be the result of cumulative exposure to multiple adversities over time or by the "biological embedding of adversities during sensitive developmental periods" (p. 2252). Through either mechanism, the risks for ill health are established in early childhood and may not be manifest until decades later. Repetti, Taylor, and Seeman (2002) found considerable evidence for the link between early exposure to adversities and many poor health and mental health outcomes, including diabetes, ischemic heart disease, chronic respiratory problems, anxiety, depression, substance abuse, and depression. Occurring more widely in disadvantaged neighborhoods and communities, exposure to significant stressors and adversities widen and sustain many socioeconomic and ethnic/racial health disparities, which suggests that reducing exposure to early adversity can be important to reducing health disparities (Braveman & Ergerter, 2008).

Furthermore, the evidence for early-age onsets of mental disorders has given an empirical boost to family-focused preventive interventions that aim to curb the intergenerational transmission of multiple risk factors for mental disorders. This does not, however, negate the individual and societal benefit to be derived from preventive interventions that target individuals at elevated risk throughout the lifespan. Regrettably, infants, young children, and older adults have been excluded from prevention trials, so research is greatly lacking (Castro, Barrera, & Martinez, 2004).

Translating prevention science into community-level interventions that reduce risk exposures, improve parenting, and promote safer and more nurturing physical environments will require an infrastructure for community engagement and participation involving numerous stakeholders. Mercy and Saul (2009) propose an infrastructure for the broader dissemination of health promoting and preventive interventions that requires three interrelated systems:

1   developing effective interventions that are accessible and user-friendly for practitioners;
2   building organizational capacity for community-level engagement in evidence-based prevention and promotion activities; and
3   delivering high-quality evidence-based interventions at the national, state, or local levels.

Zylke and DeAngelis (2009) describe the already widespread acceptance of health promotion and disease prevention approaches to child development. Starting in utero, pregnant women take prenatal vitamins, refrain from drinking alcohol or smoking, breastfeed during their children's infancy, and select healthy foods, and participate in exercise. Pediatricians in turn administer vaccines and monitor for healthy developmental milestones. However, advancing beyond individual behavior choices and doctor-patient interactions toward implementation of a broader framework for health promotion and disease prevention requires significant political and economic investments. Policy makers and program planners must recognize the long-term value of broad, interdisciplinary investments in the support and stability of children and families and thier consequences for long-term health. The inclusion of mental health concerns, mental health promotion, and mental illness prevention into an integrated public health model that fully recognizes the interrelationships of physical and mental well-being will be key to advancing effective and cost-effective interventions for the greatest societal benefit. Clearly, a research agenda for an integrated health/mental health promotion and illness prevention framework is needed to identify the public policies and the real-life community practices that will best advance 21st century public health.

References

Avenevoli, S., & Merikangas, K. R. (2006). Implications of high-risk family studies for prevention of depression. *American Journal of Preventive Medicine, 31,* 126–135.

Beardslee, W. R., & Gladstone, T. R. (2001). Prevention of childhood depression: Recent findings and future prospects. *Biological Psychiatry, 49,* 1101–1110.

Beardslee, W. R., Gladstone, T. R., Wright, E. J., & Cooper, A. B. (2003). A family-based approach to the prevention of depressive symptoms in children at risk: Evidence of parental and child change. *Pediatrics, 112*(2), e119-e131.

Beardslee, W. R., Keller, M. B., Lavori, P. W., Staley, J. E., & Sacks, N. (1993). The impact of parental affective disorders on depression in offspring: A longitudinal follow-up in a nonreferred sampled. *Journal of American Academy of Child and Adolescent Psychiatry, 32,* 723–730.

Biglan, A., Brennan, P. A., Foster, S. L., & Holder, H. D. (2004). *Helping adolescents at risk: Prevention of multiple problem behaviors.* New York: Guilford Press.

Braveman, P., & Ergeter, T. (2008). *Overcoming obstacles to health: Report from the Robert Wood Foundation to the Commission to Build a Healthier America.* Princeton, NJ: Robert Wood Johnson Foundation.

Campbell, S. B., Brownell, C. A., Hungerford, A., Spieker, S. I., Mohan, R., & Blessing, J. S. (2004). The course of maternal depression and maternal sensitivity as predictors of attachment security at 36 months. *Developmental Psychopathology, 16,* 231–52.

Castro, F. G., Barrera, M., & Martinez, C. R. (2004). The cultural adaptation of prevention interventions: Resolving tensions between fidelity and fit. *Prevention Science, 5,* 41–45.

Civic, D., & Holt, V. L. (2000). Maternal depressive symptoms and child behavior problems in a nationally representative normal birthweight sample. *Maternal and Child Health Journal, 4,* 215–221.

Cole, P. M., Martin, S. E., & Dennis, T. A. (2004). Emotion regulation as a scientific construct: Methodological challenges and directions for child development research. *Child Development, 75*, 317–333.

Coyne, J. C., Palmer, S. C., & Sullivan, P. A. (2003). Screening for depression in adults. *Annals of Internal Medicine, 138*, 767–768.

Cuijpers, P. (2003). Examining the effects of prevention programs on the incidence of new cases of mental disorders: The lack of statistical power. *American Journal of Psychiatry, 160*, 1385–1391.

Cuijpers, P., Van Straten, A., & Smit, F. (2005). Preventing the incidence of new cases of mental disorders: A meta-analytic review. *Journal of Nervous and Mental Disease, 193*, 119–125.

Cummings, E. M., Keller, P. S., & Davies, P. T. (2005). Towards a family process model of maternal and paternal depressive symptoms: Exploring multiple relations with child and family functioning. *Journal of Child Psychology and Psychiatry, 46*, 479–489.

Dixon, L., Browne, K., & Hamilton-Giachritsis, C. (2005). Risk factors of parents abused as children: A mediational analysis of the intergenerational continuity of child maltreatment (part 1). *Journal of Child Psychological Psychiatry, 46*, 47–57.

DuRocher Schuldlich, T. D., & Cummings, E. M. (2007). Parental dysphoria, marital conflict, and parenting: Relations with children's emotional security and adjustment. *Journal of Abnormal Child Psychology, 35*, 627–639.

Elgar, F. J., Mills, R. S. L., McGrath, P. J., Waschbusch, D. A., & Brownridge, D. A. (2007). Maternal and paternal depressive symptoms and child maladjustment: The mediating role of parental behavior. *Journal of Abnormal Child Psychology, 35*, 943–955.

Evans, D. L., Foa, E. B., Gur, R. E., Hendin, H., O'Brien, C.P., Seligman, M. E. P., & Walsh, B. T. (Eds.). (2005). *Treating and preventing adolescent mental health disorders: What we know and what we don't know*. New York: Oxford University Press.

Garber, J. L. (2006). Depression in children and adolescents: Linking risk research and prevention. *American Journal of Preventive Medicine, 31*(Suppl.1), S104–S125.

Gladstone, T., & Beardslee, W. R. (2009). The prevention of depression in children and adolescents: A review. *Canadian Journal of Psychiatry*, 212–221.

Grant, K. E., Compas, B. E., Stuhlmacher, A. F., Thurm, A. E., McMahon, S. D., & Halpert, J. A. (2003). Stressors and child and adolescent psychopathology: Evidence of moderating and mediating effects. *Clinical Psychology Reviews, 26*, 257–83.

Green, J. G., McLaughlin, K. A., Berglund, P. A., Gruber, M. J., Sampson, N. A., Zaslavsky, A. M., & Kessler, R. C. (2010). Childhood adversities and adult psychiatric disorders in the National Comorbidity Survey Replication I: Associations with first onset of DSM-IV disorders. *Archives of General Psychiatry, 67*, 113–123.

Horwitz, S. M., Briggs-Gowan, M. J., Storger-Isser, A., & Carter, A. S. (2007). Prevalence, correlates and persistence of maternal depression. *Journal of Womenelates an, 16*, 678–691.

Insel, T. R. & Fenton, W. S. (2005). Psychiatric epidemiology: Itrsistence of maternal depression. en*Archives of General Psychiatry, 62*, 590–592.

IOM. (1994). *Reducing risks for mental disorders: Frontiers for preventive intervention research*. P. J. Marazek & R. J. Haggerty (Eds.), Committee on Prevention of Mental Disorders, Division of Biobehavioral Sciences and Mental Disorders. Washington, DC: National Academy Press.

IOM (2009a). *Preventing mental, emotional, and behavioral disorders among young people: Progress and possibilities*. Washington, DC: National Academy Press.

IOM (2009b). *Depression in parents, parenting, and children: Opportunities to improve identification, treatment, and prevention*. Washington, DC: National Academy Press.

Jane-Llopis, E., & Anderson, P. (2005). *Mental health promotion and mental disorder prevention: A policy for Europe*. Nijmegen, the Netherlands: Radboud University Nijmegen. Available: www.imhpa.net/actionplan.

Jaser, S. S., Fear, J. M., Reeslund, K. L., Champion, J. E., Reising, M. M., & Compas, B. E. (2008). Maternal sadness and adolescents responses to stress in offspring of mothers with and without a history of depression. *Journal of Clinical Child and Adolescent Psychology, 37*, 736–746.

Kessler, R. C., Berglund, P., Demler, O., Jin, R., Koretz, D., Merikangas, K. R., et al. (2003). The epidemiology of major depressive disorder: Results from the National Comorbidity Survey (NCS-R). *JAMA, 289*, 3095–3105.

Kessler, R. C., Berglund, P., Demler, O., Jin, R., Merikangas, K. R. & Walters, E. E. (2005a). Lifetime prevalence and age-of-onset distributions of DSM-IV disorders in the National Comorbidity Survey Replication. *Archives of General Psychiatry, 62*, 593–602.

Kessler, R. C., Demler, O., Frank, R. G., Olfson, M., Pincus, H. A., Walters, E. E., Zaslavsky, A. M. (2005b). Prevalence and treatment of mental disorders, 1990 to 2003. *New England Journal of Medicine, 352*, 2515–2523.

Kraemaer, H. C., Stice, E., Kazdin, A., Offord, D., & Kupfer, D. (2001). How do risk factors work together?: Mediators, moderators, and independent, overlapping and proxy risk factors, *American Journal of Psychiatry, 158*(6), 848–856.

Kwok, O.-M., Haine, R., Sandler, I. N., Ayers, T. S., & Wolchik, S. A. (2005). Positive parenting as a mediator of the relations between parental psychological distress and mental health problems of parentally bereaved children. *Journal of Clinical Child and Adolescent Psychology, 34*, 261–272.

Lopez, A. D., Mathers, C. D., Ezzati, M., Jamison, D. T., & Murray, C. J. (2006). *Global burden of disease and risk factors*. New York: Oxford University Press.

Luthar, S. S. (2003). *Resilience and vulnerability: Adaptation in the context of childhood adversities*. New York: Cambridge University Press.

Luthar, S. S., & Cicchetti, D. (2000). The construct of resilience: Implications for interventions and social policies. *Development and Psychopathology, 12*, 857–885.

Masten, A. S., Burt, K. B., Roisman, G. I., Obradovic, J., Long, J. D., & Tellegen, A. (2004). Resources and resilience in the transition to adulthood: Continuity and change. *Development and Psychopathology, 16*, 1071–1094.

McGuire, M., & Troisi, A. (1997). *Darwinian Psychiatry*. New York: Guilford.

McLaughlin, K. A., Green, J. G., Gruber, M. J., Sampson, N. A., Zaslavsky, A. M., & Kessler, R. C. (2010). Childhood adversities and adult psychiatric disorders in the National Comorbidity Survey Replication II: Associations with persistence of DSM-IV disorders. *Archives of General Psychiatry, 67*, 124–132.

Mercy, J. A., & Saul, J. (2009). Creating a healthier future through early interventions for children. *Journal of the American Medical Association, 301*, 2262–2264.

Mistry, R., Stevens, G. D., Sareen, H., DeVogli, R., & Halfon, N. (2007). Parenting-related stressors and self-reported mental health of mothers with young children. *American Journal of Public Health, 97*, 1261–1268.

Murray, C. J. & Lopez, A. D. (1996). *The global burden of disease: A comprehensive assessment of mortality and disability from diseases, injuries, and risk factors in 1990 and projected to 2020.* Boston, MA: Harvard University Press.

National Research Council and Institute of Medicine. (2000). *From neurons to neighborhoods: The science of early childhood development.* J. P. Shonkoff & D. A. Phillips (Eds.), Committee on Integrating the Science of Early Childhood. Washington, DC: National Academy Press.

NICHD Early Child Care Research Network. (1999). Chronicity of maternal depressive symptoms, maternal sensitivity, and child functioning in 36 months. *Developmental Psychology, 35*, 1297–1310.

NIMH Prevention Research Steering Committee. (1994). *The prevention of mental disorders: A national research agenda.* Washington, DC: U.S. Government Printing Office.

Norris, F. H., Tracy, M., & Galea, S. (2009). Looking for resilience: Understanding the longitudinal trajectories to stress. *Social Science & Medicine, 68*, 2190–2198.

Pollard, J. A., Hawkins, J. D., & Arthur, M. W. (1999). Risk and protection: Are both necessary to understand diverse behavioral outcomes in adolescence. *Social Work Research, 23*, 145–158.

Repetti, R. L., Taylor, S. E., & Seeman, T. E. (2002). Risky families: family social environments and the mental and physical health of offspring. *Psychological Bulletin, 128*, 2, 330–366.

Rice, F., Harold, G., & Thaper, A. (2002). The genetic aetiology of childhood depression: A review. *Journal of Child Psychology Psychiatry, 43*, 65–79.

Sameroff, A. J., Gutman, L. M., & Peck, S. E. (2003). Adaptation among youth facing multiple risks: Prospective research findings. In S.S. Luthar (Ed.), *Resilience and vulnerability: Adaptation in the context of childhood adversities* (pp. 364–391). New York: Cambridge University Press.

Scott, J., Varghese, D., & McGrath, J. (2010) As the twig is bent, the tree inclines: Adult mental health consequences of childhood adversity. *Archives of General Psychiatry, 67*, 111–112.

Shonkoff, J. P., Boyce, W. T., & McEwen, B. S. (2009). Neuroscience, molecular biology, and the childhood roots of health disparities. *JAMA, 301*, 21, 2252–2259.

Sroufe, L. A. (2005). Attachment and development: A prospective, longitudinal study from birth to adulthood. *Attachment Human Development, 7*, 349–367.

Substance Abuse and Mental Health Services Administration. (2007). *Promotion and prevention in mental health: Strengthening parenting and enhancing child resilience* (HHS Pub. No. CMHA-SFP-6–1089). Rockville, MD: U.S. Department of Health and Human Services.

Susser, E., & Morabia, A. (2006). The arc of epidemiology. In E. Susser, S. Schwartz, A. Morabia, & E. J. Bromet (Eds.), *Psychiatric epidemiology: Searching for the causes of mental disorders* (pp. 15–24). New York, NY: Oxford University Press.

U.S. Public Health Service (1999a). *Mental health: A report of the Surgeon General.* Washington, DC: U.S. Public Health Service.

U.S. Public Health Service (1999b). *The Surgeon General's call to action to prevent suicide.* Washington, DC: U.S. Public Health Service.

U.S. Public Health Service (2000). *Mental health: Culture, race, and ethnicity.* Washington, DC: U.S. Public Health Service.

Valenstein, M., Vijan, S., Zeber, J. E., Boehm, K., & Buttar, A. (2001). The cost-utility of screening for depression in primary care. *Annals of Internal Medicine, 134,* 345–360.

Vanderbilt-Adariance, E., & Shaw, D. S. (2008a). Conceptualizing and re-evaluating resilience across levels of risk, time, and domains of competence. *Clinical Child and Family Psychological Review, 11,* 30–58.

Vanderbilt-Adriance, E., & Shaw, D. S. (2008b). Protective factors and the development of resilience in the context of neighborhood disadvantage. *Journal of Abnormal Child Psychology, 36,* 887–901.

Waddell, B., Shannon, M., & Durr, R. (2001). *Using family resource centers to support California's young children and their families.* Los Angeles, CA: Center for Healthier Children, Families and Community, University of California.

Wang, P. S., Berglund, P., Olfson, M., Pincus, H. A., Wells, K. B. & Kessler, R. C. (2005). Failure and delay in treatment contact after first onset of mental disorders in the National Comorbidity Survey Replication. *Archives of General Psychiatry, 62,* 603–613.

Weissman, M. M., Warner, V., Wickramaratne, P., Moreau, D., & Olfson, M. (1997). Offspring of depressed parents: Ten years later. *Archives of General Psychiatry, 54,* 932–940.

Weissman, M. M., Neria, Y., Gameroff, M. J., Pilowsky, D. J., Wickramaratne, P., Lantigua, R., Shea, S., & Olfson, M. (2010). Positive screens for psychiatric disorders in primary care: A long-term follow-up of patients who were not in treatment. *Psychiatric Services, 61,* 2, 151–159.

Wolchik, S. A., Wilcox, K. L., Tein, J. Y., & Sandler, I. N. (2000). Maternal acceptance and consistency of discipline as buffers of divorce stressors on children's psychological adjustment problems. *Journal of Abnormal Child Psychology, 28*(1), 87–102.

World Health Organization. (2004). *Prevention of mental disorders: Effective interventions and policy options, summary report.* Geneva: World Health Organization.

Zylke, J. W., & DeAngelis, C. D. (2009). Health promotion and disease prevention in children: It's never too early. *JAMA, 302*(21), 3370–2271.

Index

Note: Page numbers in *italics* denote tables, those in **bold** denote figures.

10/90 gap 175

absenteeism 30
absolute poverty 177
academic competence, and
    developmental competence 228
access to care 4, 33, 70, 155; children
    226; expansion 87; immigrant
    populations 72; inner-city families
    295; insurance status 80, 82;
    urbanization 58
Accountable Care Organizations
    (ACOs) 202
acculturation 72
Achenbaum, W. A. 267–8
*Achieving the Promise: Transforming
    Mental Health Care in America* 169
Action for Mental Health 123
actionability 213
Adelman, H. S. 228
adolescents: community violence
    288–9; effects of parental depression
    347–8; *see also* young people
Adverse Childhood Experience study
    218
adversities, effects of early exposure
    352
advocacy 150, 165
African American mental health 73–4
age: health disparities, U.S. 80; and
    suicide 314
Agnew, Robert 53
Aguilar-Gaxiola, S. 4
Alegria, M. 71, 72, 73, 75, 81
Alim, T. N. 293–4
almshouses 120
Alonso, J. 17

Alzheimer's disease 250–5; effect on
    caregivers 253–5; interventions 252;
    prevalence 251
American Association of Geriatric
    Psychiatry (AAGP) 255
American Psychiatric Association (APA)
    2, 285
American Rehabilitation Act, 1973 164
Americans with Disabilities Act (ADA)
    105, 106, 151–5
Anthony, William 165–6
anti-stigma education 103–4
antidepressants 129, 178
anxiety disorders, societal costs 9
Araya, R. 180
Asian American mental health 74
assisted outpatient treatment (AOT)
    143–5
Association between severity of
    12-month DSM-IV/CIDI disorders
    and days out of role *26*
Atkins, M. 235
attitude rebound 103
autonomy, reclaiming 167–8
Avenevoli, S. 347

Beard, J. R. 264
Beardslee, W. R. 346, 348–9
behavior, contagion theory 54–5
Beinecke, R. H. 175, 178
Bell, C. 288
Bellack, A. S. 167, 171
Ben-Zeev, D. 4
bias, case control studies 43, 46
Bierman, A. 264
bio-psychological characteristics, older
    people 265

Blazer, D. 58
Bleuler, E. 161
Bogat, G. A. 290
Bolton, P. 178
Bostrom, A. G. 312
Bourdon, K. H. 2
Brady Handgun Violence Prevention
    Act 149
Brazelton, T. B. 181
Breslau, J. 73
British doctors study 40–2
Buchanan, R. 236
built environment 56–7, 262–3
Burton, V. S. 100
Bush, George W. 131

Cabin, W. 5
Caine, E. D. 5
Call to Action to Prevent Suicide 303
care delivery model 267
Care Monitoring Initiative 214–15
care-seeking: future research 107; and
    stigma 99–100
caregivers, cognitive impairment and
    Alzheimer's disease 253–5
Carter, G. 312
Carter, Jimmy 125
carve outs 196
case control studies: bias 43, 46; design
    42–3; mortality due to mental
    disorders 43–4; Russian mortality
    study 44–6; validity 43
case management programs 129
case reviews 214
category fallacy 71
Center for Mental Health Services
    (CMHS) 84
Center for Political and Economic
    Studies 69
Centers for Disease Control and
    Prevention (CDC) 1, 206, 303
Chang, S. M. 21
Chicago School of Social Ecology 51,
    58
child abuse 294
childhood adversities (CAs) 346
childhood obesity 237
children 4–5; access to care 226;
    community violence 287–8; effects of
    intimate partner violence (IPV) 292;
    effects of parental depression 347–8;
    mental health 226; mental health and
    learning 227–8; morbidity/mortality
    176; population-level data 212;

resilience 289; stigma 98; *see also*
    school mental health
Children's Health Insurance Program
    88
Chile, primary healthcare clinics 180
chronic disease, and depression 256–7
Cicchetti, D. 350
CIDI 10, 16–17
City Health Information 215
civil commitment 142; outpatient
    143–5, 146
civil rights 100, 142
Claeson, M. 185
Clark, C. 290
clinical drug trials 128
clinical recovery 166–7
clinical remission 166–7
clinician payees 146
Clinton, Bill 200
clubhouses 164
coercion 150–1
cognitive behavioral treatments (CBT),
    and stigma reduction 104–5
cognitive impairment 250–5; effect on
    caregivers 253–5
cognitive therapy-based intervention,
    Pakistan 179–80
Cohen, N. L. 5, 57
Cohn, J. F. 186
cohort studies 39–42; British doctors
    study 40–2
Cole, P. M. 347
collaborative care: Alzheimer's disease
    252; and stigma reduction 104–5
Collaborative Psychiatric
    Epidemiological Surveys (CPES) 71,
    75–80
community care and treatment 121–2,
    152–4
community health workers 179–80,
    181–2
community innovations 203
community leaders, anti-stigma
    education 104
community-level interventions 352
Community Mental Health Centers
    Act, 1963 122–4, 163, 197
Community Mental Health Centers
    (CMHC) 123–4, 163, 202
community-oriented approach, suicide
    prevention 312–13
community program model 123
community provision, for multiple
    needs 125

community science approach 236
community/service environment 265
community support 348
community support program (CSP) approach 163
community surveys 2
community tenure 145
community violence: adolescents 288–9; children 287–8; intimate partner violence 290–2; overview 283, 287; partnership working 295; resilience 289, 292; strengthening "at-risk" families 294; traumatic stress studies 283–6; women 289–90; *see also* trauma; violence
comorbidity 17, 27, 76, 174–5, 256–7, 287, 305
comparative health valuations 27–9
comparative studies, dearth of 9
complementary and alternative medicine sectors 195
complex PTSD 284
compliance 93
compositional effects 264–5
compounded community trauma 287
confidentiality 86
conservation of resources (COR) theory 293
consumer movement 164, 165
contact, and stigma reduction 104
contagion theory 54–5
contextual influences 217
continuum housing models 163
contributory factors 133
Conwell, Y. 5
Cooper, A. 99
Cooper, J. L. 237–8
Cooper, P. 181–2
coordination of care, deficiencies 129
coping process research 292–3
coping resources, availability of 54
correlates, measures of 10
Corrigan, P. W. 4, 100–1
cost-effectiveness 32
costs 128, 175
courts, diversion 147
Cramer, J. A. 93
crime 4
crime and delinquency 53
criminal justice system 146–8
criminality, and stigma 98
criminalization 125
Crisis Intervention Training (CIT) 147
Cuijpers, P. 345

culture 85
Curry, A. D. 264

dangerousness 98, 143, 149
Daniels, K. 4
data analysis, health disparities, U.S. 75–80
Davidson, L. 166, 167–8, 169–70
day treatment 163
days out of role 17, 25–7
DeAngelis, C. D. 352
Deegan, Patricia 165
deinstitutionalization 4, 124–7, 143, 162
DeJonghe, E. 292
dementia 250–5
dementia praecox 161
demographic characteristics 265–6
demographic structure, United States 71–2
Demyttenaere, K. 3
depression: Chile 180; and chronic disease 256–7; comorbidity 174–5, 176, 256–7; dysfunctional parenting 347–8; maternal 179, 186, 347; older people 255–8; Pakistan 179–80; parental 347–9; public health approaches 216–17; and resilience resource depletion 293; targeting 345–6; treatment 129; Uganda 178–9; youth prevention approach to 346
Depression in Parents, Parenting, and Children: Opportunities to Improve Identification, Treatment, and Prevention 347
descriptive psychiatry 2
Detroit Area Survey of Trauma 285
developmental competence, and academic competence 228
diagnosis, delays in 343
Diagnostic and Statistical Manual of Mental Disorders (DSM-III) 2, 10
diagnostic criteria, lack of clarity 2
differential vulnerability hypothesis 53–4
disability 105–6, 341–2
disability-adjusted life year (DALY) 3, 213
Disability Advocates v. *Paterson* 154–5
disability-related work leave 31
discrimination 96, 149
disorder severity 10, 16
disorder-specific disability 21–5

Disorder-specific global Sheehan Disability Scale ratings *24*
disorders of extreme stress, not otherwise specified (DESNOS) 285
disorders, World Mental Health Surveys classification 16
distal risk factors 329, 330
diversion, from criminal justice system 147
Doll, R. 40
domestic violence *see* intimate partner violence
downstream causes 210
drug courts 147–8
Druss, B. G. 4, 99
Dunham, H. 2, 58
DuRant, R. H. 288
Durkheim, Emile 2, 51, 219–20
dysfunctional parenting 292, 347–8

early-age onsets 352
early child development 218
early childhood programs 232
Early Development Index 212
earnings, and mental health 17, 31–2
Echeverry, J. J. 75
ecologic (systems) model, suicide prevention 324, **325**
ecological developmental model, suicide prevention 324
economic outcomes 267
education, and stigma reduction 103–4
educational policies 85–6
educators, and school mental health 234–5
Elbogen, R. B. 145
elderly people 5
electronic health record (EHR) systems 215–16
emerging trends and policy initiatives 200–3
employment, Americans with Disabilities Act (ADA) 152
empowerment 104, 164
Endicott, J. 16
endophenotypes 304
environmental stress model 56
Epidemiologic Catchment Area (ECA) study 2, 4, 58, 92–3, 305
epidemiological measures 4
epidemiology: case control studies 42–6; cohort studies 39–42; overview 38–9; uses in public mental health 46–8

Evans, G. W. 57
evidence-based practices 235
expenditure 131
Experience Sampling Methods (ESM) research 107
exploration of models 233–4
exposés, of mental health care 121

Fahs, M. C. 5
families, at risk 294–6
family-based preventive interventions 348–9, 352
family-centered interventions, global mental health 185–7
family-focused service delivery 295–6
family resource centers 348
family support programs 232–3
Faris, R. 2, 58
fatal outcomes in early adulthood **331**
Federal Action Agenda 169
Federal Employees Health Benefits Program 200, 201
federal entitlement programs 124–5
federal government, in mental health care 122
Felix, Robert H. 122, 123
firearms, access to 149–50, 323
Fitpatrick, K. 264
follow-up 295
Fountain House 164
four core dimensions of care 85
fragmentation of care 85, 125, 129–30, 133, 140, 326–8
Frank, R. G. 127, 131
Frese III, F. J. 169
Frieden, Thomas 206
functional disability, remission criterion 167
funding: low- and middle-income countries 175; mental health services 87, 88; research 86; suicide prevention 331

Galea, S. 4, 52
Gallo, W. T. 5
Garrett Lee Smith Memorial Act 303, 308
gatekeeper training 317–18
gender 266; and earnings 32; health disparities, U.S. 76, 80; late-life depression 255; posttraumatic stress disorder (PTSD) 285
General Accounting Office 124, 125
general medical/primary care sector 195

general physicians, changing role 128
general strain theory 53
gentrification 56
geography, and suicide 318–19, 324
Gitlin, L. N. 254
Gladstone, T. 346
Glied, S. A. 127
Global Assessment of Functioning (GAF) 16
Global Burden of Disease estimates 251
Global Burden of Disease Study 1, 341, 345
Global Forum for Health Research 175
global issues 4
global mental health: barriers to improvement 177–8; depression 175–7; family-centered interventions 185–7; interventions in low- and middle-income countries 177–82; lessons learned 182–3; low- and middle-income countries 174–5; Millennium Development Goals (MDGs) 175–7; needs and future prospects 186; obstacles to effective programs 183; overview 174; and poverty 177; task shifting 183–5; worker shortages 183–4
globalization 60–1
Goffman, E. 94
Goldmann, E. 4
Gotland, suicide prevention 312
government oversight 206
Greenberg, P. E. 9
Greene, V. W. 1
Grob, G. N. 4
group interventions 178–9
guardianship 145–6
Gun Control Act 149
gun violence 149
Guo, J. J. 231

Harvey, P. D. 167
health behaviors 266
health care: four core dimensions 85; fragmentation 85
health care reform 201–2
health disparities, U.S.: African American mental health 73–4; age 76, 80; Asian American mental health 74; collaborative psychiatric epidemiological surveys (CPES) 75–80; comorbidity 76; data analysis 75–80; disparities in mental healthcare 74–5; disparities in

prevalence 80–1; gender 76, 80; healthcare reform opportunities 87–8; immigrant populations 72–3; implications for policy and practice 83–7; income 82–3; Latino mental health 73; logistic regression models of past-year mental health service use 79; overview 69–71; Pacific Islanders' mental health 74; past-year mental disorder prevalence 75–80; possible responses to 70; prevalence of past-year mental disorders for U.S. adults by ethnicity and nativity 77; prevalence of past-year mental health service use among those with past-year disorders 78; quality of care 83; race/ethnicity 69–70, 76; treatment disparities 81–2; workforce diversity 84; *see also* United States
health home 88; *see also* medical home
health outcomes 267
health valuations 17, 27–9
healthcare reform law, U.S. 70
healthcare reform opportunities 87–8
Hemmens, C. 100
Herman, J. L. 284
high-risk approach 308–9
Hill, B. 40
Hobfoll, S. E. 293
homelessness 143
Horowitz, K. 287
housing, contingent on treatment 145
housing-first programs 145
human capital approach 31
human services sector 195

illness prevention 208
immigrant paradox 72–3, 74, 81
immigrant populations 72–4
impairment and disability, and physical illness 3
in recovery 167–8
incarceration 4, 129, 146
income, health disparities, U.S. 82–3
incompetence, judgments of 105–6
independent living movement 164
India, Manas project 182
indicated prevention 345
individual-level approaches 209
individual-level condition-specific estimates of predictive associations 28
individual rights, and public risk 140
inequality 61

infrastructure, schools 228
inpatient care 129
Institute of Medicine (IOM) 303, 341, 343, 347
institutional care 119–20
insurance benefits, access to 99
insurance status, access to care 80, 82
intentional structural stigma 100
inter-group comparisons 209
intergenerational cycle of violence 288
International Classification of Disorders (ICD) 10
International Study of Schizophrenia 162
interpersonal group therapy (IPT), Uganda 178–9
interventions: Alzheimer's disease 252; community level 352; early, and prevention 231–3; family-centered 185–7, 348; group interventions 178–9; low- and middle-income countries 177–82; modular 233; obstacles to effective programs 183; prevention-oriented 341; preventive 348–9, 352; in school-based setting 233–4; timing-dependent 326
intimate partner violence (IPV) 290–2
investment, personal, political and economic 352–3

Jackson, J. S. 75
Jackson, P. B. 86
Jenkins, E. J. 288
Jenkins, R. 184
Joint Commission of Mental Illness and Health (JCMIH) 123
Julius, R. 93

Kaplan, G. A. 264
Karpati, A. 4
Kazak, A. E. 238
Kennedy, John F. 123
Kessler, R. C. 3, 4, 10, 30, 93, 305, 345, 349
Kilpatrick, D. G. 289
Kim, J. 264
Knox, K. L. 5, 308, 312–13
Korean Epidemiologic Catchment Area (KECA) Study 21
Kraemaer, H. C. 343–4
Kraemer, H. 315
Kraepelin, E. 161
Kuzbansky, L. D. 263

label avoidance 94, 102–5

labeling, and stigma 95
Lady Health Workers 179
LaGory, M. 264
Lang, M. 316
Last, J. M. 207
Latino mental health 73
Latkin, C. A. 264
LaVeist, T. A. 69
law: access to firearms 149–50; civil commitment 142; mandated treatment 143–5; money and housing mandates 145; outpatient civil commitment 143–5; overview 139; response to abuses 142; role of 140–1; summary and conclusions 155; *see also specific legislation*
lawsuits 142, 143
leadership, suicide prevention 331
Leaf, P. J. 99
learning, and mental health 227–8
Leffert, N. 229
Lehman, A. F. 93
Lehmann, U. 184
Leighton, A. H. 2, 51
Leon, A. C. 16, 44
lessons learned, global mental health 182–3
Levendosky, A. A. 292
leverage, tools of 140–6
Levin, J. S. 267–8
Lewis, G. 316
life course studies 39–40
life expectancy 1, 248–9, **248**
Lin, N. 54
Link, B. G. 98, 99, 101, 266
Liska, A. 108
local jurisdictions 147
logistic regression models of past-year mental health service use 79
long-term adverse effects 29–30
Lopez, A. D. 1, 345
low- and middle-income countries 174–5; barriers to improvement 177–8; interventions 177–82
Luthar, S. S. 350
Lynch, M. 289

MacArthur Network on Mandated Community Treatment 151
mainstreaming 1, 342
maladaptive family functioning (MFF) 346
managed behavioral care organizations (MBHOs) 196

managed care 130–1, 196–7
Manas project, India 182
mandated treatment 4, 143, 146–8
Mann, J. 308–9
Margolin, G. 289
Masten, A. S. 350
maternal depression 179, 186, 347
maternal distress 292
maternal morbidity/mortality 176
Mathers, C. D. 3
Max-Neef, M. 185
McGuire, T. G. 81
McKay, H. 53
McKay, M. M. 295
Mechanic, D. 4
mediational model 344
Medicaid 84, 87–8, 124, 125, 133, 197,
　201–2; managed care 130–1
medical home 86, 202; *see also* health
　home
medicalization 128
Medicare 84, 87, 124, 125, 196, 251
Medicare Improvements for Patients
　and Providers Act 201
medication, compliance 93
mental disorders: ages of onset 342–3;
　long-term adverse effects 29–30;
　severity of 20–1; societal costs 9
mental health: and culture 85; public
　health significance 3–4
*Mental Health: A Report of the Surgeon
　General* 342
mental health care: disparities in 74–5;
　future of 133–5; integration with
　health and social insurance 134;
　"second-class status" 84; utilization 4
mental health consumer movement 164
mental health courts 147–8
*Mental health: Culture, race, and
　ethnicity – A supplement to mental
　health* 82
mental health disparities, U.S. *see* health
　disparities, U.S.
mental health insurance parity 101, 108
mental health outcomes 267
mental health parity 127, 200–1
Mental Health Parity Act (MHPA) 101
Mental Health Parity and Addiction
　Equity Act 101–2
mental health policy, U.S.: community
　care and treatment 121–2;
　Community Mental Health Centers
　Act of 1963 122–4; contributory
　factors to illness 133;

deinstitutionalization 124–7;
　expansion of services 127–9; federal
　government involvement 122;
　institutional care 119–20; managed
　care 130–1; opportunities, risks, and
　prospects 133–5; overview 119;
　patterns of patient care 129–30;
　recent trends 131–3; and social policy
　126–7; *see also* services
mental health promotion 86, 228–9,
　350–1
mental health services: community
　innovations 203; cultural and
　linguistic appropriateness 70;
　expanding access and use 87; family-
　focused service delivery 295–6;
　funding 87, 88; general medical
　sector 198–200; health care reform
　201–2; as patchwork 195; policy
　initiatives and emerging trends
　200–3; private sector 196–7; public
　sector 197; recovery-oriented
　169–70, 171; sectors of 195; specialty
　workforce 198; states' role 202–3;
　summary and conclusions 203;
　underutilization 92–3; *see also* service
　utilization, U.S.
Mental Health Systems Act, 1980 126
Mercy, J. A. 352
Merikangas, K. R. 17, 27, 347
Merrell, K. W. 236
Merton, R. 53
midstream causes 210
Midtown Manhattan Study 2
migration 59–60
military screening 2
Millennium Development Goals
　(MDGs) 175–7
Mills, C. 4
Miranda, J. 81, 176–7
Mistry, R. 295, 348
Mittelman, M. 254–5
moderational model 344
modular interventions 233
Mojtabai, R. 93
money, control of 145–6
monitoring health status 210–12
morbidity, and mental health 3
mortality due to mental disorders, case
　control studies 43–4
Moscicki, E. K. 305
Moses, A. 288–9
mother–infant relationship 181–2
Motto, J. A. 312

Mueser, K. T. 4
Mulloy, M. 4
multilayered approach, suicide
  prevention 309
multilevel assessment 343
multilevel ecological models 249
multilevel growth models 324
multiple needs, community provision
  for 125
Muntaner, C. 82
Murray, C. J. 1

National Annenberg Risk Survey of
  Youth 99–100
National Association of School Based
  Health Care (NASBHC) 231
National Comorbidity Survey (NCS)
  2–3, 4, 58, 93, 99, 129, 199, 305
National Comorbidity Survey
  Replication (NCS-R) 75, 93, 127–8,
  218, 250, 305, 342–3, 345, 349
National Instant Criminal Background
  Check System Improvement Act
  (NICSIA) 149
National Instant Criminal Background
  Check System (NICS) 149
National Institute of Mental Health
  (NIMH) 122, 123, 126, 341
National Latino and Asian American
  Study (NLAAS) 75
National Mental Health Act, 1946 122
National Research Council and
  Institute of Medicine 228–9
National Stigma Study for children
  (NSS-C) 98
*National Strategy for Suicide
  Prevention* 303, 330
National Suicide Prevention Lifeline 308
National Survey of American Life
  (NSAL) 75
National Survey of Early Childhood
  Health (NSECH) 295, 348
national surveys 211–12
National Women's Study 290
natural disasters 293
needs, identification and resource
  provision 164
neighborhood disorder model 56
neighborhood-level determinants 217,
  262
Neonatal Behavioural Assessment
  Schedule (NBAS) 181
New Freedom Commission on Mental
  Health 131–2, 169, 303, 308

Norris, F. H. 350
Nugent, J. K. 181
NYC DOHMH 206, 211, 214–16, 217

Obama, Barack 133, 201
Ødegård, Ø. 51
O'Donnell, D. A. 289
older people 262; bio-psychological
  characteristics 265; care delivery
  model 267; cognitive decline 250;
  cognitive impairment and Alzheimer's
  disease 250–5; community/service
  environment 265; conceptual
  framework 258–9; conceptual
  framework for public health, mental
  health **260–1**; conceptual model
  259–67; demographic characteristics
  265–6; depression 255–8; health
  behaviors 266; neighborhood-level
  characteristics 262; physical/built
  environment 262–3; prevalence of
  mental disorders 250; and primary
  care providers 257; social
  environment 263–4; social support
  264; summary and conclusions 267
Olmstead v. *L.C.* 132, 152–4, 210
Omnibus Crime Control and Safe
  Streets Act 149
opportunities and rights 105
opportunities, risks, and prospects
  133–5
organizational responsibility 84
organizational/structural variables 75
Ormel, J. 21
outcomes 267
outpatient civil commitment 143–5,
  146
over-focus 328

Pacific Islanders' mental health 74
Pakistan, cognitive therapy-based
  intervention 179–80
paradigm shift 224–5
parental depression, children's health
  and development 347–8
parenting, dysfunctional 292, 347–8
parole 148
partial hospitalization 163
partnership working: community
  violence 295; school mental health
  234–5, 237–8; suicide prevention 330
past-year mental disorder prevalence
  75–80
Patel, V. 176–7, 178, 182

patient autonomy 140; psychiatric advance directives (PADs) 150–1
patient care, patterns of 129–30
Patient-Centered Medical Homes (PCMH) 202
Patient Protection and Affordable Care Act 84, 87, 201–2
Patient Self-Determination Act (PSDA) 150
patient variables 70, 75
patterns of patient care 129–30
Paul Wellstone and Pete Domenici Mental Health Parity and Addiction Equity Act 201
Penn, D. L. 99–100
personal recovery 167–8
Pescosolido, B. A. 98
Petrila, J. 4
pharmaceutical companies 128
Phelan, J. 266
physical environment 56–7, 262–3
physical healthcare, and stigma 98–9
physical illness, and impairment and disability 3
policy 4
policy initiatives and emerging trends 200–3
policy reforms, United States 84
Pollard, J. A. 344
population aging 248–9; *see also* older people
population approach 208–9
population-based research, lack of attention 1
population-based studies 2
population density 58
population mental health, emergence of 2–3
population-oriented approach, suicide prevention 329
positive behavior supports 230
post traumatic stress disorder (PTSD) 55, 283–7, 293
poverty 58, 82–3, 176, 177
power problem 345–6
pre-booking diversion 147
prejudice 95–6, 97
prescriptions 128
President's Commission on Mental Health, 1978 125
prevalence 2; Alzheimer's disease 251; amongst arrestees and inmates 146; amongst older people 250; depression, older people 255;

disparities in 80–1; global 174; intimate partner violence (IPV) 291–2; suicide 305–6
prevalence estimates, World Mental Health Surveys 17–20
prevalence of past-year mental disorders for U.S. adults by ethnicity and nativity 77
prevalence of past-year mental health service use among those with past-year disorders 78
Preventing Mental, Emotional, and Behavioral Disorders among Young People 228–9
Preventing Mental, Emotional, and Behavioral Disorders Among Young People: Progress and Possibilities 343
prevention and early intervention 208, 231–3, 345, 352–3
prevention/health promotion research agenda 341
prevention-oriented interventions 341
preventive cardiology 309
preventive gerontology 268
preventive interventions 348–9, 352
preventive science approach 341
primary care 214–15
Primary Care Information Project (PCIP) 215–16
primary care providers, and older people 257
primary care screening 349
primary healthcare clinics, Chile 180
Primm, A. B. 81
Prince, M. 3
principle of exclusion 72
priority-setting 212–13
private insurance sector 130
private mental health services 196–7
proactivity, care delivery 267
probation 148
professionals, anti-stigma education 103
Proposition 63 132
prospects, risks and opportunities 133–5
protected approaches 163
protection, loss of 129
protective factors, need for research 86
protest, and stigma reduction 102–3
psychiatric advance directives (PADs) 150–1
psychiatric epidemiology 38; broadening scope 48; emergence of 2–3; new models and approaches 1

psychiatric medication 122, 124, 128–9, 162, 178, 197, 198–9, 349
psychiatric rehabilitation 164–5
psychiatric will 150
psychiatry, changes in thinking 121
psychosocial resources 292–3
public education 86
public health: conceptual domains 208; definition 207; essential services **207**; hazard investigation 213–15; surveillance 210–12; tools and strategies of 1; unified approach 206–7
public health approaches: challenges and limitations 219–20; overview 206–7; suicide prevention 313–28
public health practice, integrating mental health 207–12
public mental health: integration into public health context 4; new directions 216–18; priority-setting 212
public mental health systems, shift in focus 4
public risk, and individual rights 140
public sector services 197
public stigma 94, 96, 102–5

QPR 317–18
quality of care 70, 83, 199–200; assessment and improvement 233; school mental health 235–6; and stigma 101

race/ethnicity 4, 266; disparities in prevalence 80–1; health disparities, U.S. 69–70, 76; intimate partner violence (IPV) 291; and patient variables 70; spatial segregation 55; treatment disparities 81–2; United States 71–2; workforce diversity 84
Rahman, A. 176, 179
randomized controlled trials 47
Reagan, Ronald 126
record keeping 86
recovery 132, 165–8, 208; challenges to concept 170–1; elements of 168; recovery from/clinical recovery 166–7; in recovery/personal recovery 167–8; resilience and social support 294
recovery from 166–7
recovery-oriented services 169–70, 171
recovery practice standards 170

Reducing Risks for Mental Disorders: Frontiers for Preventive Intervention Research 341
Regier, D. A. 92–3
relational revictimization 291
relative poverty 177
relief-from-disabilities programs 149
religion, and mental health 51
religious services 195
remission 166–7
Repetti, R. L. 352
Report on Mental Health, 1999 169
representative payees 145–6
research: in community care and law 141; focus 345; funding 86; macro-to-micro 108; prevention/health promotion agenda 341; stigma 106–8; suicide prevention 306–7, 330
research-to-practice gap 233
residential neighborhoods 51
residential stability 264
resilience: children and adolescents 289; need for research 296; promoting 349–50; resources 292–4
resource protection and recovery 293
Resources for Enhancing Alzheimer's Caregiver Health (REACH) project 254
response trajectories 350
revictimization 291
revolving-door admissions 143, 163
rights and opportunities 105
Rihmer, Z. 312
risk: contextual 209; intergenerational transmission 348; prospects and opportunities 133–5
risk factor epidemiology 343
risk factor studies 47
risk factors 315, 343–4
Roe, D. 4, 166, 167–8
role disabilities, mental and physical disorders 21–5
role impairment measure 16–17
Rose, Geoffrey 208–9
Rose's theorem 308, 329
Ross, C. E. 264
Rotheram-Borus, M. J. 186–7
Rothman, K. J. 43
Rowan, A. B. 291
Russian mortality study 45–6

Sameroff, A. J. 344
Saraceno, B. 177
Sartorius, N. 21, 25

Satcher, D. 303, 330, 342
Saul, J. 352
Scale of Perceived Stigma 99
Scales, P. 229
schizophrenia 161–2, 162
Schizophrenia Patient Outcome
   Research Team survey 93
school-based health centers (SBHC)
   230–1
school connectedness 229–30
school mental health: challenges and
   opportunities 225, 234–6; childhood
   obesity 237; community science
   approach 236; development 226–8;
   early childhood prevention and
   intervention 232–3; evidence-based
   practices 235; exploration 233–4;
   health promotion 228–9; integrating
   public health approaches 228–34;
   interventions in school-based setting
   233–4; missed opportunities 225;
   next steps 237–8; overview 224–6;
   partnering with educators 234–5;
   partnership working 237–8; positive
   behavior supports 230; prevention
   and early intervention 231–3; quality
   of care 235–6; school-based health
   centers (SBHC) 230–1; school climate
   229–30; screening and early detection
   230–1; *see also* children
schools, anti-stigma education 103
Schumm, J. A. 294
screening and early detection 230–1,
   253, 315–16, 349
segregation 56
selective migration 72–3
selective prevention 345
self-efficacy 96
self-esteem 96
self-prejudice 96
self-stigma 94, 96, 102–5
senility, redefinition 120
sentencing, and treatment 148
service planning and delivery,
   immigrant populations 72
service utilization, U.S. 195; *see also*
   mental health services
services: decentralization 125;
   expansion 127–9; *see also* mental
   health policy, U.S.
severe mental illness (SMI): challenges
   to concept of recovery 170–1;
   conceptualizing 161–5; consumer
   needs 162–3; deinstitutionalization

162; overview 161; recovery 165–8;
   recovery-oriented services 169–70,
   171
severity, of disorder 10, 16
sex role hypothesis 266
Shah, A. A. 175, 178
Shaw, C. 53
Shaw, D. S. 350
Sheehan Disability Scale (SDS) 16–17;
   disorder-specific disability ratings 24
shelter-based care 295
Shonkoff, J. P. 352
Silverstein, S. M. 171
Simon, G. E. 25
Sirey, J. A. 99
site-population approaches, suicide
   prevention 320–2
Skeem, J. 148
Slade, M. 166, 167, 168
slums 58
small relative risks 47
social and environmental factors 4;
   crime and delinquency 53; developing
   influences 57–61; globalization 60–1;
   levels of 52; mechanisms of influence
   52–7; methodological challenges
   61–2; migration 59–60; older people
   262–5; overview 51–2; physical
   environment 56–7, 262–3; social
   contagion 54–5; social disorder 264;
   social disorganization or strain 52–3;
   social environment 263–4; social
   resources 53–4, 56; social strain 52–3,
   56; spatial segregation 55–6;
   summary and conclusions 62;
   urbanization 57–8; useful concepts 52
social class, and mental health 51
social contagion 54–5
social disintegration, and mental health
   51
social disorder 264
social disorganization 52–3
social disorganization theory 53
social environment 263–4
social isolation 264
social networks, suicide prevention
   328–9
social policy, and mental health policy,
   U.S. 126–7
social-psychiatric epidemiology 141
social resources 53–4, 56
social skills training (SST) programs 164
social strain 52–3, 56
social strain theory 53

social support 54; and migration 60; older people 264; resilience and recovery 293–4
socioeconomic position (SEP) 52, 53–4, 55, 263–4
sociology of deviance and social control 141
South Africa, mother–infant relationship 181–2
spatial segregation 55–6, 59–60
special housing 145
specialty medical sector 195
spending priorities, suicide prevention 328
Srole, T. 2
Starfield, B. 85
State Care Act, 1890, New York 120
State Children's Health Insurance Program (SCHIP) 133
state hospitals 142
state legislation, structural stigma in 100–1
Stayton, C. 291
Steenland, M. 52
stereotypes 95, 97, 149
stigma 4, 71, 149, 186; age-related 258; as barrier 94; and care-seeking 99–100; children 98; collaborative care 104–5; contact 104; and criminality 98; educational programs 103–4; future research 106–8; harm 97–100; as individual process 94–7; in individual treatment seeking and utilization 97; manifestations 94; mental health insurance parity 101; minimizing 102; overview 92; and physical healthcare 98–9; protest 102–3; and quality of care 101; reducing 102–5; as societal phenomena 100–2; in state legislation 100–1; *see also* structural stigma
Stirling County Study 2, 51
strain theory 53
stress, and migration 59
stress research 292–3
structural stigma 94, 100–1, 105–6; *see also* stigma
Substance Abuse and Mental Health Services Administration (SAMHSA) 84, 88, 93, 168, 206
substance abuse disorders, mental health insurance parity 101–2
suburban neurosis 58
suicide 5, 176, 219–20; and age 314;

comorbidity 305; and geography 318–19, 324; language of prevention 310–11; prevalence 305–6; rates 314; risk factors 304; and unemployment 314, 326
suicide contagion 55
suicide prevention: from 2004 307–13; approaches to 308–9; community-oriented approach 312–13, 330; control and restriction 323; current perspective 305–7; developmental model of increasing risks 327; ecologic (systems) model 324; ecological developmental model 324; ecological model 325; effective public health approaches 313–28; false negatives 317–18; funding 331; gatekeeper training 317–18; Gotland 312; high risk groups 316–17; identifying "true cases" 314–17; individual-level developmental frame 326; initiatives and treatment 306; lack of coordinated strategies 326–8; lack of evidence base 303–4; lack of knowledge 323–6; leadership 331; means control 309; overview 303–4; population-oriented approach 329; protective factors 323; public and policy attitudes 307; reaching people 318–23; research centers 308; research limitations 330; research needs 306–7; risk identification 306; screening and early detection 315–16; site-population approaches *320–2*; social networks 328–9; spending priorities 328; summary and conclusions 328–31; two-fold purpose 304; U.S. Air Force (USAF) 312–13, **313**; use of risk factors 315; young people 312, 315–16, 330
Suicide Prevention Resource Center (SPRC) 306
suicide-specific developmental framework 324
support services 105–6
support system, two tier 54
supported approaches 163–4
Supreme Court *Olmstead* decision 132
Surgeon General Reports on Mental Health (US) 1
surveillance 210–12
surveys: assessment of mental disorder 2; public mental health 211–12; *see also individual surveys*

Susser, E. 1, 2, 4, 43
Swanson, J. 4, 151, 152
Swartz, L. 4
Swindle, R. 127
synthetic estimation 211
Szasz, Thomas 150

Take Care New York (TCNY) 212–13, 213, 215
targeted policies 84
targeting 209
Tarricone, R. 31
Tarrier, N. 93
Taylor, L. 228
Taylor, S. 58
teachers, and school mental health 234–5
The Prevention of Mental Disorders: A National Research Agenda 341
therapeutic courts 147–8
therapy, new models and approaches 121, 122
Tohen, M. 2
Tomlinson, M. 4
tools and strategies, of public health 1
trauma 285–6; *see also* community violence
traumatic stress studies 283–6
treatment: adherence 93, 140, 155; barriers to 199; as condition of sentencing 148; confidence in 103; cost-effectiveness of 32; day treatment 163; discontinuity 140; inadequacy 129
treatment disparities 81–2

Uganda, interpersonal group therapy (IPT) 178–9
underutilization 92–3; *see also* utilization of services
unemployment, and suicide 314, 326
unintentional structural stigma 101
United States: demographic structure 71–2; health disparities *see* health disparities, U.S.
United States Psychiatric Rehabilitation Association (USPRA) 164
University of Michigan surveys 127
upstream causes 210
upstream interventions 210
urbanization 57–8
U.S. Constitution 142
U.S. government, mental health policy 84

U.S. Surgeon General, *Report on Mental Health*, 1999 169
USAF Suicide Prevention Program 312–13, **313**
use of services, health disparities, U.S. 76
Üstün, T. B. 10, 21, 25
utilization of services: barriers to 258; expansion 87; future research 107; *see also* underutilization

validity, case control studies 43
Vanderbilt-Adriance, E. 350
Vaux, A. 293
Vega, W. A. 72–3
violence 149; *see also* community violence
Visual Analogue Scale (VAS) 27–9
voluntary support sector 195–6
voting rights 100

Waldman, R. J. 185
Walter, K. H. 293
Wandersman, A. 236
Wang, P. S. 4, 32, 33, 93, 127, 199
Web-based Injury Statistics Query and Reporting System (WISQAR S™) 319
Weiden, P. J. 93
Weissman, M. M. 349
Weist, M. 4, 230
Wellstone-Domenici Mental Health Parity and Addiction Equity Act 127
Werther effect 55
WHO Collaborative Study on Psychological Problems in General Health Care (PPG) 21, 25
WHO Composite International Diagnostic Interview (CIDI); *see* CIDI
whole-person knowledge 85
Williams, D. R. 74, 86
Willis, A. G. 93
Wilson, H. W. 289
women: community violence 289–90; intimate partner violence 290–2; maternal distress 292
women and families 5
work performance 31
worker shortages, global mental health 183–4
workforce 84, 198
workplace costs 30–1
World Health Organization (WHO) 94, 303
World Mental Health sample

characteristics by World Bank
Income Categories *11–15*
World Mental Health Surveys 3;
classification of disorders 16;
comparative health valuations 27–9;
comparative role disabilities 21–5;
days out of role 25–7; diagnostic
interview 10; earnings 17; health
valuations 17; individual-level
condition-specific estimates of
predictive associations *28*; prevalence
estimates 17–20; purpose 10; severity
of 12-month DSM-IV/CIDI disorders
and days out of role *26*; severity of
disorders 20–1; summary and
conclusions 33; Twelve-month
prevalence of DSM-IV/CIDI disorders
18–19; Twelve-month prevalence of

DSM-IV/CIDI disorders by severity
22–3; *see also* CIDI
World War II, influence on mental
health care 121

Yen, I. H. 264
young people: fatal outcomes in early
adulthood **331**; suicide prevention
312, 315–16, 330; *see also*
adolescents
youth prevention approach, to
depression 346
Youth Risk Factor Survey 315–16

Zaridze, D. 43–4
Zolneirek, C. D. 176
Zylke, J. W. 352

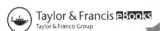